DIVIDE AND CONQUER

DIVIDE AND CONQUER

A Comparative History
of Medical Specialization

GEORGE WEISZ

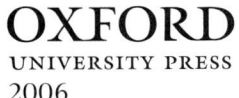

OXFORD

UNIVERSITY PRESS

2006

OXFORD
UNIVERSITY PRESS

Oxford University Press, Inc., publishes works that further
Oxford University's objective of excellence
in research, scholarship, and education.

Oxford   New York
Auckland   Cape Town   Dar es Salaam   Hong Kong   Karachi
Kuala Lumpur   Madrid   Melbourne   Mexico City   Nairobi
New Delhi   Shanghai   Taipei   Toronto

With offices in
Argentina   Austria   Brazil   Chile   Czech Republic   France   Greece
Guatemala   Hungary   Italy   Japan   Poland   Portugal   Singapore
South Korea   Switzerland   Thailand   Turkey   Ukraine   Vietnam

Published by Oxford University Press, Inc.
198 Madison Avenue, New York, New York 10016

www.oup.com

Oxford is a registered trademark of Oxford University Press

Library of Congress Cataloging-in-Publication Data
Weisz, George.
Divide and conquer : a comparative history of medical specialization / George Weisz.
p.   cm.
Includes bibliographical references.
ISBN-13 978-0-19-517969-9
ISBN 0-19-517969-2
1. Medicine—Specialties and specialists—History.
[DNLM: 1. Specialties, Medical—history—Europe. 2. Specialties, Medical—history—United
States. 3. Government Regulation—history—Europe. 4. Government Regulation—history—
United States. 5. History of Medicine, 19th Cent.—Europe. 6. History of Medicine, 19th Cent.—United
States. 7. History of Medicine, 20th Cent.—Europe. 8. History of Medicine, 20th Cent.—United
States. 9. Specialism—history—Europe. 10. Specialism—history—United States. W 90 W433d 2004]
I. Title.
R729.5.S6W45 2004
610'.9—dc22   2004019793

9 8 7 6 5 4 3 2 1

Printed in the United States of America
on acid-free paper

For Zeeva, Talia, and Jonathan

Acknowledgments

Writing a book of this scope requires many things, including money. I have been unusually fortunate in obtaining generous funding that allowed me to do research in four countries. The Social Sciences and Research Council of Canada provided two long-term grants that supported a major part of my research. Associate Medical Services (Toronto) offered support through Hannah research grants at critical moments of my research program. The Burroughs-Wellcome Fund granted me a career award that allowed me to spend a year without teaching responsibilities and made extensive travel possible. This fund also provided funding for two visits to London, where I was based at the Wellcome Institute, under the sponsorship of Bill Bynum. The Max Planck Institute for the History of Science in Berlin welcomed me for a month as a visiting scholar in the unit directed by Hans-Jorg Rheinberger; this stay substantially advanced my research on the German sections of this book. At the Philadelphia College of Physicians and Surgeons, I was a Wood Fellow for several weeks, an experience that enriched the American sections of this work. I wish to express my deepest gratitude to all of these institutions whose support made this book possible It is simply not feasible to mention all the helpful people in all the libraries, archives, and data banks who provided me with material. This book would have been impossible without their expertise and assistance.

I have been equally fortunate in having colleagues who generously gave of their time to read all or parts of the manuscript. Rosemary Stevens read the entire manuscript and shared her encyclopedic knowledge of the subject while offering suggestions and criticisms with her customary graciousness. Thomas Schlich spent what must have seemed like a large part of his first year in North America reading a first (and considerably longer) draft of this book, offering insights and correcting errors. I wish to express my thanks to both of them as well as to the following colleagues who read and commented on specific chapters: Isabelle Baszanger, Cornelius

Borck, Roger Cooter, Elsbeth Heaman, Chris Lawrence, Harry Marks, Arleen Tuchman, and Uhlrich Tröhler.

Finally, special thanks to Zeeva, Talia, and Jonathan, who patiently put up with my long absences and my preoccupation with a project that was all-consuming and seemingly never-ending.

Contents

Introduction, xi

Part I: The Emergence of Medical Specialization in the Nineteenth Century

    1: The Rise of Specialties in Early Nineteenth-Century Paris, 3

    2: Specialization and Its Opponents in London, 26

    3: Specialization in the German-Speaking World, 44

    4: The Rise of American Specialties, 63

Part II: Regulating and Standardizing Specialist Practice, 1890–1950

    5: Regulating Specialists in National Medical Directories, 87

    6: Regulating Specialists in Germany, 105

    7: Regulating Specialists the American Way, 127

    8: The French Style of Regulating Specialists, 147

    9: Regulating Specialists in the British Manner, 164

Part III: Medical Specialties in Comparative Perspective

    10: From Divisions of Medicine to Specialties, 191

    11: Division, Unification, and Competition, 210

General Conclusions, 227

Epilogue: Specialists and Generalists in the Era of Biomedicine, 231

Appendices, 257

Notes, 261

Index, 347

Introduction

Medical specialization is now a fact of life in all Western nations. The experience of medical care has been dramatically transformed not only because we now see many specialists for our ills (our ancestors changed physicians with greater frequency than we think), or because individuals suffering from multiple problems may now have difficulty receiving integrated care (undoubtedly true), but primarily due to the fact that specialization has simultaneously produced and been the product of the massive changes that have created high-technology "biomedicine" practiced in hospitals, financed (usually) by third-party payers, and expanding regularly into new domains of human life.

State authorities are now involved in medical affairs to a far greater degree than ever before and significantly encroach on the autonomy of medical professions. Everywhere nations struggle to balance a traditional free-market approach to health care with one based on administrative regulation. One of the key areas of government involvement is medical research, which has assumed massive proportions; it has become increasingly biology-based, even as large-scale clinical trials based on statistical reasoning have assumed a dominant position in evaluating therapies. Health insurance provided by the state or private carriers has affected the conditions of medical practice in most nations. The development of new technologies has vastly increased the scope of possible interventions and, in the process, raised the costs of medical care beyond a level considered affordable by most governments. The aging of populations throughout the Western world has exacerbated the apparently boundless need for and expense of health care.

Specialization in medicine has been at the heart of most of these changes. The division of medical labor is in many ways emblematic of contemporary medicine: of its successes as well as its failings; of its ability to transplant organs; and of its purported inability to deal with "whole" patients or provide personalized care. It is not that specialization has been the unique cause of all of the phenomena, both positive and negative, that we associate with biomedicine; rather, it has been a central and constituent element in their development.

It is thus rather astonishing that the major synthetic treatment of the subject dates from the mid-1940s.[1] Excellent national studies of specialization in Germany,[2] Britain,[3] and the United States[4] were written between the mid-1960s and the early 1970s. In the years since, there has been no attempt to reexamine a central feature of contemporary health-care systems, although recent publications[5] suggest that a revival of interest may be in the works. What we do have in abundance are books and articles that have extended our knowledge of the history of individual specialties in specific countries. Several sociologists have presented sociological "models" of specialization[6] that have highlighted previously underemphasized factors and forces. In the wake of this recent work, it is now possible to offer an empirically based survey and analysis of the development of specialization in historical and comparative perspectives. This is what I attempt to do in this book.

Specialization appears in many ways to be a self-evident necessity of medical science whose existence requires little explanation. This commonsense perception cannot be dismissed out of hand. By the end of the nineteenth century, at the latest, medical science had, largely as a consequence of specialization, developed to the point where the impossibility of mastering all of it seemed obvious. Furthermore, during the past centuries, the evolution of modern Western societies had moved so vigorously in the direction of increasing specialization of labor, knowledge, and expertise that it would be quite astonishing if medicine had failed to follow this path.

Nonetheless, the apparent inevitability—or, as sociologists say, "overdetermination"—of medical specialization still leaves us with many historical questions that are not in the least bit self-evident. Why did medical specialization first emerge when and where it did? Why and how did it come to appear as inevitable—though not necessarily unproblematic? Why did it take certain directions and not others? Did it evolve in pretty much the same way everywhere? These are the kinds of questions that I hope to answer in this book. The comparative nature of this study allows me to examine different national patterns of development and to search for both common features and variations in national specialization processes. I hope in this way to determine the degree to which specialization was an international phenomenon cutting across national boundaries and the extent to which it developed out of specific institutional and intellectual conditions in each nation. My chronological frame will be a long one, close to two centuries, and I will examine in detail four very different national cases: those of France, Britain, Germany, and the United States. Collectively these nations largely determined the shape of medical specialties as we know them.

The Existing Literature

In pursuing this study I have built on a significant body of existing work. The oldest, and the one most closely approximating my own efforts, is a book by George

Rosen published in 1944. Like any book of that vintage, it is in certain respects out of date. It can also be faulted for not making necessary distinctions among nations or historical periods and for generalizing a bit too much from the single case of ophthalmology. It nonetheless remains an impressive work full of astute insights that are still pertinent at the beginning of the new millennium. Although I disagree with Rosen on specific points of interpretation, I nonetheless consider his views as a natural starting point for my own work. I will be wrestling with his interpretations for much of the first half of this book.

Rosen contended that two factors were at play in the emergence of specialties during the course of the nineteenth century. First there was the "decisive influence exerted by social and economic forces"; then there were "to a not inconsiderable degree . . . antecedent and contemporary medical factors."[7] The discussion of the latter constitutes the most original part of Rosen's argument and is usually emphasized by historians.[8] (I myself discuss it below.) The tendency of historians to ignore Rosen's account of the social factors behind specialization is due to the fact that our understanding of the "social" has changed since the 1940s. For Rosen a key social development behind specialization was urbanization. Here he borrowed directly from Durkheim the idea that division of labor was a consequence of population density in cities. Another "social factor" that Rosen emphasized had to do with the movement of people and ideas. Immigration, as well as the spread of shipping and communication, accelerated specialization by fostering international social and intellectual contacts.

Rosen's concept of the "social" is surely pertinent to any understanding of specialization in medicine. In the 1970s, however, the dominant meaning of that term in the history of medicine and science shifted increasingly from broad social processes such as urbanization and immigration to the efforts of professional groups to raise their social and economic status and, more generally, pursue individual and collective interests within a "market" for medical services. This rather impoverished notion of the social is not missing from Rosen's account. But rather than being constitutive of specialization, it is treated as a secondary factor. By the 1970s, Rosen himself had become thoroughly fluent in the vocabulary of professional markets and mobility, which he utilized in his account of the history of American medicine. In this later work, he presented in this idiom many insights about specialization in the American context[9]; nonetheless, he did not attempt to recast his earlier comprehensive analysis of specialization.

After Rosen, the major studies of specialization focused on particular national contexts. Two works by Rosemary Stevens, written in 1966 and 1971, and treating Great Britain and the United States, respectively, have justifiably become classics.[10] Both are cast in the language of policy analysis, with the emphasis on current organizational problems and their solutions. In these studies, specialization was presented as both inescapable and clearly beneficial: "it was an inevitable and desirable accompaniment of scientific advance."[11] This tone is partly a product of the period in which it was written, but also follows from Stevens's chronological focus. Each book briefly discusses nineteenth-century developments but is emphatically about medicine in the twentieth century. By the beginning of the latter century, the advantages of specialization indeed appeared self-evident even to those who deplored the consequences; the great challenge was to find acceptable forms of organization for specialties within existing systems of medical institutions. This is the process that Stevens so skillfully analyzes in her two books.

Both of Stevens's books remain remarkable achievements, masterfully synthesizing huge bodies of material. As a cursory perusal of my notes makes clear, they remain invaluable accounts of specialization in Britain and the United States. One reason for their continued relevance, it seems to me, is that Stevens's emphasis was absolutely correct. The most interesting question about specialization is not why it succeeded—because there were in fact so many reasons for that success. If specialization was not inevitable, it was certainly overdetermined to an extraordinary degree. It is far more interesting and fruitful to focus on how specialization was integrated into existing networks of national medical institutions.

One last book that dates from 1970 is Hans Eulner's monumental study of medical specialties in Germany. This relates exclusively to specialties in the academic context, and pretty much ignores specialty practice (which the author discussed briefly in a separate article).[12] Each chapter focuses on an individual specialty, an approach that makes it difficult to understand the way in which the entire system of academic specialties evolved. Nonetheless, this work is a treasure house of information. And the decision to focus on specialization in the academic context makes perfect sense because, as I will argue shortly, specialization was, for much of the nineteenth century, understood primarily as a function of medical research and teaching.

Since the early 1970s, historians and sociologists have characteristically focused on individual specialties in a single country and, frequently, during a relatively limited time period.[13] Providing a broader context for these studies—when these are not narrowly empirical—is one of several theoretical perspectives.

The most common of these perspectives is the result of several decades of work in the sociology of professions. Professionalization theory has a long history among sociologists and has been cast in a variety of different ways. But among its leading practitioners, including Everett Hughes,[14] Elliot Freidson,[15] Magali Larsen,[16] and Andrew Abbott,[17] specialties do not usually loom very large.[18] Segmentation, to be sure, is usually treated as a common tendency among professional groups.[19] But when specialties are not seen as a barrier to the professional unity required by professions to achieve success in their endeavors, they are treated pretty much as miniature professions engaged in much the same activities of collective social mobility and competition for power and resources as larger professional group.[20] Many sociologists and historians have utilized professionalization theory to study medical specialties. (Among historians, theory sometimes gets lost; specialists simply pursue rather vague "interests.") Sometimes the theoretical framework is fairly simple, a matter of greedy individuals seeking power and wealth. But more sophisticated works in this vein have made an important contribution to our understanding of specialty development.

Sidney Halpern's excellent study of American pediatrics[21] begins with an analysis of specialization in the language of sociological theory. Here a "model" rather than a historical account provides a general framework for understanding the specialization process. Halpern adds important insights to Rosen's pioneering account: the centrality of public health concerns as a focus for professional activity; the role of institutional innovation in creating a division of labor that serves as a basis and stimulant for specialty development. Perhaps most useful is her argument that specialties are dynamic and constantly changing, recasting their activities and identities at regular intervals. Much the same can be said about the overall system of specialties.

Less common are studies inspired by other theoretical perspectives. Some follow the late Michel Foucault in examining how specific specialties subject individuals to "surveillance," "discipline," and "normalizing judgment."[22] Social interactionist accounts offer rich analyses of the "social world" of certain specialties in the contemporary era, which are observed directly and in minute detail by the sociologist.[23] (Historians by definition never have access to this level of detail.) Studies inspired by work in the sociology of science examine how scientific and technological innovations and their clinical applications are constructed, understood, and/or appropriated by different specialist groups.[24] Finally, a very few sociologists, political scientists, and policy analysts have undertaken comparative studies that contrast aspects of contemporary specialization in different countries.[25]

Each of these theoretical approaches emphasizes different aspects of the complex development of specialization; each provides insight for specific kinds of issues. I make occasional reference to most of them at one point or another in my account but do not restrict myself to any single one. I utilize instead an open-ended historical perspective that attempts to be sensitive to theoretical work without being handcuffed to it. My text is built around change through time and national comparison.

The Scope of This Work

Historians are trained to look for movement through time, so it is not surprising that specialization is in my account constantly in process. I have built my narrative around a fundamental distinction between the specialization of the nineteenth century (running to roughly 1890, and about 1900 in Britain) and the decades that followed (to roughly 1950). During the earlier stage, specialization was organized primarily around the tasks of clinical research and training for general practitioners. It was largely a local phenomenon advanced by individuals or small groups. The major locus of competition during this period was the combination of medical school and teaching hospital. Specialist private practice and market conflict among specialists for control of specific domains certainly existed, but were usually perceived as secondary phenomena; they became serious issues of contention only sporadically and in a few places. This initial stage of medical specialization provides the subject for the first section of this book.

During the later phase, extending from the last decade of the nineteenth century to the years before and after the Second World War, specialization continued to provide a significant framework for research and general medical education; but it simultaneously became the dominant form of medical practice, raising in the process new problems of specialist training, certification, and jurisdictional boundaries. It evolved from a largely local to a national phenomenon, producing new kinds of specialist associations, transforming the institutions of the larger medical profession, and, in some cases, becoming an issue for political authorities. From an individual career choice, it became a matter for national regulation. This second phase provides the subject matter for the second section of this book. My chronological end point differs somewhat from one nation to the next, according to the point when each worked out a system of regulation: the 1920s and 1930s in Germany and the United States, the late 1940s in France and Britain. After 1950, the consolidation of formal specialist training and certification, the spread of health insurance, the remarkable expansion of both state-sponsored medical research and the pharmaceutical industry, the rise of new modes of clinical testing, the appearance of myriad new medical technologies, and the rise of international standardization all combined to usher in a third era of specialization that continues to this day. I discuss the transformation of specialty systems since 1950 in the epilogue.

If the sections of this book are determined by chronology, they are simultaneously built around different national experiences. My account focuses on four countries: France, Britain, Germany, and the United States. Germany did not exist as a nation during the early stages of specialty development. Consequently, in discussing events during the nineteenth century, I usually refer to the German-speaking world, and particularly its great cities, Vienna and Berlin, where specialization was most developed. For the period that follows the unification of Germany, however, I focus on that country.

I argue throughout the book that there are major national variations in the development of specialization. These divergences are illuminating because they allow us to see clearly that certain characteristics that we tend to view as immutable and inherent in the very nature of medical specialization are in fact local and contingent. Nonetheless, we must be equally attentive to parallels and common features that cut across national boundaries. This is not always easy, because work based on comparison tends to be biased toward finding difference. What, after all, is the point of the exercise if one nation's history pretty much recapitulates that of another? Nonetheless, we must account for the fact that we find striking similarities among nations with very different medical traditions and histories. These may reflect common structural conditions or direct international influences.

From time to time, and especially in part III, I discuss the histories of individual specialties. But for the most part I am concerned with the larger "specialization" process. The latter can be understood as a semifictitious term that allows us to generalize about the collective experiences of many specialty groups, or it can be conceptualized as a more or less real entity or "system" in which elaborate rules determine how a complex game is played by a diverse group of actors. My own preference is for the latter view, although most of the arguments in the chapters that follow are not dependent on this preference.

In talking about national "systems" or 'networks" of specialties, I am entering territory made familiar by Andrew Abbott's now famous idea of "the system of professions." Because Abbott argues that his notion can be applied to medical specialties and presents a case study to prove it, it is necessary to distinguish clearly my use of the term "system" from his. It should be obvious that "systems of specialties" differ in fundamental ways from "systems" of professions. The fact of belonging to a larger professional group has significant consequences that no one would dispute. But the more serious difference in the way I use the term has to do with focus. For Abbott, a system applies to a particular area of social activity or need—the personal problems jurisdiction, for instance, that is dealt with at length in his book. In Abbott's telling, different groups have competed and negotiated to control this social domain. Psychiatrists, neurologists, clergy, and psychologists have all, at one time or another, contested this social terrain and their activity has constituted it. Abbott's approach works well if one examines a reasonably well-defined area of activity. But how does one deal with different specialties that do not in fact share domains? What is the nature of the relationship between psychiatry and ophthalmology, for example? What, in other words, is the nature of the "system" that holds together and shapes all the different specialties?

I have two responses. The first is that specialists spontaneously divide the evolving world of medical work into categories within which they distribute themselves. They do so in collaboration with the individuals who are their patients and the groups and institutions that constitute their social environment. As we shall see in part III, the contours of such specialty worlds may differ in substantial ways from one country or city to the next. In this sense, "system" is an abstract analytic term that attributes some degree of social logic and coherence to the particular local profiles discerned by the historian. (There is a "systemic" reason why gynecologists were so numerous in nineteenth-century Paris while there were so few pediatricians in Germany.) This meaning of the word "system" plays only a minor role in the account that follows. Far more central is a second meaning of the term that is more tangible and that has to do with concrete decisions and actions. Specialties do not differ from professions only in belonging to a larger professional group that confers advantages and forces compromises. Like professions, specialties gradually become subject to rules and models of behavior—some implicit and others quite explicit— that regulate and standardize the sometimes chaotic forms of activity that initially prevail and that determine the scope and nature of intraspecialty competition.

The rules and models imposed on systems of specialties have, until recently, been notably more constraining than those which govern relations among different professions; this is because medical professions successfully imposed a significant degree of control over the processes of internal segmentation that only the state is capable of imposing on the "system of profession." Certainly the medical profession has not operated in a vacuum. Political authorities, the legal system, economic interests, and public opinion occasionally (and increasingly over time) act directly and decisively on particular specialties; for most of the period under consideration, however, medical actors have determined the general parameters within which professional self-government has taken place. The forces that collectively mold and regulate specialties—and that are in turn transformed by these same specialties—are located in networks of institutions: medical schools, elite hospitals, national medical associations, public health agencies, and insurance authorities. It is in this specific sociological sense that specialties have come to constitute "systems." The gradual emergence of such systems in different national and professional contexts constitutes one of the major themes of this book.

One need not share the view that specialties constitute "systems" to agree that it is worth analyzing the larger historical development of specialization that cannot be reduced to the history of individual specialties. To be sure, individual specialties appear regularly throughout my account, and part III compares the way a handful of specialties have evolved in the four countries under consideration.[26] Nonetheless, I do not attempt, even in these chapters, to provide a comprehensive history of the specialties discussed. Here, as throughout this book, my goal is to account for the broader history of specialization.

This focus on "specialization" rather than individual specialties has determined certain research choices. While I have utilized a wide variety of historical sources, I have focused particularly on those in which specialists and specialties address the wider medical profession (and sometimes the public) in order to negotiate their positions within wider institutional networks. These forums include medical directories, national associations and journals, medical schools, and scientific academies and societies. I have utilized only selectively the specialist journals in which specialists address their peers. This is in part a survival strategy since there is no possible way to read even a small part of the immense literature generated by specialists in four countries. But my choice also reflects a methodological principle: one can best understand the general system of specialties through sources that describe public struggles for recognition and self-definition that take place in larger professional arenas.

The Emergence of Specialization: An Overview

Specialist healers existed long before medical specialization as we know it. There is evidence that they practiced in ancient Egypt, where, it has been argued, each body part was considered a separate entity; according to this view, the spread of systemic humoralism put an end to such conceptions of the body.[27] Nevertheless, specialization was, according to Galen, common among the Roman doctors of his era.[28] One can find other examples of this sort, but specialist practice did not loom large in the history of Western medicine until the nineteenth century. During the eighteenth century, low-status if occasionally well-remunerated practitioners specializing in particular manual procedures—including tooth extraction, cutting for the stone, couching cataracts, childbirth, and treatment of venereal diseases—existed in most Western nations. In France many of these practitioners were known as *experts;* in Germany, as *operateurs.* Among them were itinerants with little education; doctors possessing medical diplomas or licenses frequently viewed them as "charlatans" and "quacks." Increasingly during the course of the eighteenth century, small numbers of those with formal credentials, particularly among the surgeons, began offering some of the services provided by *experts* and *operateurs.* Surgeon-dentists, surgeon-oculists, and, above all, man-midwives were among the most visible. Such activity, however, occurred on a small scale.

In the chapters that follow, I will attempt to account for the emergence of specialization on a larger scale in the nineteenth century. First, I will suggest, as George Rosen did, that the commonsense explanation for the emergence of medical specialties—that the rapid expansion of knowledge forced doctors to specialize—is incorrect, at least as an explanation for the early stages of the specialization process. I agree with Rosen and Erwin Ackerknecht that a fundamental transformation of intellectual perspective lay behind the rise of specialties. Nonetheless, I do not, as they did, attribute primary responsibility to the rise of pathological anatomy, with its emphasis on organic localism, and then to new technologies. These factors, at most, provided an axis along which certain specialties were able to develop.

Instead, I argue that a fundamental precondition for these developments was the unification of medicine with surgery, both as categories of professional practice and, more important, within institutions of training and research. Only within an understanding of medicine as a unified domain did division into subfields make very much sense. Furthermore, I emphasize that specialization can best be viewed as part of the much wider change that gradually produced "professional" scientists and disciplinary communities in many different fields of knowledge. Historians call this process, which occurred roughly from 1775 to 1830, the "Great Transition."[29] Medicine was a highly idiosyncratic but integral participant in the Great Transition. An emerging imperative to pursue clinical research of various sorts encouraged specialization that allowed for the rigorous empirical observation of many cases that had become a requirement of all serious medical science. Finally, I suggest that specialization was closely linked with emerging notions of administrative rationality in the nineteenth-century nation-state. One could, it was widely thought, best manage large populations through proper classification, gathering together individuals belonging to the same class and separating those belonging to different categories. The institutions that resulted allowed specialist medicine to emerge. All of these conditions emerged first in early nineteenth-century Paris.

Professional unity, scholarly commitments to research, and administrative enthusiasm for classification and division were thus intertwined; in fact, they can all be seen as part of the development of the nation-state in search of practical strategies and new knowledge to better fulfill its expanding commitments. This link goes beyond the obvious efforts of the state to create institutions capable of producing useful knowledge. A deeper-level symbiosis was at work; both state administrators and knowledge producers were pursuing similar strategies to gain control over vast and chaotic domains. Each group was increasingly carving up its respective sphere into smaller, more manageable categories within which it could impose order and some degree of standardization and uniformity. Division permitted conquest of many different sorts.

Specialization also depended on and reflected long-standing traditions of scientific work in each country. Loraine Daston has argued that claims to specialized learning had far more salience in France than did claims to universal and synthetic knowledge. The Paris Academy of Sciences, during its formative years from 1666 to 1699, chose an orientation featuring specialized expertise, at least in part because it was a public institution devoted to, among other tasks, satisfying the practical needs of the state. The Royal Society of London, in contrast, was a private institution that long held on to "gentlemanly" notions of scientific work and resisted specialization in the name of polite learning. The situation in Berlin stood somewhere between the Parisian and London extremes.[30] Such national attitudes would influence the reception accorded to specialization.

Growing public interest in specific health issues encouraged the emergence and development of particular specialties. Such interest could be expressed through governmental action in the form of public health measures or the creation of state institutions; but it could also be expressed, as was the case in Britain and the United States, through private philanthropic activity. Public concern to reduce infant mortality was a potent stimulus to the early development of obstetrics and pediatrics as specialties. The emergence of such public "causes" led typically to the construction of new institutions within which specialties could develop. By the end of the nineteenth century, few specialties did not make at least some appeal to the public interest.

Underlying the rise of specialties were more basic changes in public attitudes. Numerous societal forces made specialization appear natural and advantageous. The increasing economic complexity of capitalist societies provided one notable example and generated the concept of the "division of labor," mobilized frequently to defend medical specialties.[31] From the middle of the nineteenth century, the theory of evolution was used to justify specialism and complexity as higher forms of structure. Few aspects of life in Western societies, in fact, did not in one way or another legitimate specialization. But it was, I suggest, the developing natural and physical sciences that provided the most striking models of specialized work. These were particularly pertinent for a domain in which practitioners thought of themselves as belonging to the larger community of science.

Specialization, I suggest, gained its initial and primary justification as a form of knowledge production and dissemination rather than as a type of skill or form of practice. It is no accident that Carl Wunderlich referred to specialties he encountered in Paris as "diese einzelnen Branchen der Wissenschaft."[32] There was, however, no sharp distinction in medicine between specialization as a form of knowledge and specialization as a form of practice; the two were inseparable because most medical teaching and research took place not in laboratories but in institutions devoted to clinical practice. Superior skill was sometimes invoked in favor of specialists; and the early entry into general hospitals of certain specialists and the creation of specialized hospitals reflected belief that these specialists could perform useful, even life-saving, procedures beyond the skills of general physicians and surgeons. Some types of institutions, notably lunatic asylums, were numerous and distinctive enough to generate specialist identities that were, in certain countries at least, independent of serious commitment to clinical research. Many sought commercial advantages from specialized practice. The successful specialist-innovator was almost always viewed as most competent to deal with difficult cases and could expect to develop a lucrative private practice. Not all or even most of those who claimed specialties were innovators or even serious researchers. Nonetheless, the public acceptance and rising status of specialization depended on the innovators and on the increasing identification of specialists with research and medical progress.

The handful of isolated specialists practicing in major cities at the beginning of the nineteenth century gradually grew in numbers and became a recognizable social category. The process began in Paris in the 1830s, moved a decade or so later to Vienna, and then to other cities in Europe and North America in the 1850s and 1860s. Specialization developed as well in Britain, but in a distinctive and uniquely troubled way. During much of the nineteenth century, debates and battles surrounding specialization usually took place in the arena of elite institutions, notably medical schools, hospitals, and medical associations and congresses, where each category battled for full acceptance. Only sporadically did specialist practice inspire controversy. By 1890 (and a decade or so later in Britain), the general battle for the acceptance of specialties in elite institutions was largely won. Individual specialties would continue to struggle for acceptance or improved position in elite institutions. But increasingly, as more and more doctors began to call themselves specialists, the battleground spread to the arena of medical practice.

That these developments occurred internationally was due in large measure to the fact that doctors everywhere faced much the same societal realities: intense professional competition, growing public faith in scientific expertise, increasing intervention by public authorities in the field of health care. But an equally important consideration is that medicine was probably the first large profession to develop a truly international culture not unlike that of the scientific disciplines to which it was closely connected. There was a striking parallelism in the timing of major developments in all the countries under consideration that can be explained only by the fact that medical elites observed closely and communicated regularly with one another. Events abroad might serve as either a model or a foil. But specialization, like the related development of medical education,[33] was characterized by a significant degree of international contact that did not preclude striking differences among our four nations.

Paris was the first city to develop specialties on a significant scale. The basis for this development, I argue in chapter 1, was the emergence of a new kind of medical research community around the teaching institutions and hospitals of the city. It was the scale of this development, rather than any monopoly of the new tendencies, that made the French capital unique. The vast majority of French medical academics initially were opposed to clinical specialties; but specialization, along with laboratory experimentation (and much less problematically), became emblematic of a new vision of medical science that captured the attention of medical reformers after midcentury. The appointment of a leading academic reformer as dean of the Paris Faculty of Medicine allowed junior positions for specialists to be created in that institution in 1862. The consolidation of the Third Republic in the late 1870s put reformers firmly in charge and also made new funding available to institutions of higher education. Consequently, specialties became solidly established at the Paris Faculty of Medicine. However, institutional rigidity and chronic underfunding characterized French higher education at a time when expanding universities were everywhere becoming the driving force behind medical specialization and scientific research more generally. One consequence was the relative neglect of institutions in provincial cities. As a result, medical specialization in France was until the twentieth century a predominantly Parisian phenomenon.

My account continues with the case of London, where specialization was accepted relatively late and halfheartedly. Because the British capital lacked most of the institutional conditions that existed in Paris, we can more fully grasp the circumstances that promoted specialization elsewhere. Despite London's huge size and great medical resources, it lacked an integrated medical research community. Consequently, specialization developed during the first half of the nineteenth century as a relatively low-status career option oriented primarily toward practice and based on direct appeals to the nonmedical public rather than to medical elites. Even after specialization became identified as a necessity of science in other countries, the British medical elite resisted it. Like British academic elites more generally, it continued to be wedded to ideals of general knowledge in teaching and practice. This resistance could not block the development of specialization in Britain, but it did limit its scope to a significant degree and gave it a character rather different from the one it acquired in other countries.

Vienna early in the nineteenth century contained many of the same resources that allowed Paris to become the first center for specialties. But the size of its academic medical community was considerably smaller and political conditions were unfavorable; this explains why specialization did not initially develop here on a significant scale. However, once specialization became identified as an integral element of the new medical science that was emerging internationally, size came to matter less and Viennese institutions moved with remarkable speed to make the city a leading center of specialism and a magnet for foreign doctors and medical students. Equally significant was the fact that the university was part of a large network of German-language universities that underwent significant expansion in the second half of the century, allowing for disciplinary specialization in all areas of knowledge. Far more than in France, medical specialization in nineteenth-century Germany was centered in universities. Building upon the competition among many institutions for students and scientific prestige, and financed generously by multiple state authorities that recognized the benefits—at once practical, symbolic, and ideological—of investments in scientific research and higher education, the German-speaking world was by the late nineteenth century widely perceived as the dominant international center of scientific and medical research. Specialties were the beneficiaries of these developments, although they were not quite so well developed outside Vienna as French reformers liked to claim.

Almost none of the conditions that prevailed in Paris and Vienna existed in the United States. Yet despite some virulent opposition, the American medical elite embraced specialization with remarkable speed and enthusiasm after 1860. American doctors flocked to Europe to become specialists. The primary cause of this development was the especially low public status of American medicine, which provoked an intense desire to raise the standing of the profession through the embrace of science. Specialization was fully associated with the new medical science but was nonetheless accessible and practice-oriented in a way that was not true of laboratory disciplines such as experimental physiology. Furthermore, the plethora of small, private medical schools competing for students, clients, and patrons, and far less bureaucratic and elitist than those of continental Europe, made it both necessary and relatively easy to introduce specialties into academic medicine. Since such institutional openness produced a medical elite that was less clearly distinguished and less prestigious than its European counterparts, it was harder in the United States to discriminate between scientific justifications for specialization and the purely commercial motives of many practitioners. The United States was thus the first country where specialist practice was directly challenged. The ongoing conflict between medical elites favorable to specialization and rank-and-file practitioners who were frequently hostile to it was actively mediated by the American Medical Association.

Regulating and Standardizing: An Overview

For much of the nineteenth century, specialization was primarily about producing and teaching specialized knowledge necessary to train general practitioners. It was locally organized and, for many, a highly individual career choice. From the mid-1880s on, however, the number of specialists began to rise precipitously; most of them made no pretense to being teachers and researchers, and claimed instead expertise in specialist practice. They did so because by now private specialist practice seemed to offer substantially greater economic rewards and professional status than general practice. Patients were demanding attendance by specialists, who were increasingly identified with scientific progress. Everywhere, developments in science, from electrification of cities to the germ theory of disease, promoted popular faith in the scientific expert. Furthermore, rapidly expanding networks of institutions dramatically augmented the sum of medical and scientific knowledge that could be taught and mastered. Medical schools in every nation faced major difficulties in organizing and imparting the mounting glut of potentially relevant information and skills.[34] For perhaps the first time, specialists could plausibly argue not only that it was more effective to specialize than to learn everything, but also that there was no longer an alternative, since it was impossible to learn everything. Specialties thus became national in scope, and they raised critical policy issues for organized medical professions and, occasionally, for governments.

Many forces propelled these developments. Population growth in large cities and new modes of transportation that facilitated travel over longer distances made specialty practice increasingly viable. Medical professions everywhere expanded rapidly during these decades, intensifying competition that encouraged doctors to differentiate themselves in order to survive economically. Humanitarian and public health issues assumed ever greater significance as governments became involved in new areas of health care. The development of mass media and novel techniques of publicity allowed fashionable objects of public concern to spread quickly and widely. Consequently, more and more specialties benefited from public campaigns on behalf of specific types of patients. Such public interest created new needs and new institutions, so that, in the words of one twentieth-century orthopedist, "very large numbers of cases have become available for clinical and teaching purposes."[35] New social metaphors became available as justifications of specialization. To the traditional "division of labor," and later ideas of evolutionary complexity, was now added the notion of "industrial organization of production."

Individuals and even entire specialties could differ substantially in the degree to which they adopted a professional identity based on specialist practice or held on to the nineteenth-century idea of specialties as domains of disciplinary research. Academic physicians remained especially attached to the latter view. Overall, however, a major shift in both identity and practice did occur. To the characteristic nineteenth-century concern that specialization might have negative consequences because it promoted intellectual narrowness and "one-sidedness" were added new worries about the explosive expansion of specialists. Would general practitioners survive? How could specialists themselves support so much competition? What were legitimate categories of specialization, and which types of practitioners could perform what sorts of procedures? Above all, it was asked, how could one ensure that specialists were in fact competent?

There were many possible responses to this last question. For a dwindling minority, allowing individuals to define themselves in such venues as medical directories, business cards, and door plaques was acceptable because the public was capable of making decisions about medical competence. Elitist specialist societies frequently set conditions on membership that implicitly or explicitly reflected definitions of specialist status. One very common condition of membership was full-time practice as a specialist and renunciation of all forms of general practice. Another was selective election based on the premise that the specialist was someone recognized by his or her peers to have exceptional knowledge and experience in a particular sphere. Or a specialist could be defined as someone who held a particular kind of post in a hospital or medical school, as was becoming the case in Britain.

If determining who was a specialist was a relatively new problem, an older question—what constituted a specialty?—took a new twist. The nineteenth-century test of an acceptable academic specialty was whether it was generating substantial new knowledge and practices. On this basis, only a few specialties might merit full chairs and a place on examinations, but almost any promising discipline could be represented by relatively cheap junior faculty. However, once specialties became forms of practice, fears of professional fragmentation intensified. There was general agreement everywhere that the number of specialties should be kept small. But how was one to choose from among the many that were in fact emerging? It was at this point that doctors began discussing whether there were abstract principles that might define a legitimate specialty. Did fields that treated specific populations, such as children, have as much justification to specialty status as those based on specific organs or hard-to-master technologies? And what about those based on social needs, laboratory procedures, or specific therapeutic modalities? One of the reasons for the persuasiveness of George Rosen's claim that the rise of specialization was based on organic localism and new technologies is that many doctors in the early twentieth century sought to delegitimize certain existing specialties by arguing that "real" specialties were defined by these very features.

Medical directories served as a major forum for the working out of such definitions, and are the subject of chapter 5. After presenting a history of these publications that sought to display the medical world of a city, region, or entire country, we examine the various ways they struggled to come to terms with increasing numbers of physicians now calling themselves specialists. One option that was available to directory editors was to attempt to control the specialty categories used by individuals for purposes of self-identification. The French made little effort to do so, a decision foreshadowing their later lack of interest in trying to define specialist competence. In the three other countries under discussion, organized medical professions first tried to suppress the use of specialty designations in directories, on the grounds that these constituted a form of unethical advertising. The British never fully abandoned this position because they viewed such published information as a threat to their developing system of patient referral. Although the British Medical

Association (BMA) was grudgingly forced to recognize the ethical legitimacy of specialist self-identification, the practice did not in fact spread to the leading national medical directory. German and American directories, in contrast, reflected the evolving positions of their respective national medical associations and repealed the ban on specialist self-identification during the first years of the twentieth century. However, they predefined and significantly limited the specialty categories that doctors were permitted to mention. This prefigured their response to the issue of certification.

The editorial policies of medical directories constituted a telling but relatively small part of professional struggles to regulate the expanding domain of specialties. The central and most difficult task had to do with finding formulas for identifying specialists on the basis of formal training and certification. One had to decide whose right to practice could be restricted in this way and by what agency or body. A related problem had to do with resolving intraprofessional disputes about which groups could perform what medical acts. How the struggle over certification unfolded in our four nations is the subject of chapters 6 through 9. It was resolved in different ways in each country, depending in large measure on the nature of national medical associations and their attitude toward professional regulation more generally. My central argument is that those countries with strong national medical associations committed to wide-ranging professional reform were the first to resolve the issue of specialist certification. My second argument is that governments and state agencies (except in the United States) played an important but indirect role in inspiring these developments by setting up the health insurance systems that distinguished between generalists and specialists in matters of fees, thus necessitating precise definitions of who was who. Governments also created the larger political and institutional conditions within which this could occur and occasionally intervened in direct ways. Nonetheless, the process of specialist certification was by and large led by organized medical professions and reflected their beliefs and values.

Debates over certification first emerged in Germany at the end of the 1880s. This occurred primarily because a national medical body representing both specialists and GPs was in a strong position at an early stage to confront and debate the difficult issues that were arising in this domain, as in many others. The chief of these problems, and a major impetus for regulating specialties, was the creation of a state health insurance system in 1883. That the Prussian government, with its tradition of intervention in the regulation of medical training and care, took an active interest in the question of specialists helped to precipitate matters. The United States followed suit, soon after the reorganization of the American Medical Association (AMA) made that body a far more representative and effective national association. Given both the direct influence of German medicine in America and similar structural conditions in the two countries—regional decentralization and vigorous competition from unlicensed or irregular healers—it is not coincidental that both medical professions opted for systems of specialist training and certification controlled by organizations representing the medical profession. The mechanisms set up for this purpose, however, were quite different in the two nations. In Germany, specialty certification was the responsibility of bodies representing the entire medical profession in a particular locality. In the United States, the national representative bodies of specialists themselves played a determining role, with the AMA and several other national groups struggling to bring coherence and more uniform standards to the patchwork of specialty programs that was being set up.

In France, the medical profession lacked an effective national representative body until well into the twentieth century. Consequently, specialization provoked remarkably little debate and the profession was slow to consider the issue of specialist certification. When it finally did so, at the end of the 1920s, it opted very characteristically for a national, state-controlled system of certification. The enormous difficulties of successfully implementing such an ambitious project in the French political milieu produced long delays. The French system of specialty certification was set up more than two decades after those of Germany and the United States began to function.

The situation in Britain was fundamentally unlike our other cases. Various sorts of short, low-level, specialty training programs were introduced in the early twentieth century but, with only a few exceptions, certification never became a widespread professional demand. The pressure for specialist training that developed in the 1930s and '40s was not linked to medical desire to curb unbridled specialist practice, as was the case elsewhere, but reflected the need to provide well-trained specialist personnel for a health care system desperately in need of reform. The traditional definition of specialists in terms of appointment to hospital posts through largely informal modes of peer selection was congruent with a technocratic vision of a unified, coordinated, and "efficient" health system that began to spread during the interwar period. The introduction of the National Health Service after World War II confirmed and extended this view of specialties. For those building a new health-care system, the purpose of organizing specialty training was to produce many more specialists in order to meet the nation's needs.

Certification was not a necessary condition for jurisdictional battles over control of medical practices. Specialists were often in the front lines of early conflicts pitting the medical profession against competing nonmedical occupations, including opticians, dentists, radiological technicians, nurse-anesthetists, and physical therapists. They might also take on those controlling specific kinds of institutions, as did American neurologists who criticized asylum superintendents. Nor did it require the existence of formal certification for specialists to try to convince hospital administrations that special wards with appropriately recruited staff should be established. But once certification in one form or another was introduced, the question of what medical activities were appropriate to each sort of practitioner became highly contentious; these disputes were intensified by the establishment of various kinds of health insurance schemes.

From its origins, we have suggested, specialization was connected to notions of bureaucratic rationality. For those responsible for vast numbers of clients, dividing these into rational categories seemed like an imperative of effectiveness and order. In the twentieth century, as the role of public authorities increased, such pressures toward bureaucratic rationality multiplied. Everywhere health insurance agencies, either public or private, were set up. Their need for clear definitions of specialist status in matters of coverage and payment served as a major stimulus to certification. The world wars of the twentieth century were especially important in diffusing notions of bureaucratic rationality that legitimated the advance and regulation of specialties. Those responsible for rapidly setting up medical services for huge numbers of military personnel seem to have been particularly susceptible to the attractions of specialization.[36] In addition, specific military manpower needs provided considerable support for the development of particular specialties, including cardiology, orthopedics, and psychiatry.

Nonetheless, notions of bureaucratic rationality could be flexible and adapted to local cultural and professional values. The National Health Service in Britain could live without formal certification of its specialists; insurance agencies in Germany could accept specialist accreditation based on training credentials rather than written examinations; in France nothing less than national certification under the aegus of the state following formal studies and examination was acceptable. Norms of bureaucratic rationality could also be utilized to argue that specialization had gone too far and that the health system now needed more GPs or new forms of practice to compensate for the narrowness of the specialist practitioners. Bureaucratic rationality was a highly elastic concept.

The 1920s and 1930s, the decades that witnessed the nearly total victory of reductionist medicine founded on specialization, also gave birth to a holistic revival that reviled narrow specialists and that looked to a new "synthetic" medicine more sensitive to the total human being. Various institutional proposals were suggested to compensate for the perceived narrowness of specialist practice, including revitalization of general practice, group practice, and gathering together specialized institutions within a single medical center. Many specialties now cast their claims to significance and resources in more holistic terms: the growing emphasis on psychosomatic factors in illness and healing gave new life to psychiatry.[37] Even organ-based specialties frequently emphasized that their organs provided a gateway to the entire "constitution" of individuals. An ugly variant of the anti-specialist impulse during these years was to blame nefarious Jewish influences for the continuing spread of specialization. This was of course only one of many evils for which Jewish doctors were held responsible. The identification of specialization with Jewish doctors was especially prevalent in Germany but was not restricted to that nation.

The international culture of medical science became even more influential during these years. International associations of every sort proliferated and contributed to a common medical culture. To be sure, extreme political conditions in Germany led to extreme, indeed hideous, medical ideas and behavior that eventually took that nation's medical profession well beyond the international pale. And neither cultural nor institutional differences among nations disappeared. Nonetheless, one is struck by many similarities of development among our four national cases. During the 1930s, one international association undertook large-scale inquiries into the ways that different nations were dealing with such major issues as specialization, illegal practice, and national health insurance. Emerging from these surveys, it suggested, was the following conclusion:

> Whatever may be the form of government, the medico-political and medico-social problems are identical in all countries. . . . Secondly we find that they are being resolved in every country by methods which are either identical or analogous; our discussions and annual conferences have therefore always been of a practical nature. We have tried in each case to formulate conclusions which could be quoted as evidence of international medical agreement, and have nearly always been unanimous.[38]

Such purported agreement, however, did not prevent the emergence of major differences in the way specialties came to be organized in each country.

National patterns and characteristics are not the only perspective from which to view all the forces and issues that were at play. The final chapters in part III shift focus, and examine the formation and development of a number of specialties in comparative perspective. Some, such as surgery and internal medicine, were the original divisions of medicine that had been recast as specialties. Many others gradually assumed their modern form as they split off from or combined with other specialist groups. A few, such as gynecology, developed in a particularly complex environment and faced particularly intractable problems. Yet others, notably stomatology, gradually lost their positions as fields of medicine in at least some of the nations under discussion. Taken together, these studies demonstrate how different nations worked out tensions between the forces favoring international standardization and national variations, in the context of evolving institutional arrangements, and shifting balances of power among contending groups.

Conclusion

The title of this volume, *Divide and Conquer*, highlights some important features of specialization. First, it expresses a fundamental intellectual strategy: dividing problems into smaller and more manageable units in order to solve them more easily. This strategy has become the hallmark of modern science and has produced almost unimaginable advances. It also has serious limitations about which we are regularly reminded by proponents of more "holistic" or synthetic intellectual strategies. Second, it represents a way of dividing people into smaller and more manageable groups based on common attributes in order to facilitate their management in every sense of the term. It is this quality, more than anything else, that explains the very close links between specialization in medicine and state administration. Third, it describes what has happened to medical institutions and the medical profession that in the space of a century were literally divided and conquered by new forms of organization based on a novel kind of expertise. In some ways this has been the most spectacular conquest of all. Finally, it portrays what we now experience as patients: we are allocated to special wards or hospitals so that specific parts of our bodies can be treated. One consequence is that our diseases are more predictably cured or at least controlled than at any time in the past. Another is that our autonomy and capacity for informed judgment in the face of huge, segmented institutions have been severely curtailed. The triumph of specialization has involved painful trade-offs.

Part I

THE EMERGENCE OF MEDICAL SPECIALIZATION IN THE NINETEENTH CENTURY

Chapter 1

The Rise of Specialties in Early Nineteenth-Century Paris

Medical specialization emerged in large cities. It first did so in Paris during the 1830s as a result of three processes: the unification of surgery and medicine, the rise of a novel sort of medical research community in the capital, and the spread of a new kind of administrative rationality within the municipal hospital system. The initial emergence of specialties is best understood as part of the process of professionalization in science that took place throughout Europe during this period. After midcentury, specialties were gradually admitted to the Paris Faculty of Medicine, despite substantial opposition, because they represented the innovative forms of medical science that were sweeping the Western world and that the Paris Faculty, as France's showcase institution and chief claim to international stature, could not ignore. The spread of specialist clinical chairs was facilitated by the coming to power of a new generation of Republican politicians and a new generation of academics leaders, both equally committed to the reform of scientific and educational institutions as a symbol of national renewal.

Specialists in the Eighteenth Century

In France during the ancien régime, medical practitioners were divided into three distinct professional groups: physicians, surgeons, and apothecaries. While their medical activities were gradually merging, practitioners remained divided by distinct institutions and conflicting aspirations and self-images. Outside the medical mainstream, at the margins of surgery, there existed a group of practitioners called *experts*—specialist healers who performed particular operations on specific parts of the body; these included dentists, oculists, midwives, hernia surgeons, bonesetters and lithotomists (who performed surgery for the stone). These were distinguished by mastery of specific manual techniques. Their procedures were often "secrets" transmitted through oral tradition and practical example. They occupied a relatively low position in the medical hierarchy; many were untrained or unlicensed itinerants, and they were treated by surgeons as charlatans. But they performed procedures that surgeons were ordinarily unwilling to undertake because these were considered either undignified or too dangerous. From 1699 *experts* began to be integrated into the regulatory system of the surgical guilds; they were required to pass special examinations and were subject to regulation by master surgeons, at least in part so that they would not compete against surgeons. But by the end of the eighteenth century, according to Matthew Ramsey, most surgical bodies refused to certify *experts* since surgeons themselves were increasingly claiming the entire human body as part of their normal sphere of activity.[1]

The status of *experts* was gradually undermined by the successful efforts of French surgeons to raise their own social and intellectual status. As part of this effort, Toby Gelfand has shown, the surgeons introduced formal teaching and promoted research.[2] This raised their status by marking them as an educated and theoretically informed occupational group, as opposed to one utilizing mere manual skills; it thus undermined the claims of physicians to regulate their activities. Surgeons were now, like physicians, trained in "theory"—in this case, anatomy—as well as in practical surgical techniques. They also increasingly invaded the territory of *experts*, taking on surgery for stones, eyes, mouth, and teeth, as well as childbirth and repair of hernias. Some master surgeons even specialized in these procedures, "in effect assuming the function of the *expert*."[3]

Among the first surgical specialists were *accoucheurs*—specialists in birthing. The calling in of a male midwife to deliver the child of Louis XIV's mistress launched a fashion that intensified during the next century—first among the privileged classes, then increasingly among the less affluent.[4] There was surprisingly little French opposition to male midwifery or to the use of the forceps that distinguished male work from that of midwives. A Reims surgeon, Pierre Robin, earned very significant sums from his obstetrical practice, which involved approximately 200 births a year, among women of all social strata. The royal *accoucheur* Julien Clément was ennobled in 1711, as was one of his successors, N. Puzos, in 1751. The need to provide both doctors and midwives with obstetrical training (made pressing by government concern to encourage population growth) led to considerable teaching activity; many private courses were available in Paris. Courses were introduced in most surgical colleges (in Paris in 1747) and at the medical faculties in Strasbourg (1728) and Paris (1745).

Chairs of ocular surgery were established in 1765 at the Paris College of Surgery and at the Medical Faculty of Montpellier in 1788.[5] A key development in this field was the work of Jacques Daviel, who developed the method of removing cataracts through excision. This practice distinguished licensed surgeons from the itinerant cataract *experts*, who merely lowered them.[6] A group that emerged without benefit of academic credentials was the *dentistes*, specialists in the mouth and teeth. These body parts became objects of concern within the royal household and among the privileged classes due in part to the growing importance of personal appearance at the royal court.[7] As Roger King has demonstrated, operations on the teeth, long seen as a normal part of surgery, disappeared from surgical treatises early in the eighteenth century and were replaced by a body of literature devoted exclusively to dental surgery.[8] The authors of these works constituted a new breed of prestigious surgical specialist, the *chirurgien dentiste*. The first and most eminent of these was Pierre Fauchard, who invented many apparatuses and interventions, but whose writings were also full of anatomy and medical theory.[9] Several surgeon-dentists were ennobled by the middle of the eighteenth century, some, such as Étienne Bourdet in 1767, in large measure due to the quality of their writings.[10]

As the century progressed, surgeons in other fields also became known as specialists. One of these was the hernia expert François Pipelet.[11] Those who taught specific surgical procedures in Paris or the provinces might also become known as specialists. A medical directory of 1776 included the dean of the École Royale de Chirurgie, Le Blan, who was listed as lithotomist of the Hôtel-Dieu Hospital in Orléans, while Louis Deshayes Gendron was described as an oculist as well as royal demonstrator for eye diseases at the École de Chirurgie.[12] There is also evidence of surgical specialists outside Paris, in major cities such as Lyons and Bordeaux.[13] A handful justified medical specialization in their published works.[14]

While most specialists came from surgery, a few physicians also developed specialist interests, especially in the fields of obstetrics and ophthalmology.[15] If the problem for surgeons was making surgical procedure something more than manual activity, a product of "theory" and science, the challenge faced by physicians was to disengage from purely speculative theories in order to base medical knowledge on empirical science. The embrace of anatomy was for many a key requirement. For a very few individuals, advancing medical knowledge demanded the limitation of practice to a specific domain or specialty. The most notable of these was Jean-Emmanuel Gilibert, a young graduate of the Montpellier medical school who went on to become professor of botany at the College of Surgeons in Lyons.[16] In 1772 he wrote a three-volume work that criticized surgeons and apothecaries and specified the kind of knowledge that physicians required in order to improve their art. The next-to-last essay in the book defends the principle of specialization among medical practitioners. It is followed by an essay outlining a program of research in the author's chosen field, pediatrics.[17]

If surgical specialization reflected the aspiration of educated surgeons to take over existing and potentially lucrative procedures that had once been performed by *experts*, the specialization of physicians involved the creation of new medical categories (such as pediatrics) whose main justification was not a particular therapeutic practice but the need to advance medical knowledge by amassing extensive information and experience in a restricted sphere. The difficulty was that such specialization, unlike surgery for cataracts or the stone, did not necessarily correspond to real patient demand. Gilibert, for instance, complained that pediatrics was not lucrative because parents did not care enough about their children to pay doctors for their care. This may be one reason why he, like the Scot, John Cheyne, and the Swiss, Christoph Girtanner, two other physicians who attempted to practice pediatrics during this period, eventually abandoned this specialty.[18]

The Appearance of Modern Specialties

The reorganization of medicine during the Revolutionary and Napoleonic periods fused medicine and surgery, treated as two branches of practice with a common knowledge base. The new system of medical education had a generalist orientation; consequently, obstetrics was the only clinical specialty that appeared in the curriculum. Courses in ophthalmology that had existed during the ancien régime were not reestablished. Nor was there any provision for *experts*, with the exception of midwives, who were subjected to a system of education and licensing. *Experts* continued to practice in small numbers,[19] but among licensed doctors at the beginning of nineteenth century, the few specialists who appeared in directories usually represented the surgical specialties of the old regime: oculists, *accoucheurs*, hernia specialists, and dentists. Many of these had pre-Revolutionary diplomas and continued the time-honored but disparaged customs of advertising and itinerant practice.[20]

Several decades later, the situation was little changed. The second edition of an early Parisian medical directory published in 1830 showed a majority of individuals (86 percent) described as "*médecin.*"[21] In a sample of the first 436 listings, thirty-one individuals identified themselves as surgeons, and twenty as *accoucheurs.* There were five oculists, three dentists, and one specialist in hernias. A handful of individuals whose main identification was *médecin* indicated some form of special interest. One named Chamat included the phrase "occupies himself especially with scrofulous illnesses," while Chambeyron added the term "legal medicine of the insane."[22]

Overall, few specialties were mentioned by few doctors. Several individuals whom we now know were actually in the process of developing specialties, such as the psychiatrist J.E.D. Esquirol and the venereologist François Cullérier, made no reference to these activities. One could pursue a special interest without conceiving oneself as a specialist, an identity still linked in the minds of many to charlatanism and patent medicines. The only significant exception was obstetrics, a unique field. It had a specialized clientele, parturient women, receiving attention from a state concerned with the size of its population, and had its own hospital, the Paris Maternité, as well as maternity wards in general hospitals. Initially the rationale for specialists in childbirth was to decrease mortality in childbirth through the provision of obstetrical training for midwives and, later, doctors.[23] By the end of the eighteenth century, obstetrics had become a recognized form of medical practice. In 1830, the three national medical faculties all contained chairs of obstetrics.[24] In 1844 the subject was added to the *agrégation*— the competition that provided access to junior teaching posts at the faculty—devoted to surgery. The reorganization of the sections of the Academy of Medicine in 1829 established a separate section of obstetrics. The Parisian hospital administration began, sometime before 1850, to refer to physicians at the Maternité hospital as *médecins-accoucheurs*.

Obstetrics can thus be seen, in France as elsewhere, either as one of three general branches of medicine (the others being physic and surgery) or as the first of the nineteenth-century medical specialties. It was widely (though by no means universally) recognized to be a distinct domain, but this distinctiveness could be conceptualized in different ways. When the notion that medicine was divided into many specialties became widely accepted in the decades after 1830, this existing category was recast as specialty. In contrast to both the English- and the German-speaking worlds, where ophthalmology was emerging as an important field, Parisian oculists in 1830 seem to be a throwback to earlier patterns of medical practice. The field's major asset in the early nineteenth century was royal favor. Hubert's *Almanach général* listed two royal oculists and a baron described as a former royal oculist. Since the reign of the Bourbons came to an end in 1830 court favor proved a fragile basis for the field.[25] This situation may account for the relatively poor development of Parisian ophthalmology during much of the nineteenth century.

During the 1830s the visibility of specialists and specialties in Paris increased significantly.[26] In 1839, two journals devoted to medical specialization came into existence. Appearing in June was *L'esculape: Journal des spécialités médico-chirurgicales*. It was edited by Dr. S. Furnari, who was described in medical directories as a specialist in diseases of the eyes. The journal remained in publication for three years. A second journal, the *Revue des spécialités et innovations médicales et chirurgicales*, appeared in November 1839 and was published, with some long gaps, until the 1860s. It was edited by Vincent Duval, a specialist in orthopedics, who described himself as director of orthopedic treatments of the Parisian hospital system. (Today, his main claim to fame is the surgical procedure for clubfoot, immortalized by Gustave Flaubert in *Madame Bovary*.) Duval claimed among his contributors several well-known hospital physicians and surgeons and contended that his teacher, F. Broussais, had encouraged him to create a revue of specialties.[27]

Both journals treated the entire range of specialties, since no single specialty had enough practitioners to support its own journal. Though their broad coverage made them look much like existing medical journals, their editors proclaimed them to be new kinds of publications. Both were clearly sensitive about medical hostility to specialization. Each journal opened with an editorial essay defending the legitimacy of competent medical specialization based on a strong general medical education. Each also quoted well-known figures who had made comments favorable to specialization and listed those who had made important discoveries precisely because they specialized in a particular area of medicine.[28]

The medical encyclopedias and dictionaries that proliferated during the first half of the nineteenth century provide yet another perspective on the spread of specialties. Medical knowledge was at this time being produced at an accelerated rate, with considerable scope for conflicts of doctrine and perspective. As a result, a large number of encyclopedic works sought to summarize, classify, condense, and interpret existing medical knowledge. Some of these works were prepared collectively by large groups of doctors who were members of the Parisian medical elite. These huge collective works, unique to Paris, are wonderfully illustrative of the way communities of scholars emerged in the hothouse atmosphere of the French capital.[29]

I have come across three dictionaries published in the early nineteenth century (among six that I found in the Osler Library) with something to say about medical specialization. None of them recognizes "specialization" as a category deserving of mention. Very few specialist categories, in fact, are specifically referred to at all. The ones receiving attention come as no surprise in view of our preceding discussion. Obstetrics is discussed in a variety of ways, mostly positive[30]; but there is an essay published in 1829, taking up forty pages and written by Antoine Dugès, that denies that obstetrics is a real branch of knowledge.[31] Dugès, appointed in 1824 as the first holder of the chair of obstetrics at the Montpellier Faculty of Medicine, felt strongly enough about the low intellectual status of this field to move three years later to a chair of surgical pathology.

Other specialties fared worse in the three early encyclopedias. The *Dictionnaire de médecine,* the fifteenth volume of which appeared in 1826, published an entry on oculists by M. J. Raige Delorme, general editor of the publication; this was the occasion for a critique of specialization, which "gives rise to more abuses than it provides advantages for science."[32] The criticism of this occupation grew progressively stronger as the essay advanced. Only an entry on dentists written by J. N. Marjolin, which appeared in another volume of this work, has anything remotely positive to say about a specialist group.[33]

The situation, however, began to change somewhat in the second edition of the *Dictionnaire de médecine,* which began appearing in 1832. Although the first volume was introduced by a preface in which the editor, Raige-Delorme, criticized excessive specialization in medical science,[34] specialties began at least to be noted, if not always with approval. By 1840 and 1841, when volumes 21 through 23 appeared, there are entries for "Obstétrique" (now one of the three fundamental divisions "of the art of medicine which the specialization of studies and the necessities of practice have established most naturally")[35]; "Odontechnie" (the art of dentistry, which, it is argued, had long suffered from its practitioners' lack of medical knowledge);"[36] "Ophthalmologie," in which the author, Velpeau, criticizes medical specialization on the grounds that eye diseases could not be distinguished from maladies of the other body systems;[37] and "Orthopédie" and "Pédiatrie," the practitioners of which remain largely unmentioned. The existence of such articles indicates that the fields involved were becoming distinct, if contested, domains of medical knowledge.

By the 1840s, specialized private instruction was part of the experience of American doctors studying in Paris.[38] The change that had occurred is illustrated by two books by German doctors, written only five years apart. In 1836 Adolf Muerhy gave his impressions of French and British medicine garnered during a trip the year before.[39] Brief mention is made of several Parisian specialty clinics, notably that of Ricord in syphilology and, in greater detail, the weaknesses of ophthalmic clinics. But specialism does not exist as a relevant category in his account. In striking contrast, the visiting German physician Carl August Wunderlich (later a pioneer in the use of medical thermometry) published in 1841 his study comparing Paris medicine with that of Vienna, in which he made his much-quoted observations about the unique popularity of specialties in Paris: "Now a specialty is a necessary condition for everybody who wants to become rich and famous rapidly. Each organ has its priest, and for some, special clinics exist."[40]

One form that such visibility for specialists took in Paris was a slowly growing trade in private teaching of specialties. Among forty-four private courses listed in Hubert's *Almanach* of 1830,[41] there are only ten specialty courses, seven of them devoted to obstetrics; of the three others, Pierre-Paul Broc taught a course in andrology; Octave Lesuer, in legal medicine and toxicology; and P. S. Ségalas in diseases of the genito-urinary organs. Twenty years later, however, Meding's directory listed eighty-nine private courses being offered. Some of these were cram courses to prepare students for various exams, but thirty-nine were devoted to specialties. Once again, obstetrics led, with twelve courses. But there were also six courses devoted to diseases of the eyes, three each on venereal diseases, urology, and dermatology, and two each on mental diseases and diseases of the chest.[42]

In a book of 1845 listing about 1,500 Parisian physicians, 12 percent of the physicians were, according to Erwin Ackerknecht's calculations, described as specialists of one sort or another.[43] (This figure excludes surgeons.) In Meding's directory, published seven years later, about 8 percent of all Parisian physicians were described—probably by the author of the publication—as specialists. In yet another medical directory that appeared that same year, about 5 percent of those listed identified themselves with specialty designations.[44] More important than the numbers of specialists in each publication—which are variable and probably somewhat arbitrary—is the fact that forty-three individuals were described as specialists in both of the 1852 directories, suggesting some degree of stability in specialist identity. Equally significant is the wide range of specialties—going well beyond the surgical specialties of the ancien régime—described in these works. Clearly specialization was becoming a recognized, if not fully accepted, fact of medical life.

Most specialties, it must be emphasized, were represented by only a handful of individuals, and there was little agreement among different sources about what constituted a specialty and who was a specialist. Nonetheless, the sudden appearance and spread of specialists and specialties within such brief period of time demands an explanation. General demographic factors, notably growing density of doctors and patients in Paris, the second largest city of Europe,[45] were certainly important conditions of possibility. By itself, however, this explanation is insufficient and does not account for the fact that London, by far the largest city in Europe, was not associated with medical specialties, though it, too, had its individual specialists. That growing popular faith in specialized expertise provided a basis for new professional patterns is indisputable; but it still needs to be explained how and why such faith suddenly manifested itself and how it overcame traditional confidence in the superiority of broad general knowledge. Nor can one simply appeal to the material self-interest of doctors; there is no reason to assume that they were notably more self-interested in the nineteenth century than they had been in the eighteenth. What needs explaining surely is why specialization became within a short period of time a profitable and respectable professional option.

A plausible explanation is advanced by George Rosen as part of a complex analysis of the development of specialization (that includes social factors).[46] Specialization, he insists, was not a consequence of the accumulation of knowledge, but rather of a new conception of disease. It was specifically the influence of localist organic thinking, based on pathological anatomy and subsequently on new technologies such as the ophthalmoscope and laryngoscope, that created "foci of interest" in organ systems around which specialties could develop. Rosen's analysis is meant to explain the long-term development of specialties across the entire nineteenth century; Paris in the 1830s and 1840s is significant chiefly as the place where organic localism originated. But Erwin Ackerknecht has applied Rosen's analysis directly to the early development of specialties in Paris; in this view, the newly emergent pathological conception of disease that replaced humoral theory best explains the advance of specialism during this early period.[47] Ackerknecht, I believe, is correct to attribute causation to the unique characteristics of the Paris school of medicine. And one of these characteristics, the emphasis on organic localism, undoubtedly played a role in the development of specialties. However, this role, I would suggest, was not determinant, since many of the emerging specialties of the period were not in fact based on specific organs.

To cite just one example, *L'esculape*, one of the journals devoted to specialization, had during its first year of publication a masthead listing the medical specialties. These appear in the following order:

> *Accouchemens* [sic]; *Maladies des femmes et des enfans* [sic]; *Orthopédie; Maladies des voies urinaires; Chirurgie dentaire; Maladies des yeux; Médecine légale; Maladies du système nerveux; Chirurgie herniaire; Maladies des oreilles; Hygiène et chirurgie militaire; Hygiène publique et privée; Maladies vénériennes; Maladies de la peau; Eaux minérales.*

The list contains many categories that are organically based but also many that are not. The specificity of "Accouchement" (birthing) long predates the rise of pathological anatomy and is based both on the much earlier entry of men into the field and on public health concern to lower maternal and infant mortality. "Diseases of children" is similarly based on a particular class of patients subject to special governmental solicitude. Likewise, it may be argued that however somatic subsequent definitions of insanity eventually became, the original basis of psychiatry was the need to isolate and manage a uniquely troublesome class of patients.

Its status as a recognized specialty was largely due to the Asylum Law of 1838 as well as to the activities of Esquirol and his circle.[18] Yet other specialty categories are based on forms of treatment (mineral waters, hernial surgery), types of diseases (venereal), and social functions (legal medicine, military hygiene and surgery, public and private hygiene). Among the organically based specialties, "maladies des yeux" was, we saw, a traditional category (*oculiste*) based on specific surgical procedures. Although the field had not yet been significantly transformed by pathological anatomy, it was just then in the public eye (no pun intended) due to a new surgical technique to cure strabismus that had been discussed at some length in the Academy of Medicine. Similarly "maladies des voies urinaires" was a long-standing surgical specialty and remained closely associated with operations for the stone. It was also in the public eye due to debates about the efficacy of the new procedure of lithotomy and priority disputes among its leading practitioners. Perhaps the most surprising categories are those which we no longer think of as medical specialties: legal and forensic medicine, military hygiene and surgery, and public hygiene.

It is not credible to suggest, as Rosen did, that so many of these specialties emerged simply as by-products of specialization based on organic localism.[49] My point here is not to deny that organic localism played a role in the emergence of specialties. Rather, I want to suggest that pathological anatomy must be understood as part of a much deeper transformation that resulted simultaneously in specialization. This crux of this transformation was the creation of an unprecedented large and integrated community of doctors around an organized system of institutions and, most important, devoted to advancing medical knowledge through rigorous empirical clinical research. The study of organic lesions was only one component of this new research imperative

My argument runs as follows, in five parts.

1. The fundamental justification for specialization was not so much the improvement of skill that it engendered (though this might occasionally be invoked) as it was its necessary role in the advancement of knowledge and technique.
2. Early in the nineteenth century, Paris became a center of knowledge production based on a coordinated network of institutions whose size was unprecedented. Knowledge production was closely associated with teaching, both formal and informal.
3. The attempt to organize Parisian institutions along rational administrative lines produced divisions into intellectual categories: disciplines for the curriculum, sections of the academy, editorial subject areas in medical encyclopedias.
4. The logic of state administration was critical to this process because it resulted in creation of the institutions that allowed the advancement of medical knowledge to become central to academic activity. It was at the same time responsible for the functional specialization of hospitals that allowed for the production of specialized knowledge and the training of specialists.

5. Although its fundamental justification was intellectual, specialization was always associated with some form of specialty practice because the production of specialist knowledge was inconceivable outside the framework of clinical practice.

Let me discuss each of these points in greater detail.

First, the fundamental justification for specialization in medicine from the eighteenth century on was the commonsense idea that, given the limits of human intelligence, it was preferable to master a part of the vast medical art rather than attempting to know and do everything. In the words of Gilibert: "However vast, however extensive is the spirit of man, it loses its power in proportion to the multiplication of objects that it deals with."[50] This basic insight was reinforced by many social forces in the eighteenth and nineteenth centuries and could thus be formulated by utilizing diverse analogies and metaphors. Toby Gelfand, for instance, has emphasized the belief of Enlightenment political economists in the division of labor, especially for the crafts; this belief, he argues, proved useful to surgeons attempting to improve their status.[51] A more common analogy focused not on craft production (which had relatively low social status) but on the advancement of knowledge, and looked to specialization in the sciences for its inspiration and models. It was this formulation especially that would come to the fore in post-1830 Paris.

Specialization permitted mastery of existing medical literature in a specific domain and allowed physicians to see the large number of cases of the same type that were now deemed necessary for rigorous clinical research and serious medical training. In the eighteenth century, Gilibert made this link explicit. Only specialization, he argued, would allow medicine to progress. Universality of practice was so damaging precisely because practitioners, incapable of observing any class of phenomena in sufficient depth, were "diverted by the fatal mania for murderous theories that dishonors us."[52] Mediocre physicians would, by specializing in a limited number of diseases, improve their practical skills: "Not having received from nature this spark of genius that characterizes the doctor who discovers, they will be content to profit from the views of their predecessors."[53] But for the more gifted, specialization could lead to significant medical progress. It permitted careful, methodical observations that were informed by a vast knowledge of the subject; and it allowed the physician to reflect, judge, make connections, and generalize.[54] "Through this method all the illnesses which he [the physician] treats will furnish him with the means to enrich his art or to confirm his certainty."[55]

Underlying Gilibert's views were a variety of perspectives on the body that were then in circulation. Each demanded specialized observation. His emphasis on specialization by disease and on knowing and comparing related "species" of disease was based on the principles of nosological medicine.[56] One can also find a budding anatomical perspective in Gilibert's account.[57] Contemporary views on environmental influences on the body pointed to even greater complexity. Whatever the perspective, "our meditations should not merely be general. Let us occupy ourselves in detail and in practice in extending the limits of that part of practice for which we have the greatest preference."[58]

So it was not any particular conception of health and disease, but rather the desire to *know* "in detail and in practice," that lay behind the eighteenth-century faith in the powers of specialization. In the following century both the aspiration to pursue clinical research and the tendency to identify this aspiration with specialization spread ever more widely. The stated rationale of the two specialist journals of the 1830s was to bring the results of specialist research before the general medical public. The deeper connection between the flourishing of specialism and the rise of pathological anatomy was that both represented a concern with intellectual rigor in an empirical mode; this concern characterized a new type of medical research community that had emerged in Paris and in which many different kinds of medical investigation were being pursued.

Second, unlike historians of German science, historians of science in France rarely speak of "a Great Transition" that created professional science in that country. This is because the process occurred gradually, starting in the eighteenth century and accelerating after the Revolution, but without any single institutional innovation comparable with the rise of the German research university. Joseph Ben-David, in a classic work of historical sociology, explicitly denied that much in the way of institutional change took place in post-Revolutionary Paris, claiming that the "great upsurge of French science following the Revolution was only indirectly related to the new institutions of higher education established between 1794 and 1800, and those institutions did not constitute a beginning of organized patterns of scientific work. They were rather the culmination of eighteenth century patterns of scientific work."[59] This explains why French science, according to Ben-David and many others, began after 1830 to decline from its position of international scientific leadership. No one bothers to discuss medicine in this context. This is, I suspect, partly because it lacked the epistemological status of the physical sciences usually considered to be at the center of this shift, and also because medical research was "professionalized" in clinics rather than universities or laboratories and remained subsidized to a considerable degree by private medical practice. It would take us well beyond the scope of this book to discuss these issues in detail. I will, however, make three points. First, it is certainly the case that developments in nineteenth-century French science built on eighteenth-century attitudes and institutional patterns, not least in their openness to specialized research. Second, medicine was not just part of the milieu of amateur science from which "real" disciplines such as physics and chemistry emerged; it, too, went through a comparable process of professionalization and discipline formation. Third, however one chooses to evaluate the overall institutional system devoted to science and technology in France, Paris medicine brought into being a new institutional form that was in its way as revolutionary as the German research university, even if it proved to be less enduring.

Early in the nineteenth century, Paris became a center of knowledge production based on a network of interconnected institutions and individuals of unprecedented size and scope. The Faculty of Medicine, the Sorbonne, the School of Pharmacy, the Collège de France, and the Muséum d'Histoire Naturelle, as well as the municipal hospitals, shared students, professors, and junior staff; all became part of a common career structure for the elite that I have described elsewhere.[60] Around these institutions was a flourishing world of medical societies, private medical teaching, and medical periodicals that observed closely and often criticized harshly the elite of official medicine. Only those with formal teaching positions can be considered fully "professional researchers" in the modern sense. And even for these, as well the much larger number of individuals who did not hold posts providing substantial salaries, medical practice not only supplied the data of clinical research but also frequently subsidized it financially. Nonetheless, these limitations in no way diminish either the novelty or the vigor of this new type of research community.

A research community numbering many hundreds of individuals was unique to Paris. The Paris Faculty of Medicine, the largest medical school in the world, had more than two dozen full professors and many junior personnel. The Parisian hospital system employed several hundred doctors and surgeons. To these one must add all the ambitious students and graduates who were seeking to make their mark in the world of academic medicine. In this competitive world, nepotism thrived and some nonentities managed to achieve notable success; but it was nonetheless deemed imperative to produce new knowledge. Critics argued that many of the structural characteristics of the institutional system were counterproductive and harmful. But no one disputed that the goal was to advance knowledge. And few disputed that what was needed was "positive" knowledge, based on careful empirical observation of many different clinical cases and postmortem dissections. Some, such as Broussais and his supporters, might criticize *mere* empiricism and argue for the importance of theory in making sense of empirical observation, but no one of any stature suggested that empirical observation was less than central. As a consequence, many hundreds of individuals were, at all levels of the system, seeking to make or consolidate elite careers through various kinds of clinical research and teaching. The advantages of specialization in this struggle to produce knowledge remained as pertinent as they had been for eighteenth-century figures such as Gilibert: ability to master and keep up with the literature, and the possibility of seeing many different cases of a certain type during a relatively brief period.

Specialization was further encouraged by some of the structural characteristics of the Parisian institutional world. The close proximity of medical and scientific institutions and the overlapping of personnel among them allowed growing disciplinary specialization in the natural sciences to serve as a model for medicine. Furthermore, in the post-Revolutionary institutions of Paris medicine, the MD degree became a state diploma uniting both medicine and surgery within the same profession. A single, all-encompassing profession, defined and protected by the state, made internal segmentation appear feasible. To the extent that medicine and surgery remained distinct, a primitive form of specialization came into immediate existence; this argument was in fact made explicitly by some early supporters of specialization.[61] This set a pattern that could be easily replicated as practitioners began to cultivate new branches of medicine. Furthermore, the unity of the state diploma defused the threat that specialization would irreparably fragment medical science and the profession. In Britain, where the profession was institutionally divided, specialization was widely perceived as a highly disruptive force.

Third, that specialization was seen initially as applying primarily to medical research and teaching, and to practice secondarily, was important to its acceptance. If there were relatively few positive models for specialty practice, post-Revolutionary Paris was teeming with models of specialization in research and teaching. Even in the eighteenth century, it has been argued by Lorraine Daston, French scientists were uniquely tolerant of specialized technical knowledge, associated with the state's patronage of scientific societies that provided expert knowledge of a utilitarian nature. The Paris Academy of Sciences, which developed its institutional arrangements during the last years of the seventeenth century, had built-in structures of specialization in the form of disciplinary sections.[62]

Such tolerance for specialization increased in the nineteenth century. To a much greater extent than the small corporate institutions of the ancien régime, the huge scientific and educational institutions of Paris in the nineteenth century carved up medical knowledge into disciplinary units cultivated and taught by specialists. By far the largest single medical institution in Europe, the Paris Faculty of Medicine had twenty-six chairs representing nearly twenty different disciplinary categories, ranging from medical chemistry to obstetrics. Not everyone's commitment to a specialty was lifelong, and not all professors contributed intellectually to the subjects they taught. But there were enough who did, to provide models to younger doctors. And such models were reinforced by other institutions. In 1829 the Academy of Medicine shifted from dividing its members into three professional sections to dividing them among nine discipline-based sections. Many ambitious young candidates for the medical elite also frequented courses and laboratories in scientific institutions such as the Muséum d'Histoire Naturelle, the Collège de France, and the Sorbonne, where lifelong teaching and research commitments to a single academic discipline were the rule. Outside educational institutions, some emerging specialties were thought to require an expert editor in the medical encyclopedias that proliferated in Paris.[63] Consequently, the principle of disciplinary specialization was well established in early nineteenth-century Paris. It was not difficult to apply it to emerging subject areas growing out of the clinic.[64] Whether a field became widely recognized as a disciplinary specialty or not depended on the amount and quality of knowledge that its practitioners were thought to produce.

Fourth, the logic of state administration made specialization possible in two critical ways. First, at the heart of the Parisian community of medical scientists were state institutions. Some, such as the Academy of Sciences, the Collège de France, and the Muséum d'Histoire Naturelle, already had a long history. Others had a more recent origin. The ordinances establishing the Paris Faculty of Medicine in 1803 and the Academy of Medicine in 1820 specified that these institutions should be devoted to the advancement of medical knowledge. Leaving details aside, I will merely note here that promoting the development of medical knowledge was considered part of the public health mission of the French state.[65] In these state institutions, models of disciplinary specialization were first elaborated.

But administrative logic also operated on another plane, making possible the flourishing of research in a network of specialized hospitals. Unlike the private, semi-entrepreneurial institutions of London, these were part of an extensive municipal system that was set up after the French Revolution. Doctors who worked in them enjoyed all the prestige associated with posts in general hospitals. Some of these special hospitals long preceded the Revolution; their foundations could reflect philanthropic or administrative concerns to isolate certain types of patients in order to guard against disruption, immorality, epidemics, or promiscuity; or they might simply be efforts to innovate in the provision of charitable care. Such institutions might emerge for largely pragmatic reasons, as was true of the St. Louis Hospital for skin diseases. Built by order of Henri IV in 1607, it was designed initially to isolate plague victims during epidemics and later began taking in victims of other epidemic diseases. In the long periods between outbreaks, it admitted patients suffering from chronic skin conditions who could be quickly sent home in the event of a new plague outbreak.[66] Humanitarian values might also play a role. In 1784, Minister of the Interior Louis-August de Breteuil, visited the venereal ward at the Bicêtre and, appalled by the awful conditions in which its occupants, primarily prostitutes, were held, ordered their transfer to another institution. This led to the opening of the Hospice des Vénériens in 1792.[67]

In the years before the Revolution, the sheer size of Paris's major general hospitals suggested to reformers that hospitals should be divided into smaller and more rational categories; thus Jacques Tenon, in his famous report on the subject, proposed that the Hôtel Dieu be replaced by four hospitals: one for maternity patients, a second for the insane, a third for "fetid" diseases, and a fourth for contagious diseases.[68] (Within each hospital, the sick were to be further divided according to type of illness and type of patient.[69]) Such ideas were not uniquely a French response to the size of public hospitals. In Vienna these principles were realized when the Allgemeine Krankenhaus was established around this time with five specialized divisions.[70]

After the Revolution, the newly established municipal hospital system became characterized by the drive to distinguish and separate. This reflected the same administrative impulse that led in higher education to the creation of many specialized vocational schools rather than comprehensive universities. Almost two decades of warfare promoted the tendency to regulate populations of every sort by dividing them into manageable categories. Applied to hospitals, this practice separated the sick from the poor, women from men, children from adults, convalescents from the sick, and chronic from acute and surgical patients.[71] Thus the specialized vocations of older hospitals were confirmed.[72] The maternity ward of the Hôtel Dieu was moved and became the Maternité Hospital; in 1814 the foundling hospital associated with the Maternité was split off to become the Hôpital des Enfants Trouvés.[73] A new hospital for children, the Enfants Malades, was set up in 1802; venereal patients from throughout the system were transferred to the Hôpital des Vénériens (later to become the Midi) on the Faubourg St. Jacques[74]; similarly, the insane were transferred into special hospitals or wards. In the post-Revolutionary decades, children (Enfants Malades, Enfants Trouvés), women (Salpêtrière, Lourcine), the elderly (Salpêtrière and Bicêtre), the insane (Sainte-Anne, Charenton, special wards of the Salpêtrière and Bicêtre), and sufferers of venereal (Midi) and skin (St. Louis) diseases were some of the categories of patients segregated in special hospitals. The system was designed according to norms of administrative rationality: a central admissions bureau was supposed to direct patents to the most appropriate of many available institutions.[75]

The reasoning behind this strategy seemed self-evident and was rarely explained. The eighteenth-century concerns to get rid of those creating disorder or to assure moral propriety did not disappear. But they were supplemented by a new administrative and medical vision that was expressed clearly in a report to the Administrative Council of the Paris Hospitals prepared in 1816, contrasting the situation before and after hospital reform. In the eighteenth century, "the confusion of patients and their crowding together had very nefarious results. Fever cases, the wounded, those suffering from contagious maladies, pregnant women, the insane, epileptics, and convalescents were brought together in connecting wards, or piled one on top of the other in the same building."[76] Today, in contrast, the report continued several pages later, "every infirmity, every need, every stage of life has now, in Paris, institutions that are devoted to it. . . . those illnesses which cannot be conveniently treated [in general hospitals], which require special care and regimen, which must be isolated for the benefit of those who suffer from them and in the interest of those who do not, have special hospitals."[77] Such specialization seems to have aimed primarily to improve the quality of patient care; but it may have also had another effect, that of improving clinical teaching by ensuring that students saw a sufficient number and variety of illnesses in any specific field.

The tendency toward segmentation together with economies of scale made possible further innovations that would have been difficult in individual hospitals. In the 1830s, the hospital administration integrated some of the traditional surgical specialties into the system. It appointed an orthopedist, and a small hernia service in the central bureau became, under the direction of J.-F. Malgaigne, a full-fledged surgical clinic.[78] Hospital surgeons vigorously opposed efforts to create a special service for urinary surgery,[79] but the lithotomist Civiale was able to practice urological surgery exclusively within the confines of the Necker Hospital. Other specialties fared less well in contests with powerful vested interests. Several efforts to establish a special hospital for the eyes in Paris resulted in failure.[80]

Overall, hospital segmentation contributed mightily to the intellectual atmosphere that made choosing a specialty a possible and desirable professional option. But it did considerably more, providing a location for both training and the production of serious specialist knowledge. Philippe Ricord, for example, was a young surgeon who had never shown a particular interest in any specialty when an appointment to the Hôpital des Vénériens led him to embark on an ambitious program of research and a lifetime career in venereology.[81] When Philippe Pinel became physician in chief of the Salpêtrière, he fully recognized that a hospital treating so many women "opens a great career for new research on women's diseases that have always and rightly been considered as the most difficult and complicated of all."[82] J. L. M. Alibert, appointed to St. Louis Hospital in 1807, attempted the task of classifying skin diseases and offered the first lectures on dermatology. He sponsored important research by students including J. C. Galès (on the insect origins of *la gale*, the itch).[83] Other hospitals that played a determining role in the early development of specialties included the Salpêtrière and, later, the Charenton Asylum, where J. E. D. Esquirol established the intellectual foundations for French psychiatry; the Foundlings Hospital in neonatal care; and Enfants Malades in pediatrics. Formally outside of the hospital system but part of the Paris intellectual world were institutions such as the Institut des Sourds Muets, where J. M. G. Itard did important work on lesions causing deafness. Such institutions created a critical mass of individuals working in a given field.[84] They made it possible to produce clinical knowledge based on large numbers of clinical cases, analyzed quantitatively as well as qualitatively, and frequently complemented by data from postmortem dissections. The most determined opponents of specialization understood full well that medical specialties depended on these hospitals and would have liked to see them eliminated.[85]

Specialty hospitals did not invariably produce specialists. It was common to move from one institution to another, resulting in a complete shift of research interests. One could also view oneself as a general physician or surgeon who happened to work in a specialized hospital.[86] Finally, not all specialized hospitals generated specialist disciplines. Some of the largest hospitals in Paris, such as the Salpêtrière, were devoted to geriatric patients; but geriatrics did not emerge as a recognized domain, whether because it lacked specific therapeutic or diagnostic procedures, because diseases of old age seemed inevitable and incurable, or because the elderly, unlike children, generated little public interest.

The crux of my argument here is that emerging specialization in Paris was based on the coming together of a system of career competition based on some notion of advancing medical knowledge—which itself promoted specialization—with classificatory categories that emerged from efforts to impose bureaucratic rationality on huge institutional structures. Both these elements were promoted directly, though in quite different ways, by the French state.

Fifth, there was no sharp distinction between medical research and practice because, except for a handful of laboratory scientists or specialists in public health, research was based in clinical practice, most often though not exclusively in hospitals. Furthermore, anyone with a prestigious hospital post, whether a specialist or not, was in a position to develop a lucrative private practice because patients viewed such posts as indicators of excellence. Some individuals created small private hospitals as extensions of their public hospital practice.[87] The hospital administration set up a private venereal hospital under the direction of François Cullerier.[88] But it was not just members of the medical elite or potential producers of knowledge who called themselves specialists. Once specialties became identified with medical science and innovation, they could be claimed by practitioners like Dr. Cheneau, identified in medical directories as specializing in the treatment of nervous maladies, migraines, and epilepsy, or Dr. Dechambre, identified as a specialist in maladies of old age and the nervous system.[89]

Some of the emerging opposition to specialties targeted such claims to specialty practice. Not only did such claims lend themselves to entrepreneurial practices, but they seemed incongruent with common understanding of systemic links both within the organism and between the organism and the environment. To criticisms at this level, defenders of specialization could sometimes respond that specialization improved medical practice.[90] During the middle decades of the nineteenth century, however, the primary justification for specialties had to do with their critical role for medical research and teaching. Specialist practice advanced steadily but unspectacularly until the 1880s, and in the process provoked relatively little controversy. In contrast, the role of specialties as disciplines within the medical curriculum raised vociferous opposition.

Specialists Conquer the Paris Faculty of Medicine

Despite its many advantages for the production of knowledge, specialization remained a minority option in mid-nineteenth-century Paris and generated substantial opposition. General surgeons feared that specialists would take over lucrative operative procedures. Professors were hesitant to add new chairs and courses to the already overcrowded faculty and curriculum. Some opponents raised scientific objections. The German observer Carl Wunderlich admitted that specialization in Paris had resulted in both important discoveries and manual improvements in surgery, but argued as well that it produced intellectual one-sidedness. He cited well-known Parisian medical figures as examples of the superiority of the all-round physician over the specialist.[91]

Such attitudes were not uncommon. They expressed continued widespread belief in the systemic nature of most diseases, notwithstanding the demise of traditional humoral doctrines and the rise of pathological anatomy. They also reflected in some cases a holistic view of medical science that was expressed in 1832 by M. J. Raige-Delorme in his editorial preface to the *Dictionnaire de médecine;* Raige-Delorme targeted growing disciplinary specialization. While admitting that the advance of knowledge required that science be divided and subdivided, he nonetheless argued that usage had led to the arbitrary and harmful separation and isolation of subjects: of anatomy and physiology from medical practice; of pathology and therapeutics from surgery. It had also set up as special sciences subjects, such as public hygiene and legal medicine, that were simple applications of medical knowledge. Beneath these practical considerations lay the vision of a unified medical science available to the general practitioner and to which detailed empirical research could be related. All parts of medicine were linked, and one could not evaluate even the minutest aspect without knowing the whole, because "the science of man is one." Incomplete, partial knowledge was the chief cause of those competing "schools" that set equally false theories against one other.[92] Views of science as unity and disease as systemic have proven to be enduring and have resurfaced regularly in medicine as a protest against excessive reductionism and segmentation.

Although vocal critics of specialization were less numerous in France than in Germany or Britain, they nonetheless remained powerful until well after mid-century. By the 1850s, private courses in many specialties had become widespread enough to provoke demands that these fields be recognized in the programs of the medical faculty. Some of those making such demands had friends in high places, for in February 1859 the Paris Faculty of Medicine received a letter from the minister of public instruction asking whether it was advisable to create new chairs for the emerging specialties.[93] A commission convened to deal with the subject rejected the proposal.[94] When the issue came up for general discussion in the Faculty, opposition remained overwhelming.[95] Only one professor, Armand Trousseau, supported the admission of specialties to the Faculty, on the grounds that these important subjects were not being taught adequately. Everyone else was more or less violently opposed. Many reasons were cited: some claimed that these subjects were in fact being well taught in existing clinical courses; others pointed to the lack of any real pressure for change beyond the desire of a handful of specialists to become professors; some speakers insisted that most specialties were based on relatively little knowledge; yet others feared that once the gates were opened, a flood of demands for faculty chairs would inevitably result. But above all else, specialties represented an intellectual narrowness that appeared to the professors to be profoundly dangerous for medical science. They would fragment medical science and would "interdict the professor from any view of the whole."[96] It is no accident that opponents of specialty chairs presented an alternative demand for the reestablishment of the chair of the history of medicine (which had been eliminated in 1823). This subject represented the breadth of spirit, the attempt at a comprehensive perspective, that was thought to be vital for medical science. The unanimous vote against the creation of specialty chairs was followed by an immediate vote to request a chair in medical history.[97]

The dean of the Faculty suggested that the teaching needs of specialties could be met by elective courses taught by junior personnel (*agrégés*).[98] But in the following years the suggestion was not implemented. Hostility to specialties was so strong, in fact, that Armand Trousseau, in 1862, was roundly criticized in the Faculty assembly for allowing the venereologist Ricord to lecture in his course. His actions, it was argued, went against the unanimous opposition of the faculty to specialist teaching.[99] In the face of such hostility, the introduction of specialties into the faculty could be imposed only by force.

This occurred suddenly and quickly. In 1862 the personal physician to Emperor Napoleon III, Pierre Rayer, was named to the newly created chair of comparative medicine.[100] Since this was a new chair, there was no need to consult the Faculty about the appointment, as was the usual practice when an existing chair was being filled. Simultaneously, Rayer was named dean of the Faculty. Within a month, Rayer effectively destroyed the power of the old guard in the Faculty by eliminating a permanent administrative committee of professors. Shortly thereafter, he introduced six new "complementary" or elective courses devoted to the clinical specialties. Junior-level personnel, the *agrégés,* would teach these courses. Rayer's motives are not entirely clear, since he never bothered to explain his actions.[101] But two facts are worth noting. First, his appointment was accompanied by a second appointment, that of Paul Robin to the new chair of histology. Both nominations seem to have been an attempt by the educational administration to raise the scientific status of the Faculty. Second, Rayer was identified with a new vision of medical science that was closely associated with laboratory experimentation. He had helped to found the Société de Biologie, which would come to play a major role in French medical science. Beginning in the mid-1870s, the members of the Société whose careers Rayer had supported would seize power in Parisian medical institutions and introduce a new model of science into medical training and research. Within this model, specialization seemed an obvious necessity.

Rayer's reform was modest and could not have been otherwise; the hostility of professors could not be completely dismissed and the budgetary constraints of the period[102] would have made it impossible for the government to create a significant number of expensive new specialty chairs. Rayer's reform got around both problems. Since the courses were taught by junior personnel, they were cheap, and the prerogatives and resources of existing professors were preserved. Though a modest investment, these courses provided official recognition to the specialties involved: mental and nervous diseases, skin diseases, venereal diseases, diseases of children, diseases of the eyes, and diseases of the urinary tract.[103] From here it was a relatively short step to the status of full chairs if representatives of the specialties succeeded in demonstrating the requisite scientific vitality.

Rayer's reforms did not eliminate academic hostility to specialties. In 1868, the director of the medical school in Marseilles made some waves with a speech attacking specialization for leading to the "atrophying of intelligence." Nonetheless, it is significant that we know about this chiefly because a supporter of specialization published a pamphlet in rebuttal.[104] And the specialist courses seem to have given new life to medical publishing; during the 1860s and 1870s, many specialty medical journals were set up. Most were founded and supported by elite physicians at the Faculty of Medicine and in hospitals (or in other state institutions, such as those for the blind or the deaf). And they were predominantly in those fields on the verge of full acceptance into the medical curriculum.[105] The earliest journal to materialize was in the field of dermatology-venereology, in 1868. During the decade between 1871 and 1880, there appeared no fewer than five long-running journals of ophthalmology and four journals of obstetrics-gynecology. Even fields not yet represented at the Faculty began producing journals in order to better position themselves academically. The first journal in the emerging field of otorhinolaryngology appeared in 1875. Figures in better-established fields organized Parisian and even national specialist societies. These were parts of international networks of specialty societies that were beginning to convene from time to time at international congresses.

In the mid-1870s, pressure to transform specialty courses into professorial chairs accelerated. Reformers were particularly influenced by what they saw as the rapid development of specialist medical teaching in Germany. In fact, as we shall see, their claims in this respect were exaggerated. But this mattered little in the intense competitive climate that followed France's defeat at the hands of Prussia in 1870.[106] Creating chairs in clinical specialties was perceived as integral to a fundamental reform of medical and higher education that was gaining support among the nation's political and intellectual elites. New specialty chairs were thought necessary to maintain France's prestige within the international community of medical science; they were equally essential in order to attract the foreign doctors who had once come to France to complete their postgraduate training but were now choosing instead to travel to Austria and Germany.[107] Debate of this issue began within both the educational administration and the Faculty of Medicine in 1875. Although there was some disagreement about which subjects deserved professorial status and about the prerogatives that should be attached to these new positions, there was almost no opposition to the principle of expanding the role of specialties.[108]

In 1877, a clinical chair in mental maladies was established, the first of seven chairs in the various clinical specialties that were introduced by 1890; the others were in diseases of children, ophthalmology (1878), dermatology/syphilology (1879), neurology (1882), clinical obstetrics, and urology (1890). These were the products of international educational and scientific competition. Some Faculty reports on these matters explicitly distinguished between specialization of medical practice, considered to be of little interest, and scientific specialization, which was vitally important in the competition against foreign science.[109] "If we ask for specialized chairs, it is in order to have professors devoting themselves entirely and without second thoughts to the study of certain specialized parts of science; it is in order that French science be capable of battling in this area against foreign science."[110]

Scientific considerations played a predominant role in Faculty deliberations. With limited resources at their disposal, professors tried to determine what fields had developed sufficient knowledge to merit professorial chairs. At the head of the list was ophthalmology. Academic reports and debates referred specifically to the discoveries that the ophthalmoscope had made possible.[111] Urology was rejected in the 1870s on the grounds that it was not sufficiently advanced scientifically. Such scientific considerations, however, were not always congruent with political and public health realities. In such cases, politics usually triumphed.

In 1879, for instance, the French government established a clinical chair devoted to diseases of the skin and venereal diseases, combining two specialties occasionally but not usually practiced together.[112] This occurred in spite of earlier reports by Faculty and administrative commissions recommending that only dermatology be raised to the status of a chair, on the grounds that venereology was a distinct field of little scientific interest.[113] However, it was a subject of great public health concern for the government, which, it soon became clear, would not consider a new chair in dermatology unless venereology was included in the designation. Consequently, the Faculty capitulated quickly.[114] Furthermore, the minister of public instruction appointed to the chair, without consulting the Faculty (as was the usual practice), the venereologist Alfred Fournier. This was in fact a popular choice within the medical community, but Fournier showed little interest in dermatology, which languished during his tenure in the chair.[115] It is also likely that the creation of a chair in the diseases of children in 1878 owed more to state concern to combat infant mortality than it did to the scientific status of this field.

Almost all this institutional activity, it should be noted, took place in Paris. Provincial medical faculties were slow to obtain specialty chairs. This was largely a consequence of the motives of international competition that underpinned the reforms. Since the Faculty of Medicine in Paris was the showpiece of the French system, the institution meant to attract foreigners, it was necessary to provide it with a full range of specialty chairs. There was not much concern about provincial institutions that were invisible internationally. This was all the more true since the educational administration was engaged during this period in expanding the number of medical faculties from three in 1870 to seven by the end of the century. This process meant that funds that might have gone toward creating new chairs and courses in existing provincial institutions went instead toward developing the minimal resources required by the new faculties.[116]

Parisian hospitals evolved more slowly toward formal specialization. Specialized hospitals, of course, continued to make it possible to pursue clinical practice and research while training students in many fields. The Parisian hospital administration, the Assistance Publique, began in the 1870s to create specialized wards, and many hospital physicians and surgeons were known to be specialists, whatever their official titles.[117] Later in the century, clinicians in general hospitals could make agreements with the central admission bureau of the hospital system to direct certain types of patients to their wards, creating services that were de facto specialized. Perhaps for this reason, there was relatively little pressure to formally recognize hospital specialists.

Such formal recognition was in any case complicated to achieve. In the bureaucratized Paris hospital system, the highest form of recognition for a field was self-recruitment through special competitive examinations; this required support from the Paris Municipal Council, and thus political patronage. Certain specialist groups managed to manipulate the system to their advantage. In 1878, the Municipal Council of Paris, responding to significant improvements in infant mortality statistics in lying-in hospitals (due to the introduction of antiseptic methods and isolation), voted to create a small corps of obstetricians in the hospitals. These hospital obstetricians, appointed through their own special competition, were to be responsible for new obstetrical wards established at the major general hospitals. Despite opposition from hospital surgeons, this measure was implemented in 1881. However, surgeons exacted a high price; gynecological surgery was excluded from hospital obstetrics and remained firmly in the hands of surgeons.[118] Several years later, a special competition was introduced to recruit a special corps of hospital alienists.[119] Other efforts were less successful. On several occasions, the venereologist Alfred Fournier, trying to take advantage of growing anxiety over the spread of syphilis, failed to convince the Academy of Medicine to support the creation of hospital venereal services staffed by a corps of specialists.[120]

Near the end of the 1890s, the medical politician Paul Strauss launched a campaign within the Municipal Council of Paris to bring more specialization to the hospital system.[121] A special commission headed by the dean of the Faculty of Medicine surveyed five specialties and decided to create a corps of specialists, chosen by special competition, in ophthalmology. The regulations to this effect appeared in 1899. Several years later it was decided to establish a corps of hospital otorhinolaryngologists.[122] In other cases (gynecology and neurology), the commission decided that existing resources were adequate. Concerning dermatology-venerology, it was judged that a new specialist hospital and more outpatient clinics were required, but that a separate specialist corps was unnecessary. In 1901 a corps of dentists required to have both the medical doctorate and the dental diploma was established in the Parisian hospitals.

Specialist practice outside the elite Parisian institutions also expanded throughout this period. Initially expansion was slow. The *Annuaire Roubaud,* for instance, included 85 self-identified specialists in 1870[123] and 144 in 1880. By 1884 there were 233, suggesting that the success of specialties in finding a place in the education system was making it more respectable to identify oneself as a specialist. In the next decade, the growth of specialist practice would be exponential, as we shall see in chapter 5. The tenth volume of the *Dictionnaire encyclopédique des sciences médicales* (edited by A. Dechambre) appeared in 1881 with an entry (the first, to my knowledge) on medical specialties. The author, A. Chéreau, emphasized that, unlike the specialists of old who lacked science,

> Most of our specialists of today are graduated men, who have demonstrated knowledge, and who, while cutting up the art, do not bring the profession into disrepute. So-called special works do not impede in any way so-called general works, and analysis cannot do harm to synthesis. After all, it is specialists who have produced most of the useful inventions and, from this point of view alone, they fully deserve that we offer them a friendly and brotherly hand.[124]

Conclusion

Specialization in nineteenth-century France, we have argued, was primarily justified by its significance for medical research and teaching. Its expansion was thus closely related to its integration into the Paris Faculty of Medicine, which reflected the perceived need to regain for Paris its role of leadership in medical science and, more generally, the political desire for national renewal through the reform of educational and scientific institutions. Only after 1880 did specialist practice spread widely. Before dealing with two other countries that followed a broadly similar trajectory, we shall first deal with developments on the other side of the English Channel, and more particularly in London, where specialization developed *without* becoming closely identified with medical research and teaching. The consequences, we shall see, were far-reaching.

Chapter 2
Specialization and Its Opponents in London

London was the largest city in Europe. It possessed medical resources that were certainly as extensive as those of Paris. Among the many practitioners in the city, specialists were clearly visible. And yet, specialization as a compelling social category did not first emerge in London; and once it did appear on the scene, it faced a unique degree of hostility. In fact, almost none of the conditions that pertained in Paris applied in the British metropolis. London provides an almost exact negative image of the situation that allowed specialization to flourish in the French capital. In the British context, specialization appeared to be something less than inevitable and self-evident, and did not achieve the strong identification with medical research and innovation that existed elsewhere.

There are many reasons why specialties appeared so problematic to London doctors in the early years of the nineteenth century. Several stand out.

To begin with, during the first half of the nineteenth century, the British medical profession was divided into three occupational groups: physicians, surgeons, and apothecaries; by midcentury such corporate divisions were gradually being replaced by another division, between GPs and elite hospital consultants, though corporate distinctions remained significant. The fragmentation of licensing among the nineteen degree-granting or licensing bodies was another characteristic feature of British medicine that provoked considerable protest. From the early decades of the nineteenth century, the main thrust of efforts by would-be reformers of British medicine was to bring unity, simplification, order, and greater equality to this complex and, for some, chaotic professional context.[1] Under these conditions, specialization appeared threatening to many doctors, foreshadowing even greater professional division and conflict. And for the medical elites in the royal colleges whose power was being challenged by reformers, specialization represented yet another one of the forces that threatened to whittle away their power and privileges. Thus viewed with deep suspicion by reformers and the medical establishment, GPs as well as consultants, specialization had considerable difficulty winning medical approval.

A second reason that specialties were slow to develop was that despite its huge medical resources and population, London lacked the single unified hospital or educational system within which pressure for administrative rationalization and specialization might build up. The state in fact was largely absent from most sectors of British medicine. On the contrary, the system of competing private hospitals of varying sizes, with many also serving as medical schools, was fragmented, unwieldy, and, some said, wasteful. The staffs of even the larger teaching hospitals were small in comparison with the leading institutions in France and Germany.[2] Providing the basic necessities of medical education left little room for special interests to emerge. (In fact, since teachers were paid from student fees, there was financial incentive to exclude teachers of new subjects, with whom fees would have to be shared.) While considerable private teaching, especially in fields such as anatomy, went on in London, the relationship between private teachers and the medical elite was one of highly charged antagonism. Limited opportunities existed for movement from the private teaching domain to posts in elite London institutions.[3] For all these reasons, specialization had to emerge outside the system of elite institutions. And because of their "outsider" status, specialists could be easily dismissed as opportunistic interlopers, if not charlatans and quacks.

Third, a key distinction between Paris and London had to do with research. From the 1830s to the 1870s, many individuals in London devoted themselves to the advancement of medical knowledge; but the hospital elite as a whole did not.[4] This elite was made up predominantly of "gentlemen," usually appointed through patronage or the purchase of junior hospital posts,[5] who prided themselves on clinical skill and "gentlemanly" personal and cultural attributes rather than on the methodical, empirical research that promoted specialization elsewhere. To medical reformers who complained of the decline of medical science in London, as well as to American doctors who chose to study in Paris or Edinburgh, the London elite appeared uninterested in medical science.[6] They remained relatively remote from much of the international medical community in which specialization was developing. Such judgments need to be qualified, of course. Each London hospital had its own medical culture. Guy's, whose staff included Richard Bright, Thomas Hodgkin, and Thomas Addison, and that boasted a clinical society on the model of those existing in Paris, was clearly an institution where advancing science mattered a great deal. This may explain why it was frequently cited for its unique openness to clinical specialties. But Guy's was exceptional in the London context. The impetus toward specialization that was generated in Paris by a large community committed to research emerged in London only in localized milieus.

Fourth, the condition of medical research in London mirrored the slow and hesitant professionalization of scientific research more generally—what we have called the "Great Transition"—in the larger British context. During the first half of the nineteenth century, professional research played a relatively minor role within universities and major scholarly societies. Even prestigious institutions such as the Royal Society of London fostered a view of science as a "gentlemanly pursuit" and resisted specialization.[7] British academics, it has been argued, subordinated the demand for specialized research to "an older professional ideal of the teacher as moral guide and member of a broadly literate community of gentlemen."[8] Such views changed only slowly within the academic world during the second half of the nineteenth century. But the inexorable spread of such research ideals did not immediately provide elite London doctors with proximate models of specialized research, as the scientific institutions of Paris did for doctors there, because so much elite medical training took place in general hospitals that remained isolated from universities—even when formal institutional links existed. In countries where medical education was closely tied to other institutions of higher learning, it was difficult for elite doctors to resist new models of research and specialization that were coming to dominate education in science. Furthermore, until the last decades of the nineteenth century, voluntary hospitals were controlled by laymen who held power to appoint senior medical staff. These lay directors tended to be more interested in matters of "personality, style, and character" than in medical science or even clinical skill. Their appointees developed similar values that shaped their careers and informed their choice of junior staff.[9] Making room for medical science, and merit more generally, within the British system was one of the chief goals of reformers in the early nineteenth century; the precursor to the British Medical Association (BMA) was initially set up as a scientific organization.[10] Merit and research skills of various sorts gradually became more pertinent for elite recruitment in the latter half of the nineteenth century without, however, completely displacing "gentlemanly" criteria.[11]

This combination of factors did not prevent specialization from emerging in the early and mid-nineteenth century; but the specialization that emerged took a distinctive form. It was cultivated to a considerable extent outside of the medical elite and had a conspicuously entrepreneurial cast. It was financed by philanthropists and built around the provision of care for specific diseases rather than research.

The Emergence of British Specialists and the Rising Backlash

Britain had the usual kinds of specialists in the eighteenth century. Bonesetters, dentists, oculists, and specialists in venereal disease usually functioned outside the regular profession and were frequently considered "quacks" by doctors.[12] In the late eighteenth and early nineteenth centuries, some medical men encroached on these domains, becoming ophthalmic surgeons, surgeon-dentists, and, later, orthopedic surgeons.[13] By far the most widespread form of specialist practice, however, was midwifery. Adrian Wilson[14] has masterfully described the process that transformed obstetrical surgery in the eighteenth century. Initially a part of general surgery whose practitioners extracted dead babies from the womb, it became by mid-century a tiny specialty that dealt with complicated live births in collaboration with midwives; finally, toward the end of the eighteenth century, it evolved into a larger medical category whose practitioners dealt as well with routine births, having partially displaced midwives as providers of primary birthing care. Although midwifery in Britain was to some extent a category of teaching and knowledge production (William Smellie and William Hunter played a major role in the development of obstetrical knowledge and techniques), it appears to have become a category of private medical practice to a much greater extent than was the case in France.

This identification with private practice rather than research may explain some of the hostility that obstetrics and other specialties faced in London. The Company of Surgeons excluded midwifery from surgery, as did its successor, the Royal College of Surgeons (RCS). The Royal College of Physicians (RCP) did offer midwives a subordinate status and in 1783 introduced a license in midwifery. But this was viewed as a distinctly inferior form of practice, and in 1800 the license was discontinued. The problematic place of midwifery in the early nineteenth century—intensified by the appropriation of routine childbirth by surgeon-apothecaries—foreshadowed the peculiar difficulties faced by aspiring specialists in Britain.[15]

During the eighteenth century, specialty hospitals appeared with increasing frequency. These were usually private institutions and sought to serve those excluded from voluntary hospitals: initially the insane, parturient women, children, sufferers from fevers or venereal disease. These coexisted with and complemented the general voluntary hospitals.[16] In the nineteenth century, the establishment of such hospitals accelerated and was associated with a new form of entrepreneurship. Rather than making direct appeals to the public, often through a publication that vaunted a specialist's treatments (as had been the usual case in the eighteenth century), specialists now targeted philanthropists who might support a small, specialized dispensary or hospital; this could make a practitioner's reputation as a specialist and attract wealthy private patients.[17] Although it was based on the philanthropic model of the elite voluntary hospitals, specialization in the British context had a strong dissenting quality. It was taken up by ambitious outsiders excluded for religious, educational, or social reasons from posts in general hospitals and who consequently established competing institutions.[18] Some had studied on the Continent,[19] and a few were foreign-born and -trained.[20] Although the scientific value of special hospitals was frequently emphasized,[21] these tended to focus primarily on the provision of useful and heretofore unavailable charitable services.[22] One did not, of course, preclude the other, and certain specialists had very strong scientific interests.[23] Nonetheless, such interests were not necessarily at the center of public perceptions of special hospitals, whose development was frequently shaped by the imperatives of private philanthropy; those devoted to children were particularly subject to such pressures.[24]

During the first half of the century, twenty-seven specialist hospitals, infirmaries, or dispensaries were established in London (joining twelve that survived from the eighteenth century) and another twenty-two in provincial cities. Those devoted to diseases of the eye were especially prominent early in the century.[25] It has been argued that the Egyptian military campaign, a result of which was a major outbreak of ophthalmia among British soldiers, "galvanized British medical practitioners to investigate the eye" and led to many publications on the subject. Attention to the economic and human costs of blindness allowed philanthropists to feel that they were particularly virtuous in supporting eye hospitals.[26] This is a thoroughly plausible explanation, but since the field was also developing—albeit less spectacularly—in the German-speaking world, one must add that that there now existed procedures—cataract removal, topical substances for eye infections—that were thought to be effective and that could provide the basis for practical appeals to philanthropists and for subsequent specialty development. It is probably fair to say that in Britain, as in Germany, ophthalmology constituted the first fully modern specialty.[27]

Despite the success of eye hospitals, specialization made little impact on the profession. It has been argued that most elite physicians preferred to remain generalists because this allowed them to serve as general physicians to the wealthier classes of society.[28] But this is just another way of saying that specialized expertise did not have the same kind of attraction for the Londoners that it had on the Continent. The RCS, early in the century, had regulations to the effect that any newly elected member had to resign posts held in specialist hospitals, though this rule was ignored in the one case where it came into play.[29] The College refused to consider specialists for its new fellowships when it was reorganized in 1843, though it was forced by political pressures to back off in the case of obstetricians.[30] The RCP was even more hostile to specialists. But in some ways, the marginality of specialists stemmed less from outright hostility than from the fact that they were largely ignored; during the 1840s and 1850s, specialization was rarely discussed in a medical press that was preoccupied by the various campaigns for professional reform.

The major medical directory of the period provides another indication of how little specialization seemed to matter in the British context. In 1847 *The London and Provincial Medical Directory* allowed practitioners to specify their area of practice and to mention specialty interests. Less than 5 percent of the first 1,000 London practitioners listed identified themselves with a specialty designation.[31] The figure itself is less telling than the fact that in the majority of cases the specialty was combined with general medicine or surgery. Even more significant is how few specialties were actually mentioned. Over half of those supplying specialty designations (N=25) were practitioners of midwifery, a long-established field with lectureships in the general hospital medical schools.[32] Also well represented in the directory was dental surgery (with ten mentions), which was already becoming a partly autonomous profession. The only other groups identified were specialists of the eyes and homeopaths (with four mentions each), alienists (three), and orthopedists (one). This is a far cry from the richness of specialty designations in Parisian directories of this period.

Starting with the edition of 1849, the editor decided "[o]n mature reflection, and in accordance with the opinion of the profession generally," to eliminate any mention of areas of practice, on the grounds that listing an individual's diplomas or other qualifications was sufficient.[33] It is not clear what motivated this decision. There is no evidence of outside pressure, and even if lobbying did occur, the editor, Churchill, would several years later vigorously resist the demands of the medical profession to prohibit homeopaths from listing their honors, posts, and publications in his directory.[34] It is quite likely that Churchill viewed specialization as too insignificant to bother with.

Indifference or, in some cases, qualified support for specialization turned to vigorous hostility after midcentury as new specialty hospitals multiplied at an even faster rate. During the entire first half of the century, twenty-seven specialist institutions had been established in London and another twenty-two founded in the provinces. During the 1850s, fourteen London and twelve provincial hospitals, infirmaries, or dispensaries came into existence. In the 1860s, a further twenty-two London and twelve provincial institutions were set up.[35] Most of these were very small, but perhaps because a mobile middle class was eager to confirm its social status through new forms of philanthropy, the public response was enthusiastic.[36] Nor did these institutions lack for patients.[37] It is possible that the belief, then spreading abroad, that specialization meant better and more scientific practice was insinuating itself into British society. For this reason, perhaps, the movement provoked a major medical backlash. The resulting outcry was aimed less against specialized practice than against specialty hospitals, which were seen as a threat to the financial health of the general voluntary hospitals from which they were successfully drawing away charitable donations.

Thomas Wakley, editor of the journal *The Lancet* and a leading radical medical reformer, provides a good if rather idiosyncratic example of growing hostility to special hospitals. A virulent critic of the medical elite, he initially showed sympathy for specialists, in many cases outsiders like himself who, when denied positions in traditional institutions, set up their own. It is said that in the 1840s he encouraged one of his collaborators on the journal to become a dermatologist. In 1851, an editorial in *The Lancet* criticized rather obliquely the "management and the conduct" of the officers of a specialist institution, the Orthopaedic Hospital. Wakley began with the following statement: "It has come to be a recognized thing by the profession and the public that there shall be hospitals and dispensaries for the treatment of *special* maladies." The problem in this case was that the governors were acting according to the same corrupt, elitist principles prevalent in general hospitals.[38]

A year later, Wakley delivered a qualified endorsement of the "division of professional labour. . . . the subdividing and specializing process has continued, until in these latter days, medicine, surgery and midwifery, are little else than three great systems of specialties."[39] Initially, doctors had opposed this process, Wakley suggested, because divisions among medical practitioners ordinarily meant that specialties passed out of the hands of the profession to "the brutal [asylum] keeper and the ignorant midwife." But this danger had vanished, and "men now boldly enter upon special paths of study and practice without any fear of separating themselves from the interests or sympathies of the profession as a whole; indeed, the more special the practice, the more readily can the practitioner arrest the attention of the profession and the public."[40] Even the pure physicians and surgeons who most deprecated specialism had in fact accepted it: "Every internal organ of any consequence finds the devotee of its diseases in the roll of the College of Physicians." Many general hospitals now had "provision for special cases."[41]

Among the reasons for this development, Wakley suggested, were the "analytical spirit which is abroad in the profession" and the desires of the public that "rightly or wrongly applies to medicine conditions in industry and the mechanical arts where the subdivision of labour leads to much better quality of products." The benefits, however, were clear: specialization was the path to the advancement of medicine. Based on recent results, "we may hope that great good will eventually accrue both to pathology and treatment from the devotion of particular inquirers to particular subjects."[42] There of course existed the danger of "evil developments" due to the "rank luxuriance of specialism." But these could be minimized if the general hospitals abandoned their exclusionary policies and like Guy's, perceived as exemplary in this respect, opened themselves to specialism.

Underlying this tolerance for specialization, however, was a profound desire for professional unity. Admission of specialties into general hospitals would advance one of Wakley's pet proposals: "One Faculty," a single, comprehensive educational portal to the profession to replace the many existing portals. The desire for professional unity was the dominant theme of Wakley's professional vision and made his support for specialism conditional. Its present usefulness, he suggested, would eventually come to an end; "specialism cannot always prevail. It is assuredly only a state of transition. With proper control on the part of the profession, we may hope that hereafter, when the various parts of medicine and pathology have been improved as far as possible by specialism, all the departments of practice may unite into something like a perfect whole."[43]

Wakley's ambivalence persisted well into the decade. In 1857, responding to the appearance of a new journal devoted to ophthalmology, he wrote that by studying a narrow subject area, specialists often attributed too much significance to "particular forms of vital mutation. Hence the Science of surgery and of medicine often suffers at the hands of specialists. But it cannot be doubted that the Art has gained much from their labours. To this fact the modern progress of orthopaedic and ophthalmic surgery especially testifies."[44] A year later he welcomed the establishment of the London Obstetrical Society because it would lead to the methodical analysis of the huge number of obstetrical cases in the capital.[45]

Also in 1857, however, Wakley began to perceive specialization more critically. He was motivated, he said, by the growing proliferation of "the excrescences called special hospitals" that provoked frequent editorials in his journal.[46] Wakley was hardly alone. A steady stream of articles and letters to editors condemning specialist hospitals began appearing in the medical press. In June 1860, in response to the announcement of the imminent establishment of St. Peter's Hospital for the Stone, a committee of hospital physicians composed a statement of protest against specialist hospitals. Nineteen eminent consultants, including the presidents of the two royal London colleges and the Royal Society, signed the widely published statement.[47] Within months over 400 hospital physicians added their names.[48] Both the *British Medical Journal* and *The Lancet* ran active campaigns against specialist hospitals. Such professional unanimity was unprecedented.

Criticism centered on the damage that special hospitals wreaked on general hospitals. The former, it was charged, diverted charitable funds away from the latter.[49] This was bad for hospitals and for the poor because it deflected money away from actual care and into extensive duplication of services and facilities. Such special institutions also drew valuable clinical material away from general hospitals and threatened medical education because entire categories of cases could no longer be seen by medical students. They harmed the reputations of general hospitals by promoting the unfounded belief that these were inferior to special hospitals. They provided care to patients not requiring charity, thus damaging the interests of private practitioners. They benefited only their founders, who used these institutions to attract private patients, often through advertising bordering on quackery. Finally, by focusing on isolated organs and specific illnesses, they drew attention away from the systemic nature of most diseases and fostered an inferior form of medical practice. In Sir Benjamin Brodie's frequently quoted formulation: "Diseases generally are so connected with each other, and a knowledge of one is so necessary to a right understanding of another, that no one who limits his attention to any given disease can be so competent to investigate its nature and to improve its method of treating it, as those who have a wider field of observation and who are better acquainted with general pathology."[50]

In addition to the general argument that the "division of labor" would prove as efficient in medicine as in other spheres, there were three arguments in favor of special hospitals that opponents had to confront.[51] The first, that such institutions advanced medical knowledge, was usually rejected without much explanation. A second argument was more difficult to ignore: doctors in special hospitals performed procedures that staff in general hospitals were incapable of performing adequately or successfully. Everyone admitted that there were a few cases of this nature: ophthalmology and orthopedics were cited by many. Wakley admitted such special status only in the case of a new hospital for epilepsy.[52] But the vast majority of special hospitals, it was claimed, offered no special skills or services. The third argument was that many conditions and illnesses were in fact excluded from general hospitals, making special hospitals necessary.[53] Wakley took this point very seriously and argued that general hospitals were already changing and would have to change even more radically.

The campaign against special hospitals can be seen both as a defense of traditional systemic views of disease and as a self-interested effort by the medical elite to defend its turf; this was not different in kind from the response of professors in Paris or Berlin who initially refused to admit specialists to the institutions that they controlled. What distinguished London in the 1860s was the near total absence of powerful voices supporting specialization in the name of medical science. There were no administrative equivalents of Rayer in Paris or Ludwig Baron von Türkheim, in Vienna, who insisted on making room for specialists in elite institutions. Nor were there figures comparable with the Harvard medical professor of clinical medicine, Henry I. Bowditch, who in 1866 wrote a "Minority Report" defending specialization against the majority report of a special committee of the American Medical Association (AMA).[54]

One reason for this lack of support is the almost exclusive identification of specialization in London, and eventually all of Britain, with specialist hospitals. As a result, even reformers such as Wakley did not step in to defend specialties. To the editor of *The Lancet*, the general hospitals, reorganized and comprehensive in scope, represented the nation's only hope for the single educational portal of entry to the profession that could produce a unified medical profession. In defense of the general hospital, Wakley proposed two related strategies. One was to ruthlessly banish anyone attached to a special hospital from all posts in general hospitals. In this way special hospitals would be denied legitimacy and links to the medical elite. The second involved "the practical assertion of the unity of medicine"[55] by opening up the general hospitals to all diseases and specialties. Special departments had to be established in all the recognized fields, as some hospitals, notably Guy's, were supposedly doing.[56] In this way the rationale for special hospitals could be undermined while general hospitals would, by appointing more staff, become more democratic and representative of the profession.[57]

Throughout the 1860s, *The Lancet* appealed for more special departments while at the same time defending the progress being made.[58] Wakley argued that even traditional forms of patient exclusion were no longer justified. Segregating patients in fever hospitals, for instance, now made no sense because medical science had proven that collecting together fever patients intensified the locus of miasma; disseminating such patients throughout a hospital was the best way to prevent the spread of these diseases. The exclusion of mental patients was somewhat more justified by the special difficulties of controlling them. But the price of this segregation—that most GPs knew nothing about mental illness—was too high. The policy of segregating victims of venereal disease on moral grounds, he viewed as hopelessly old-fashioned and morally unjustified. The general hospital should include every form of disease so that it could educate the fully rounded physician[59] and create a comprehensive medical science.[60]

The Laborious Advance of Specialties

Thomas Wakley's advice, repeated frequently by *The Lancet* during the next three decades, was not followed as ruthlessly as its advocates would have liked. Consultants sought to isolate special hospitals, and in a number of well-publicized cases forced men with dual appointments to choose between a post in a general hospital and one in a special institution.[61] Such efforts, however, had limited effect. In 1866 the new editor of *The Lancet*, James Wakley (Thomas' son), cited figures, based on the most recent *Medical Directory*, to the effect that of the 170 medical officers attached to general hospitals, no fewer than 61 were also attached to one of the special hospitals.[62] By 1889 only 31 of 195 medical officers in general hospitals were *not* also attached to a specialist hospital.[63] Many of the general London hospitals did establish specialty departments; from 1855 to 1875 the number of these departments rose from twenty-three to fifty-two.[64] But many of these were not well appointed. In the words of one dermatologist, "no proper accommodation has been provided for them, as if the aim were rather to strangle the existing special institutions . . . than to grapple with the subject in any adequate manner."[65] London hospitals responded quite variably in accordance with the dominant institutional culture. At St. Bartholomew's a perceived need to provide more specialist teaching seems to have motivated the creation of many specialist posts; in contrast, at St. Mary's specialty posts were established at a desultory pace.[66]

General hospitals did not, on the whole, become central to specialist careers because they systematically appointed nonspecialists to run most specialty wards. (Obstetrics and ophthalmology were exceptions in this respect.) *The Lancet* defended this practice on the grounds that diseases were systemic and closely related, so that physicians required wide general knowledge.[67] In 1867 the editor endorsed the majority report of the American Medical Association's commission on specialties, which called for specialists to be general practitioners with an interest in a specialty. The goal was to permit "[the] general practitioner appropriating to his own use more and more of the special knowledge which accrues from the more numerous and refined means of investigation which are taught, or should be taught, in every hospital. . . . The only specific against the extension of specialism is, that the general practitioner himself shall be more special in his knowledge and his resources."[68] Such attitudes were widespread. The Liverpool physician Hugh Thomas, a pioneering innovator in orthopedic techniques, always thought of himself as a general practitioner and spoke out against the "mania for specialties."[69]

Virulent opposition to specialization was largely confined to London. A review of the *Edinburgh Medical Journal* from 1875 to 1900 found no trace of hostility to specialists. Among the many reviews of specialized books and journals that took specialization for granted, only one series of articles in this publication discussed the phenomenon; a general practitioner sought to outline the knowledge of the eye, ear, nose, and throat required by GPs in order to recognize what to treat and what to refer to a specialist.[70] There are other indications as well that specialization was a less contentious concern outside London.[71] But even in the metropolis, starting in the 1880s, it became possible to have something like a specialist career in general hospitals, while posts in specialist hospitals were becoming routine steps in the career trajectories of hospital elites. Many young men, it is true, moved from one hospital and from one specialty to another in their ascent of the professional ladder.[72]

But specialist hospitals and wards also began to produce permanent specialists who dominated the societies and journals that were being established. Many of these combined posts in specialist hospitals with appointments in general hospitals.

The idea of specialization seems to have become gradually integrated with professional aspirations for a unified and rationally organized medical profession. Although complaints about specialization continued to be expressed with great frequency, anti-specialist sentiment became less harsh and more qualified. *The Lancet* from 1875 on admitted that the subdivision of medical labor was necessary and in fact beneficial, but it distinguished between legitimate (based on wide general knowledge) and illegitimate (based on a narrow perspective) forms.[73] Rather than simply ignoring special hospitals in the hope that general hospitals would establish special departments, the journal began advocating the utilization of special hospitals in medical education and even amalgamation of some of the larger ones with general hospitals.[74] This notion would be taken up in 1892 by the Select Committee of the House of Lords on Metropolitan Hospitals.[75] The RCP remained reluctant to allow specialists to become officers.[76] However, in 1876, the Royal College of Surgeons appointed a specialist in ophthalmology to its prestigious Hunterian professorship of surgery and pathology.[77] Several years earlier, the College had accepted a donation from one of its fellows, the dermatologist Erasmus Wilson, establishing a professorship in dermatology. Wilson was then appointed to the post.[78] Possibly as a result of his generosity to the College in this and other matters (after his wife's death his considerable fortune reverted to the College), Wilson became president of the College in 1881.[79] In 1903, the ophthalmologist John Tweedy was elected president of the College.[80]

Leading specialists also contributed to a growing consensus about the limits of acceptable specialization by frequently warning of the dangers of narrow specialization and advocating the introduction of special departments in general hospitals.[81] Ideas about the unity of the body and of medicine no longer served as an argument against specialization, but rather as one for the integration of specialties into hierarchical and unified systems of knowledge and institutions.[82] The research potential of specialties was frequently seen as a resource for general medical practice. In the words of an editorial in *The Lancet:*

> With the possible exception in favour of specialisms which are based upon some extraneous branch of knowledge, as ophthalmology upon optics or otology upon acoustics, the benefit to be derived from specialism in the future is likely to be proportionate to the degree in which its researches are made to enrich medicine in its entirety and to be contributory to the increased efficiency of the general practitioner.[83]

There are three primary reasons, in my view, for the gradual if grudging acceptance of specialties.

First, the British medical elite gradually came to terms with international developments in medical education, including acceptance of a central role for clinical research, by now strongly identified with specialization. Increasingly, the British Medical Association referred to the growing number of specialized sections that comprised the major part of its annual meetings as the locus of its "scientific work."[84] Furthermore, British physicians were part of an international network of medical elites monitoring each other in the medical press and meeting regularly at international congresses. It was difficult for British doctors to resist the spread of specialization occurring everywhere without becoming marginalized internationally.

Second, growing government involvement in health care produced many of the same kinds of pressures for administrative rationalization that supported specialization in other countries; here, as elsewhere, rationalization meant division into manageable categories.[85]

Third, the thirst for professional unity that I identified earlier among reformers spread widely and encouraged compromises that everyone could live with. Both the introduction of the referral system and qualified acceptance of specialism promised conflict resolution as much as technical efficacy by reconciling the conflicting interests of elite doctors and general practitioners. Consultants would now depend on the referral of patients by GPs rather than on direct appeals to the public. But this compromise also allowed elite consultants to appropriate and eventually monopolize specialist practice.

As in other nations, the spread of specialist practice generated problems. Medical journals were filled with passionate discussions about the proper relationship between specialists (and consultants in general) and GPs. Likewise, specific procedures became objects of contention among groups. General surgeons vigorously defended their monopoly over gynecological surgery in London hospitals against the claims of obstetricians.[86] Some anesthetists sought to transform themselves from surgical adjuncts and assistants into full-fledged specialists directing special departments and having direct access to patients.[87] And the attempts of certain specialists, such as pediatricians, to take over large domains of general practice were vigorously opposed.[88] Nearly all doctors agreed that paramedical personnel such as nurse-anesthetists, opticians, and nonmedical radiologists were a very bad thing.

However, the main arena of conflict was, before the 1920s, medical education. The special hospitals began early on to offer lectures and practical training; many gradually came to be recognized as training sites for the clinical clerkships required by the Conjoint Board Examination established in 1884 [89] Such recognition was seldom explicit. The General Medical Council (GMC), when it discussed the addition of a fifth year to the medical program, rejected wording that allowed this fifth year to be devoted to clinical work exclusively "in a general hospital or public dispensary"; but it also could not accept as an alternative formulation "general or special hospitals." Instead, it settled on the ambiguous phrase "at one or more public hospitals."[90]

Special hospitals were also the main locus of specialist research and often provided the foundation for specialist societies. The Ophthalmic Society of the United Kingdom, for instance, grew out of Moorfields Hospital. St. John's Hospital for Skin

Diseases was important in the development of the London Dermatological Society in 1911.[91] Perhaps because of the entrepreneurial and individualistic orientation of pioneering specialists, specialty societies were organized somewhat later in Britain than elsewhere. A handful of societies appeared after 1850, but it was not until after 1880 that most came into existence. By 1893 *The Lancet* was referring to the "deluge" of special societies as "an evil to be repressed" because discussions of special diseases needed to be brought before general medical societies.[92] Nonetheless, sixteen specialist societies would be amalgamated in 1907 to become special sections of the newly established Royal Society of Medicine.[93]

The history of specialty periodicals is patchier because many did not survive very long.[94] On the whole they appeared considerably later in Britain than elsewhere. In 1880 a journal devoted to *all* specialties was set up, on the grounds that so few specialty journals existed. (One of the few cited as being in existence, *The Obstetrical Journal*, collapsed a year later.[95]) This new journal was no more successful than more narrowly focused ones, and soon ceased publication. After a rather slow start, however, specialist societies and journals did begin to produce specialist knowledge of one sort or another.

Although general medical directories did not usually identify specialists, they did mention special hospital affiliations and sometimes listed published work. To make up for the lack of information in such publications, several specialist directories were published around 1890. One of these with very liberal inclusion criteria drew the ire of the *British Medical Journal* (*BMJ*), which called on respectable physicians to refuse to allow their names to appear in it.[96] But two more acceptable publications were also produced. One of these provided what was purported to be a comprehensive list of all those London practitioners appointed to special hospitals or special wards of general hospitals.[97] It included 600 individuals divided among seventeen specialist categories. Diseases of children and midwifery-gynecology had by far the largest number of practitioners (seventy-six and seventy-four, respectively), followed by diseases of the chest (sixty-one), the eyes (thirty-seven), and the skin (twenty-eight).

By the end of the century, specialization was becoming visibly developed in London and in Britain more generally. In 1861 there were in England and Wales seventy-two special hospitals in addition to those devoted to maternity (twelve), tuberculosis (five), and infectious disease (seven). By 1891, 128 specialist hospitals as well as sixteen maternity, fourteen tuberculosis, and five infectious disease hospitals were functioning.[98] The number of beds in specialist hospitals more than doubled between these years, reaching a figure of nearly 5,000 in the special and maternity hospitals combined.[99] A handful of major specialties were represented in elite hospital medical schools, though not usually on licensing examinations. Diseases of the ear, the eye, and the skin, and obstetrics/gynecology were represented by special departments in virtually all of the great London general hospitals, while forensic medicine and public health were represented by lecturers.[100] These fields were also developed in major provincial hospitals.[101]

As in other nations, the acceptance of specialties seems to have been the outcome of the international tendency to increasingly introduce specialized sciences into medical education. In 1908, Guy's Hospital set up a special committee to reorganize specialist departments. Among the recommendations were that new departments be created and that "pure" specialists be appointed to head them.[102] Other hospitals might emphasize a different kind of scientific research. In 1923, the inspectors of the University of London described the situation at St. Mary's thus: "[i]t has for many years stood out prominently for its encouragement of medical research in its pathological institute. There would seem to be a tendency to develop the training in Medicine and Surgery to the disadvantage of training in the specialties."[103]

In 1908, the *BMJ* could contrast with some smugness the situation just twenty-five years earlier, when specialization had been widely identified with quackery, with an emerging recognition that it "is a necessary consequence of medical science," so that every consultant is being "driven to more or less open specialism."[104] Nonetheless, the editor admitted that "the state of things is not satisfactory" because teaching of specialties in hospitals remained in many cases inadequate and "the specialist is made, in the language of the police courts, to feel his position."[105] The British situation was peculiar in the international context in several other respects as well.

A Distinctly British Form of Specialization

There seem to have been fewer specialists in Britain than in France, the United States, and Germany.[106] Since there are no accurate statistics on this matter, this perception may or may not be factually correct, but it results from the almost exclusive identification of specialization with posts in specialist hospitals or specialty wards of general hospitals. Elsewhere specialists might or might not be associated with hospitals and medical schools; but specialists in Britain were ordinarily identified through hospital posts.[107] This may have reflected nothing more than lack of opportunities for specialists in private practice to identify themselves as such in medical directories, on doorplates, or through advertising, and the reality may not have been all that different from the situation elsewhere.[108] In those few instances when practitioners were freely allowed to identify themselves as specialists, they did so almost as frequently as doctors in Paris.[109] But public perceptions create a reality of their own, and the identification with hospitals was strengthened by the developing system of referrals that, in theory at least, left primary care to GPs, and hospitals to consultants who were appropriating specialism.[110] British consultants in any event were frequently ambivalent about their status as specialists. Britain remained the only major Western country in which, after the turn of the century, specialist identification in medical directories was rarely practiced. Even in international specialist directories, the unwillingness of many eminent British figures to be classified as specialists made British data uniquely unreliable. An international directory of laryngologists and otologists first published in 1899 complained that its listings for Great Britain were badly incomplete because it felt it could not include British practitioners without their expressed agreement.[111]

Another peculiarity of British medicine was the continued tendency to view medicine and surgery as the two basic divisions of the profession. As a result, new specialties had to develop as either medical or surgical specialties—within the context of the appropriate royal college—thus severely constraining their development. Elite physicians and surgeons also continued to value general knowledge and practice to a degree inconceivable in France, Germany, or the United States.[112] This had practical repercussions. Well into the twentieth century, some of the most innovative specialist surgeons in the country thought of themselves, and to some degree practiced as, general surgeons who happened to have a special interest in orthopedics or neurology (for example). This was as true of representatives of established specialties as of those in new fields seeking professional validation. In the latter case this attitude was a consequence of institutional realities, notably the lack of posts for new fields in general hospitals. Surgeons might work in specialist hospitals or dispensaries; but if they wanted the posts in general hospitals that guaranteed career success, relatively few were available to them outside general surgery.[113] To put it differently, the widespread practice of combining posts in special hospitals with those in general hospitals had real consequences for professional identities; it became internalized in the self-images of elite specialists.

This state of affairs had a great deal to do with the major institutions representing the medical elite and the profession as a whole. The royal colleges, for instance, resisted pressures to include specialty subjects on the examinations for general practitioners, thus denying specialists crucial professional legitimacy. Even obstetrics, a mainstay of medical practice, was not made a required part of the licensing examination until the mid-1880s.[114] Some of the provincial licensing bodies were considerably more open. Trinity College Dublin introduced a mandatory examination in ophthalmology around 1870.[115] The General Medical Council made efforts in the early years of the twentieth century to promote specialist courses in the medical curriculum; institutions that adhered to these high standards included course work or clinics in ophthalmology, anesthesia, mental diseases, and fevers, as well as the more traditional midwifery. But most specialties continued to be excluded from medical education and not all institutions abided by the GMC guidelines.[116]

One consequence of this was the increasing popularity of short postgraduate courses in specialties geared to GPs whose education had been incomplete. Such courses, said the *BMJ*, would enable the GP "with entire justice to the interest of his patients, to dispense in a great many cases with the services of a consultant."[117] The Medico-Psychological Association justified its postgraduate certificate on the grounds that every medical practitioner should have a "complete knowledge" of the subject.[118]

Despite their uncompromising position on examinations, the London colleges nonetheless attempted to co-opt specialists into their version of a united profession.

In one speech after another, leaders of the profession explained that there was a place for specialization that grew out of general practice and that did not isolate itself from general medical knowledge and from the profession as a whole. In 1905, the president of the London RCP, William Church, took a major role in the planning for a confederation of London medical societies, predominantly specialist societies, that would become the Royal Society of Medicine; the initial meetings in fact took place in his institution. Everyone agreed on the advantages of such a union: it would raise the public status of the profession; pooling resources would provide more funds for the advancement of science; travel expenses for individuals belonging to several societies would be reduced. But among the chief benefits was the creation of a center of convergence that could counter the excessive tendency toward specialization and create closer ties between general medicine and the "special branches."[119] In the words of *The Lancet*, "It is above all things in the combination of interests of those branches of medicine that tend each year to become so specialized as to lose touch with medicine as a whole that we confidently predict will be found the chief justification for the institution of the latest of all the Royal Societies and the chief warrant for its success."[120] David Innes Williams is surely correct in stating that the founding of the Royal Society of Medicine represented the belated acceptance of specialization by the British medical profession and that, as a purely learned society, it recognized specialties as categories of knowledge rather than as divisions of practice.[121] That it was also meant to combat excessive specialization is less frequently recognized.

Either because they were so marginal to the profession or because the profusion of licensing bodies and diplomas set a precedent, British specialists demanded special examinations and diplomas for themselves considerably earlier than their counterparts elsewhere. One very early antecedent was a license for surgeon-dentists created by the RCS in 1859 as a way of distinguishing surgeons practicing dentistry from the far larger number of nonmedical dentists. Dentistry, however, was too removed from medicine and surgery to serve as any sort of model. The development of positions for medical officers of health stimulated Trinity College Dublin in 1870 and Cambridge University in 1875 to create postgraduate diplomas in state medicine and public health, respectively.[122] The Royal College of Physicians in 1886 introduced a certificate in hygiene (soon changed to public health). Early in the twentieth century, public health needs of another sort prompted the Colonial Office to request a diploma in tropical medicine. In 1910 the College of Physicians established such a diploma. However, until the 1920s, both London royal colleges successfully resisted efforts by clinicians for special diplomas.[123] In the absence of diplomas granted by recognized authorities, the Medico-Psychological Association granted its own certificate from 1884, but this provided no professional advantages and does not appear to have been very popular.

The British Medical Association was closely identified with GPs and had an equally complex relationship with specialism. It participated actively in the battles of the 1860s against special hospitals; at the annual meeting of 1860, it condemned them but made the implementation of stronger measures contingent on the reform of general hospitals. A committee was formed to report on the issue of hospital reform but produced no specific resolutions.[124] In subsequent years the question of specialties disappeared almost completely from the field of vision of the BMA and from the pages of its flagship publication, the *BMJ*.[125] The reason for this apparent neglect is that the problems of specialization seem to have been subsumed under, and to some degree to have been obscured by, two more general and controversial issues: (1) the problem of free care in hospital dispensaries that competed against the paid work of GPs and (2) the need to ensure the spread of the system of referrals from GPs to consultants that the BMA was trying to promote.

In this context, specialists seemed threatening to representatives of the BMA only when their special dispensaries offered free care at the expense of GPs or when they seemed to go beyond their role as consultants and publicized their specialist interests publicly. That is why self-identification as specialists in medical or telephone directories and the provision of information in other sorts of directories regularly aroused the wrath of the BMA.[126]

But aside from these issues, the association seemed willing to live with specialists on condition that these maintained a discreet profile. In 1867, the Association introduced a system of sections for its annual meetings. Initially three sections—medicine, surgery, midwifery—were represented, but gradually the number of sections multiplied and the specialties took their place first as subsections and then as full-fledged sections. By the annual meeting of 1898 there were sixteen such sections. As in the case of the American Medical Association, achieving the status of a full section was viewed as a form of professional recognition; introductory addresses to the sections were regularly used to advance a variety of professional claims.[127] But the specialty sections of the BMA did not achieve the permanent existence and substantial power that their counterparts were developing within the AMA. Each year the choice of sections was decided ad hoc by the executive of the local society organizing the national meeting, and the arrangements committee would name section officers for that meeting only. It was not until 1934, we will see in chapter 9, that permanent specialist groups of a totally different sort were set up within the Association. By the first decade of the twentieth century, the *BMJ* was a strong advocate of specialization as a necessity of medical science. But this support remained somewhat remote because the journal, like its parent association, primarily served the community of general practitioners. Tense relations with the medical elite would persist throughout the twentieth century.[128]

Conclusion

Britain was unique among the four countries we are examining in the degree to which a profound medical mistrust of specialization was shared by *both* the organized profession *and,* more surprisingly, the medical elite. This negative attitude did not prevent the development of specialties, but shaped and sometimes limited their growth in significant ways. The nature of this restraint did not lie in the smaller number of specialists, or specialist wards and beds; quantitative differences may or may not have existed, but there is no way to tell for certain. What is clearer is that specialization in Britain was molded by a strong desire within the profession to keep specialization camouflaged and, above all, firmly integrated within a united and largely integrated profession. Specialists, it was repeated endlessly, were only generalists who through training and experience acquired special expertise that was recognized by their peers and that did not necessarily imply exclusive practice in a special field. They did not, in other words, constitute a separate category of practitioners. The refusal to put specialty identifications in medical directories or on doorplates served as a potent symbol of prevailing attitudes. Specialization should not be visible to the public, not only because such visibility made it possible to short-circuit the referral system but also because medicine needed to appear unified. The initiated could look at the *British Medical Directory* and recognize specialist competence in the initials of diplomas, special hospital posts, and publications that were listed[129]; everyone else would see only medical practitioners with greater or lesser accomplishments.

Similar considerations explain both the refusal of the BMA to set up specialty sections on a permanent, self-governing basis, as the AMA did, and the importance attributed to bringing specialist societies together in the Royal Society of Medicine. The identification of specialists with hospital posts led to an understanding of specialties as specific *institutional functions* rather than as fundamental divisions among types of medical practitioners. Given all these reservations, it is hardly surprising that public demand in Britain does not seem to have functioned in the way it did elsewhere; it does not appear to a have provoked a massive medical migration toward specialties by doctors in search of lucrative practices; and it certainly did not propel the exclusive specialist practitioner to the apex of the professional pyramid.

Chapter 3
Specialization in the German-Speaking World

In comparison with events in Britain, the development of specialization in the German-speaking world confronted relatively few intractable obstacles. Following their emergence in Paris medicine, specialties appeared in rich profusion in Vienna, capital of the Austro-Hungarian Empire, and somewhat more slowly in the largest university cities of what would become the German Empire. Throughout the German-speaking world, early specialties evolved around state systems of medical education. Even more than in France, specialization here was originally perceived and justified as an academic activity that was central to medical teaching and research. It can be seen as the medical variant of the more general transition that produced professional scientific careers and specialized disciplinary communities within the German research university. The university-centered character of medical specialties reflected the high status of state-administered medical schools and the relatively unimportant role of municipal hospitals (at least those without university affiliations) as independent loci of scientific investigation. Despite the identification of specialties with teaching and research, a powerful ideal of general, synthetic knowledge had to be overcome before specialization could become widely accepted; and this generalist ideal in turn modified and helped domesticate the specialty system.

The Emergence of German Specialists

Specialization was never limited exclusively to Paris. The German-speaking states in the eighteenth century had the usual numbers of oculists, bonesetters, lithotomists, hernia specialists, and teeth pullers; these were sometimes called *operateurs*.[1] Many were itinerants who required authorization from the local *collegium medicum* (board of health) in order to practice. The *collegium medicum* of Braunschweig-Wolfenbüttel allowed such practice in ordinances promulgated in 1721 and 1747, on the grounds that certain operations "like the couching of cataracts, lithotomy, the surgical correction of cleft palates" were so infrequently performed that "regular surgeons [could] lose their touch"; it thus granted special licenses to "skilled operators" who offered these "needed services."[2] Despite general recognition of their usefulness, it was not always easy to distinguish such practitioners from disreputable itinerants and dispensers of patent medicines.

Although they dealt with many of the same body parts as did the *operateurs*, surgeons rarely specialized in their fields.[3] As in other countries, specialists in birthing emerged early, directing the growing number of lying-in hospitals where midwives served as birthing personnel. One of these was Johann Jakob Fried, who directed the lying-in ward at the hospital in Strasbourg, which served as a model for wards and lying-in hospitals established during the second half of the eighteenth century throughout the German-speaking world. The motivation for creating these new institutions was the mercantilist idea that population was the basis of a nation's wealth and strength. Unlike the situation in other countries, however, many of these hospitals were connected to universities, setting a precedent that would shape specialization in the German-speaking world.[4] Medical personnel in these institutions had far more power than their equivalents in French lying-in hospitals, and some of them, such as F. B. Osiander in Göttingen, set out to train skilled obstetricians. Nonetheless, even though an examination in obstetrics was officially required of medical students in certain German states, few male practitioners practiced midwifery.[5] In the early nineteenth century, a variety of new, more academically oriented specialties appeared in the German-speaking world. However, nothing like the Paris model of urban specialization emerged until after 1850. The obvious question is Why not?

The simple answer I will suggest is that no city in the German-speaking world had at that point created the kind of research-medical community that existed in Paris and that was capable of producing self-conscious specialists. Much of this was a consequence of population size. Both Berlin and Vienna had about one-third the population of Paris, and the number of scientists and doctors was relatively small. As the founder of the national association of scientists and doctors (Versammlung der Deutschen Naturforscher und Ärtze), Lorenz Oken, lucidly remarked: "We have in Germany no Paris and no London; we have no place where hundreds of natural scientists and doctors live together."[6] Consequently, the elements of specialization that emerged in the early nineteenth century—and which were in important ways even more advanced in Vienna than in Paris—did not immediately produce a critical mass of individuals who considered themselves members of an emerging category of practitioners distinct from general physicians and surgeons.

Medical education and certification in the German states, as in France, were controlled by the state. In Prussia, reform of examinations in 1825 brought medicine and surgery closer together by allowing students to choose whether to be tested in medicine alone or in both medicine and surgery. Most students seem to have chosen the latter option.[7] A few medical faculties in the German-speaking world were fairly large, though none came close to matching the Paris Faculty of Medicine in size. Heidelberg in the early nineteenth century offered twenty-six courses and Berlin, twenty-nine.[8] Overall, the number of full professors in the states that would eventually constitute Germany remained small: there were only seventy altogether in 1820, although this number grew rapidly in the following decades.[9] In contrast, the university medical school in Vienna had sixteen professors, exclusive of junior staff.[10] In that city there was also a second school for surgeons, the Joseph's Academy, with fourteen professors.

The relatively small size of cities and institutions meant that emergent elements of specialization remained isolated. Unlike the situation in Paris, independent, non-university hospitals were few in number and did not play a major role in education or research. Berlin, for instance, had only three hospitals in the early nineteenth century: just one of these, the Charité, was of significant size; a fourth (Catholic) hospital was established in 1846.[11] Medical faculties thus loomed larger in the German medical context than in France, where municipal hospital systems in the large cities served as relatively autonomous loci of research and teaching. Until the 1830s, Johanna Bleker has argued, there was little support for utilizing hospitals—which treated the poor—for training German doctors whose future careers would be based on private practice among the more affluent.[12] Once this opposition began to dissipate, university clinics and hospitals would become the chief domains of medical research and training.

All German medical schools taught obstetrics early in the century.[13] Courses offered in 1828 in Berlin included pediatrics, psychiatry, ophthalmology, and venereal diseases.[14] Private orthopedic hospitals proliferated everywhere.[15] Several specialized clinics were established at Berlin's Charité Hospital around 1828. These were small; the children's clinic had thirty beds, as opposed to 500 or so at Enfants Malades in Paris. But these clinics closely connected certain specialties to the medical faculty. Volker Hess has described how spatial differentiation into more specialized wards went hand in hand with the growing role of clinical research at the Charité.[16] A university clinic in obstetrics was established in 1817, and in 1828 a university eye clinic was set up, justified by the emergence of such clinics in London and Paris.[17] In 1838, S. Barez, head of the children's clinic, was named extraordinary (equivalent to associate) professor of pediatrics. And six years later the Elizabeth Children's Hospital was established. Academic clinics even in smaller towns fostered specialized interests; Göttingen had a long tradition of ophthalmic specialization under Carl Himly.[18] But such developments remained isolated and did not generate a sense of specialist identity during the early decades of the nineteenth century.

In addition to the size of its population, several other factors contributed to the relative lack of medical specialties in Berlin. One had to do with the fact that the city's largest hospital, the Charité, was used for the training of military physicians and was not much available to the medical faculty for clinical training purposes.[19] Another was a strong proclivity among doctors and scientists for pure, nonapplied knowledge that was comprehensive and organically unified. Such views had been influential enough to prompt the Berlin Academy of Sciences of the eighteenth century (in striking contrast to its Parisian counterpart) to hold only full meetings of the entire institution rather than allowing meetings of the individual sections that composed it. This may also explain the fact that the last three decades of the eighteenth century saw a substantial rise in the number of general intellectual journals at the expense of more specialized journals.[20] Such beliefs underpinned the humanistic reforms of higher education in the early nineteenth century that emphasized the unity of all knowledge (*Wissenschaft*).[21]

Perhaps the most strident expression of this striving for unity was *Naturphilosophie*, that current of biological thinking associated with the philosopher Schelling. But it went considerably further. Timothy Lenoir has masterfully analyzed the fruitful tradition of biological research he has termed "teleological mechanism" and that was associated with researchers of the caliber of Karl Ernest von Baer and Johannes Müller. Representatives of this tradition eschewed narrow specialization and were "guided by a comprehensive program for constructing a unified science of life."[22] When it was created in 1822, the peripatetic Versammlung der Deutschen Naturforscher und Ärtze (VdNÄ) was organized around the expressed aim of unifying all knowledge. Despite the fact that in 1828 it introduced separate meetings for each of the organization's disciplinary sections, the rhetoric of wholeness continued to be widely utilized in subsequent years. This resistance to fragmentation may be one reason why, until the 1850s, this institution contained a single section of medicine that lumped together internists, surgeons, and obstetricians.[23] A significant caveat, however, is in order. Belief in the unity of knowledge was real, but one should not overstate its consequences, given the speed with which the entire German university system embraced disciplinary specialization after 1840.[24]

Vienna in the early nineteenth was the urban center with the most significant medical-scientific community in the German-speaking world and had the most developed medical specialties. Not incidentally, it was also a city where there had arisen a close relationship between medical institutions and state administration. Under Gerhard van Swieten in the eighteenth century, innovative university teaching clinics were set up. These were moved to the General Hospital (Allgemeine Krankenhaus) on that institution's establishment in 1784.[25] Although Vienna was the scene of significant activity in pathological anatomy, the city did not, during the first half of the nineteenth century, produce a medical research community to rival that of Paris. Nonetheless, its institutions were in significant ways even more open to specialized clinical subjects than were those of the French capital.

Some subjects developed within the university. In 1808, H. X. Boer became the first lecturer (*Privatdozent*) in women's and children's diseases.[26] From 1821, Georg Caraballi was "extraordinary" professor of dentistry.[27] Other specialties emerged from one of the several specialist hospitals that had been established, as in other nations, in response to public health and philanthropic concerns. The Vienna Maternity House for unmarried mothers, established during the reign of Joseph II, became a major maternity clinic whose head, J. Boër, also became extraordinary professor at the university, where he taught "expectant" obstetrics with minimal technical intervention.[28] Obstetrical teaching clinics were also founded in such other German cities as Göttingen, Hannover, and Berlin.[29] In addition to the usual foundling home (which became a major center of pediatric research in the 1840s and 1850s), a private dispensary for sick children was founded in 1787, becoming the Institute for Sick Children in 1794; this would also serve as a significant center of clinical research. The most important development, however, was the private founding of the St. Anna Children's Hospital in 1837. This was the third major pediatric hospital to be established in Europe.[30]

The most successful academic specialty in Vienna during this period was certainly ophthalmology. It became a clinical and teaching subject in 1773 (in association with anatomy) largely due to the interest shown by Empress Maria Theresa in the work of the oculist Baron Michael de Wenzel. Teachers of the subject were granted two small wards in the Allgemeine Krankenhaus upon its completion in 1784.[31] Demonstrating much the same philanthropic and public order concerns manifested elsewhere, the government established an outpatient ophthalmic department for indigent patients as a means of reducing the incidence of blindness. In 1812, an "extraordinary" professorship in this field was established at the university for Georg Joseph Beer, alongside a hospital teaching clinic that became the preeminent locus of ophthalmology in Europe. In 1818, ophthalmology was raised to full, "ordinary" status and the subject was made compulsory.[32] A second chair in the subject existed at the Joseph's Academy.

Vienna's large public hospital system manifested many of the tendencies toward rationalization through classification and division that were visible in Paris. The huge Allgemeine Krankenhaus was divided into five sections: internal diseases, external diseases (surgery), diseases of the eye, venereal disease, and obstetrics.[33] A sixth division, devoted to chest diseases, was opened in 1840. There were in addition wards devoted to specific conditions including skin diseases, bladder problems, and breast cancer.[34] Nonetheless, despite such developments and several more mentioned in his book, Carl Wunderlich made it clear after visiting France in 1841 that nothing like the Parisian proliferation of medical specialties existed in Vienna or elsewhere in the German-speaking world.[35] Wunderlich was perhaps not taking the most recent expansion in Vienna into consideration, but he was probably correct in his general appraisal. There were several reasons for the apparently less extensive development of specialties in Vienna.

The first had to do with size; Vienna, like Berlin, was considerably smaller than either Paris or London and lacked the medical density that permitted specialist communities to emerge. Second, the profession remained divided between medicine and surgery, even if the latter was by now a recognized part of medical education. Divided among several institutions, academic surgeons in Vienna had less opportunity to develop the surgical specialties that played such a significant role in Paris medicine.[36] Furthermore, such institutional divisions made it difficult to perceive medicine as a single entity made up of subunits.[37] Third, and most important, were the political conditions surrounding medical education. In early nineteenth-century Vienna, professors had little power to pursue their own special interests because the faculty was linked administratively to the collegium of practitioners in the city and dominated administratively by the emperor's first physician and proto-medicus, Joseph Andreas von Stifft. This deeply conservative figure strongly oriented the university medical school toward the production of medical practitioners with textbook knowledge and proper moral qualities.[38] Although subjects such as chemistry, state medicine, and ophthalmology were made compulsory, clinical research did not become a major concern and the faculty did not become the center of a wider medical research community on the Parisian model.

Conditions began to change after the death of von Stifft in 1836.[39] Ludwig Baron von Türkheim, who had been a student of Johann Peter Frank, assumed leadership of the faculty, and in the ten years before his death took it resolutely in a more scientific direction that emphasized the new anatomical pathology. At the same time, he encouraged the development of new specialties. In 1837 he was instrumental in founding the Vienna Society of Physicians, which published several journals. And he rewarded the most promising exponents of the new medical science with positions at the Allgemeine Krankenhaus. In 1840, a department devoted largely to chest diseases was created for Joseph Skoda. Two years later, Ferdinand Hebra began to offer clinical courses on skin diseases in the dermatological department. Soon after, a gynecological ward was opened under the direction of Eduard Mikschik, and in 1846 a neurological department was founded for Ludwig Türck.[40] During this period, a succession of bright young men was sent to Paris to learn about the latest medical developments in the French capital. They included Skoda, Rokitansky, Hebra, Schuh, Sigmund, and Türck.

Many were rewarded with positions at the medical faculty. In 1844, Rokitansky was appointed full professor of pathological anatomy, and a stream of young men were appointed lecturers in specialized subjects; they included Ludwig Wilhelm Mauthier in pediatrics, Ernst von Feuchtersleben in psychiatry, Moriz Heider in dentistry, Hebra in skin diseases, and Ignaz Gruz in otology.[41] A reform plan, which von Türkheim developed and which was promoted during the Revolution of 1848, was partially implemented in the following years. This gave Austrian professors a large degree of autonomy in the management of their affairs and thus indirectly encouraged the specialization that was emerging in the academic world.[42] In 1850 the St. Anna Children's Hospital became a university clinic, and a year later its founder, Ludwig Mauthner, was appointed extraordinary professor of children's diseases.[43] He was one of several appointments at this level; among other extraordinary chairs established were those devoted to skin (1849, Hebra), venereal diseases (1849, Carl Sigmund), and histology (1853, Wedl).[44] These were soon turned into full chairs.

Despite all this academic activity, a list of 387 doctors in Vienna in 1848 that was part of a survey of medicine in that city[45] contained no information about the specialist interests of the doctors mentioned. Considering the specialist resources that existed by then, it is likely that at least some of the differences between Vienna and Paris had to do with self-perception: men working in specialty areas did not yet see themselves as "specialists" somehow distinct from colleagues in internal medicine and surgery. Wunderlich himself had suggested that there was a special ethos in Vienna that opposed specialization. If this was the case, such views were not sufficiently powerful to prevent the rapid emergence of self-conscious specialists in Vienna after 1850. A more plausible explanation has to do with the small size of the medical community—387 doctors in the list of 1848 mentioned above, and 437 as calculated by Erna Lesky for that same year. These numbers compare with about 1,600 doctors listed in Parisian medical directories at this time. Vienna certainly contained individuals engaged in the same kinds of specialist activities that were taking place in Paris. But because their numbers were small and they remained relatively isolated, they did not necessarily think of themselves as members of a new medical species.

Less than a decade after the appearance of Wunderlich's book, specialties were in fact better integrated within official medical education in Vienna than in Paris. And this new reality was beginning to be recognized by foreign medical students, who came to the city in increasing numbers to take advantage of new clinical opportunities in the specialties. The outstanding organization of the ophthalmology clinic, for instance, was one of the major attractions for British doctors who came to Vienna to supplement their education.[46] And the desire to serve the foreign students beginning to flock to Vienna added to the continuing pressure to recognize new specialties with hospital and teaching posts. Some Viennese specialists developed enough of a reputation to attract patients even in the French capital. The medical press published accounts of Viennese doctors who spent a part of each year practicing successfully in Paris.[47]

Consequently, the specialization of medico-academic disciplines in Vienna was quite advanced by the early 1850s. It had been fostered by administrative fiat, reflecting the commitment of key administrators to the new scientific and research orientation that had emerged in Paris. Early specialization in Vienna, and eventually other cities of the German-speaking world, was predominantly academic in character, and was linked to the rise of university "disciplines" rather than specialist practice. Hans-Heinz Eulner has suggested that the first reference in any German dictionary to the word "specialist"—dating from 1879—emphasized the specialization of knowledge (*Wissenschaft*) in medicine.[48] And many of the men appointed to academic positions during these years did much to advance their respective disciplines. Except for psychiatry, where the creation of hospitals and asylums usually preceded teaching needs, the pattern was for professors or lecturers to set up either private clinical facilities or specialized wards in large urban hospitals in order to satisfy clinical teaching requirements.[49]

Even more than in Paris, much of the specialist work in Vienna was based on the new pathological anatomy represented and promoted by Rokitansky and Skoda. This may well be the source of George Rosen's opinion that specialization was a product of localist organic thinking.[50] But, as the Paris example suggests, specialization was compatible with other modes of medical thought. And without denying the influence of organic localism, it seems more useful to see the simultaneous rise of pathological anatomy, the research imperative, and specialization in Vienna as a historically contingent development based on specific local conditions.

Certainly, similar processes were occurring simultaneously in nonmedical units of German universities, in disciplines where anatomical localism was not at issue. Steven Turner has described the transformation of Prussian universities during the first half of the century from local, collegial institutions devoted to pedagogy to integral parts of a system of national, scientific disciplines in which research and publication were major activities. Increasingly, such publication consisted of monographs and articles intended for small communities of specialists rather than the public.[51] In all fields of knowledge, pressure to advance knowledge and pursue research was leading to greater specialization. Particularly after 1848, the spread of the research ideal throughout universities expressed itself in institutional growth, differentiation of disciplines, and the creation of new specialties.[52] The emergence of medical specialization in Germany is thus best understood in this context of institutional change rather than as the consequence of any specific research model. Medical reformers themselves explicitly made the link between specialization and academic needs.

In 1848, an article in Rudolf Virchow's newly established journal *Die medizinische Reform* argued for the establishment of specialty clinics in university hospitals, on the grounds that general clinics were useless for teachers and students.[53] Only specialty clinics would allow teachers to develop the necessary expertise in their field and students to see enough cases of each type to acquire the comprehensive, anatomically based knowledge now required for competent medical practice. In defense of his position, the author of this article appealed to the increasing specialization that characterized the natural sciences. Although he devoted most of his article to the needs of medical education, he concluded it with a section arguing for the importance of specialist clinics for medical research. As a field developed more knowledge, sharper and narrower questions were posed; "and the sharper the question, the more clear, the more certain is the answer."[54] The article concluded with the painful contrast between the success of French and British medical research and the dreadful situation in Germany.

> Here [abroad] numerous monographs, rooted in a multitude of the most accurate and truest observations with the most weighty consequences for diagnosis, prognosis, and even if frequently only indirectly, for therapy; among us, innumerable textbooks and handbooks, in part cobbled together from unrecognizable fragments of foreign treasures, in part containing arbitrary and fanciful opinions, whose basis rests on a scanty, incomplete practical experience [*Erfahrung*]. The few men among us who have also produced real facts have been able to do this likewise only because they restricted their energies to a confined domain.[55]

There were many reasons for this growing enthusiasm for academic research and specialization. It is probably not a coincidence that the rapid emergence of specialties in the German states followed the unification of medicine and surgery in 1852 in Prussia. The relationship of these two developments is not necessarily causal. Both processes reflected a new political and administrative will manifested first in Prussia, and then spreading to other German states, to intervene actively in order reorganize professional and educational institutions along what appeared to be more rational and productive lines.[56] Desire to join the brave new world of international medical science, as well as rivalry among academics, disciplines, and institutions, also undoubtedly account to a large extent for these developments. But all this activity was made possible by the significant interventions and financial investments of political authorities.[57] Some of this reflected the competition among German states for prestige and student enrollment, which forced governments to vie for the services of the most celebrated researchers.[58] Governments were also motivated by the belief that "science" promised practical technological, therapeutic, and economic benefits, as well as modes of thinking useful to all professionals; and for those not willing to leave civic education to traditional religions, science was also thought to provide the basis for the political and moral values needed to hold together complex societies.[59] Timothy Lenoir has suggested that the ideal of scientific research was linked to the emerging class-consciousness of the rising German middle classes.[60]

Whatever its origins, increasing specialization and division of medical labor were widely perceived as an outgrowth of the scientific expansion of German universities and a new, empirical research orientation.[61] Academic specialization spread gradually after 1850 throughout the German-speaking world. The VdNÄ, within which speeches about the unity of knowledge never ceased to be a regular feature, fragmented increasingly along specialized disciplinary lines. During the first half of the century a single section included doctors, surgeons, and obstetricians. This uniformity was breached when a section of psychiatry was established in 1846, and again in 1856 when surgery and obstetrics broke into separate sections. From then on, there was no looking back. By 1874, twelve of the VdNÄ's twenty-two sections were specialized medical sections, and in 1893 the figure was nineteen of thirty-one.[62] And this evolution of the VdNÄ was itself connected to the growth of autonomous specialist societies that occurred during the same period.[63] Despite the rhetoric of wholeness they cultivated, the leaders of this association understood that unless they adapted to the prevailing scientific ethos, they would lose their members and influence to specialist societies.

The Pattern of Specialty Development

Increasing specialization did not translate automatically into university professorships, the pinnacle of academic legitimacy for new disciplines. Medical schools in the German-speaking world established, on the whole, fewer specialty professorships than did the Paris Faculty of Medicine; and those in what was becoming the German Empire invested later and less heavily in such chairs than did those of the Austro-Hungarian Empire. The number of full professorships even in Vienna was not great; among eighteen ordinary professors in 1884, six represented specialties (excluding surgery), but three of these were in obstetrics or obstetrics-gynecology and two were in ophthalmology. (The other was in psychiatry-neurology.) Berlin had four full professors in the same three specialties.[64] And some specialties were introduced surprisingly late. In ophthalmology, which achieved early academic recognition in Vienna, there was only one professorship in German medical schools (in Leipzig) until the second half of the century. (In Berlin, the chair of ophthalmology was established in 1866.) Dermatology, which received a professorial chair in Vienna in 1869, did not get its first Prussian chair until 1904 (in Rostock); Berlin had to wait until 1911 for one.

Specialty chairs spread surely but slowly and selectively among the medical schools of the German-speaking world. And they tended to spread as a block. Once a specialty was raised to the status of a chair in one major medical school, the process was likely to be repeated in other schools during the following decades.[65] The success of Viennese specialists and widespread commitment to the most advanced modes of medical research drove this process inexorably. Those universities without chairs of obstetrics were provided with them after 1840. In the laboratory sciences, chairs of physiology and pathology spread to all the universities from 1840 to 1875. From 1865 on, pharmacology and bacteriology expanded widely. In the clinical sphere, chairs of ophthalmology became commonplace in German universities after 1859. Typically, a private eye clinic would be opened in order to provide training in the new diagnostic procedures for students and postgraduates; eventually it would win recognition as a university clinic and, later still, a professorial chair for its director.[66] Chairs of psychiatry were established in one university after another from 1865 on. These were followed around the turn of the century by new chairs at about half of the universities in dermatology-venereology and pediatrics; in most of the remaining medical schools, pediatrics remained tied to internal medicine.[67]

Overall, fewer specialties were represented by ordinary professorships than was the case in Paris. Compounding the relative paucity of professorial chairs was the fact that specialized positions and wards were not commonplace in German municipal hospitals. Manfred Stürtzbecher has argued that municipal hospitals in Berlin at the end of the nineteenth century had no specialist wards and relied on outside consultants to handle difficult cases.[68] Specialization in hospitals was meant to serve the training needs of medical students; consequently, only university-linked hospitals had specialists.[69] Overall, it would seem that French reformers of the 1870s who built their arguments for recognition of specialties on events in Germany probably exaggerated the development of specialty chairs in German universities.

Several factors contributed to the relatively slow pace of specialty diffusion. First, university professors in Germany were notoriously conservative politically, which may have played a role in their resistance to innovation.[70] Professors in established disciplines were also not eager to share power, students, and, especially, fees with new colleagues despite strong contrary pressures from state governments.[71] Second, German universities, particularly those of Prussia, invested heavily in the laboratory sciences, creating not just new chairs and courses in these fields but also "institutes," for which no equivalents existed in France. This left fewer resources for clinical specialties.[72] While it is not clear how much the ideology of disinterested and unified scientific knowledge came into play, it is clear that basic laboratory sciences—despite their increasingly specialized and technical character—were easier than clinical specialties to defend, in the traditional terms of general education (*Bildung*), as the intellectual underpinnings for a unified medical science. Third, whether such ideological influences were significant or not, there was clearly an institutional "style" at work in the German Empire. In both the basic sciences and clinical specialties, German universities created professorships in relatively small numbers of conventional and well-established subjects: physiology, pathological anatomy, obstetrics, and ophthalmology. In contrast, Parisian institutions showed much greater variation and even idiosyncrasy; in the basic sciences, for instance, the Paris Faculty of Medicine had, since the early 1860s, chairs in histology and comparative medicine, which had no equivalents in Germany. This French style would be transferred to provincial medical faculties when these began to expand at the end of the nineteenth century. A further limit on the number of chairs in Germany was the practice of combining disciplines such as neurology and psychiatry or obstetrics and gynecology in a single chair, whereas they tended to be divided into separate chairs in French medical schools.[73]

A final reason for the apparent reluctance of faculty administrators to establish too many specialty chairs may have been a laudable belief that specialty clinics needed to be properly installed and financed, to a degree that went far beyond the mere cost of professorial salaries that was frequently the primary investment in Paris. In the basic medical sciences and a few specialties, the establishment of expensive "institutes" served as an alternative to new specialty chairs. In Germany as a whole, 173 institutes were established between 1860 and 1914.[74] A survey of German universities cited statistics to the effect that the University of Berlin in 1890 had ten medical scientific institutes that cost the state the huge sum of 618,000 marks, nearly 75 percent more than the cost of the fifteen institutes in the natural sciences.[75] It was widely thought that large amounts of money were required for each new clinical chair. A critic noted in 1892 that administrators seemed to believe that each faculty clinic needed its own building, classrooms, amphitheater, laboratories, and library, and were thus understandably reluctant to introduce many new specialty clinics into medical schools. (This may also explain why foreigners were so favorably impressed by those German specialty clinics that did exist.) He suggested that it made more sense to fully integrate specialist wards into general hospitals, where they could share resources with other hospital divisions.[76]

The relative affluence of existing specialty clinics points to the danger of generalizing hastily from the number of specialty professorships to the state of specialties in German medical schools. For one thing, it was relatively easy to introduce junior positions into German medical schools. Thus otology, a subject that does not show up on lists of university chairs, was nonetheless well represented in junior positions. In 1879, fourteen universities in the Kaiserreich had a total of seventeen teachers in the field, nine of them extraordinary professors.[77] At the institutional level, one must also take account of the impressive development of specialist clinics at certain universities. In addition to Vienna's six specialist chairs in the 1880s, there were thirteen specialist clinics (excluding those in surgery and internal medicine), each directed by an extraordinary professor and having from one to four assistants.[78] To these one could add a large number of university-affiliated wards, sections, and outpatient clinics. More than professorial chairs, it was these institutions and posts that largely accounted for Vienna's reputation as a center of specialist teaching and research in the latter decades of the nineteenth century. This situation was not without critics. The famous surgeon Theodor Billroth acknowledged that specialty clinics encouraged research and attracted foreign students. But he believed that having too many of them damaged the general education of medical students, who needed to see the widest possible variety of cases within the unified context of medical and surgical wards. There was, he observed dryly, "much superfluous money for unimportant subjects, . . . "[79]

Universities in the German Empire were less richly developed in this respect. The largest one in Berlin had ten clinics, polyclinics, or institutes relating to clinical specialties, while the others had significantly fewer resources.[80] Clinical specialties were also less well represented in the medical curriculum. One writer calculated in 1906 that German universities on average devoted nearly 45 percent less clinical time weekly to specialties than did those of Austria.[81] Nonetheless, a key feature of the German system was significant flexibility and permeability between private and public institutions. To a considerable degree this compensated for the reluctance of medical academics to fully recognize all specialties. Ophthalmology, orthopedics, and psychiatry were specialties especially rich in private hospitals and clinics. Many of these private clinics were profit-making establishments exploiting the growing desire of the German middle classes for a new kind of medical care. Others were charitable institutions. Both types, however, frequently focused as well on teaching and research.

In Berlin, private hospitals and clinics were particularly significant for the development of ophthalmology, orthopedics, and dentistry.[82] Albrecht von Graefe in 1851 opened a private eye clinic that became the dominant site of ophthalmic training and research in the city in spite of the existence of an eye ward at the Charité Hospital. In 1868, after the retirement of the incumbent, Johann Jüngken von Graefe was finally named to head the Charité ward. More immediately successful in his academic career was Julius Wolff, named director of the university polyclinic in orthopedic surgery in 1890, only five years after opening own his private clinic.[83] Private hospitals for psychiatry and "nervous diseases' were commonly geared toward those families who could not care for loved ones but refused to consider state asylums. Nonetheless, they might assume considerable importance for clinical research. Heinrich Laehr's sanatorium for nervous disorders, founded in 1853, played a significant role in the eventual development of academic psychiatry in Berlin.[84] As specialties became more widely accepted, success could be even more striking. Kurt Burkner, for instance, was the first academic representative of otorhinolaryngology in Berlin. After he received his *Habilitation* in 1877, which allowed him to teach, he set up a private polyclinic in his specialty. In 1884, this institution was recognized as a university institute, and a year later Burkner was named extraordinary professor in the medical faculty.[85] This was one of many cases in which the establishment of private clinics led eventually to university recognition of a specialty.[86] Sometimes the order was reversed, and specialists with academic appointments went on to work in private clinics as well. The number of private clinics in Berlin rose from eleven in 1873 to seventy-three at the turn of the century.[87] According to Wilfried Teicher, by 1914 about one-third of all Prussian specialists worked in private hospitals or clinics.[88]

There is one final and critical point to be made about the state of specialties in German academic medicine. Resources to support specialties in Germany were spread around to nearly all of the nation's twenty medical schools, including some that were very small. In contrast, the creation of specialty chairs in France took place overwhelmingly in Paris until the end of the century. The provincial medical schools of France were very few in number (six at the end of the nineteenth century), and until the first decades of the twentieth century they possessed even fewer specialty chairs than did their German counterparts. Let me cite just one example of this contrast, involving the geographically related institutions of Alsace and Lorraine. The comparison is a little unfair since the Kaiser-Wilhelms-Universität in Strasbourg was admittedly one of the most "progressive" and best-endowed in the German Empire because it was designed to be a showcase of German medical science. It was founded in 1872 with a chair in dermatology/syphilology and two chairs of obstetrics. There were in addition extraordinary professorships in psychiatry and in ophthalmology; the former was turned into a full chair in 1876 when the incumbent, Jolly, was offered a chair in Leipzig, an offer that the university administration matched in order to keep him. Two years later, ophthalmology was transformed into a chair on the grounds that most other universities already had chairs in this subject. Extraordinary professorships were founded in pediatrics in 1876, in otorhinolaryngology in 1882, and in dentistry in 1894. In contrast, the medical school at Nancy, which had a similar symbolic role of representing French medical science in this region and which was typical of provincial universities generally, had only two specialist chairs during this period, one in obstetrics and gynecology and another in obstetrics and pediatrics. And when one of the chairs was transformed into a chair of histology, the other became devoted exclusively to obstetrics.[89]

To sum up, if German universities recognized fewer specialties with professorial chairs than did the Faculty of Medicine in Paris, the existence of certain specialty professorships in every university, of junior personnel and university and private clinics in fields lacking chairs, the specialties indeed had an imposing collective presence in the German universities. In 1901 a reform of the examination regulations (*Prüfungsordnung*) in Germany made a semester of attendance at the major specialty clinics a requirement for all medical students.[90] A similar reform would be introduced in France only a decade later.

As was the case elsewhere, the rhetoric of academic advancement in Germany justified specialization as an imperative of both research and the need to train competent general practitioners.[91] The more common and socially disruptive the illnesses covered by a specialty, the easier it was to make this latter case.[92] Specialties competed for space within the medical curriculum and examinations, and for recognition as sections in general scientific societies (such as the VdNÄ). Alongside the informal flexibility provided by private teaching clinics, there existed an enormously complex formal framework within which specialties could gain legitimacy and a piece of the teaching program. As important as were chairs, clinics, and junior positions, the pinnacle of success was representation as a required subject on examinations, particularly the state *Prüfungsordnung* required for state medical licenses. A field could be integrated into a more general medical or surgical examination (a *Prüfungsfach*) or, even better, become the subject of an independent examination (*Prüfungsabschnitt*) drafted and graded by representatives of the relevant specialty. Obstetrics achieved a place on the *Prüfungsordnung* throughout Germany by 1852; a reform of the ordinance regulating these examinations in 1883 introduced hygiene as an examination subject and required one semester of attendance at the ophthalmology clinic. It also specified that psychiatric diseases had to be included in the examination for medicine.[93] It was above all the reform of regulations in 1901 that consecrated the major specialties by requiring all doctoral candidates to attend medical, surgical, and obstetrical clinics for one year, and clinics of ophthalmology, pediatrics, psychiatry, otolaryngology, and dermatology/venereology for half a year; these subjects were at the same time accorded a place on the *Prüfungsordnung*, with ophthalmology and psychiatry becoming self-contained *Prüfungsabschnitte*.[94]

Medical schools and examinations did not provide the only arena in which specialties operated. As in other countries, specialist societies and journals carried the main burden of establishing scientific legitimacy. And there was, as one would expect, great richness of specialist societies and journals in the German-speaking world. These emerged in waves: those in psychiatry and ophthalmology appeared at mid-century; in gynecology, in the 1870s and 1880s; and in dermatology/venereology mainly in the 1880s and 1890s (although the very first journal dates from 1869).[95] In the last domain, Eulner's list of major developments gives some idea of the international impact of German research; it includes the isolation of

Gonococcus by Neisser in 1879, development of light therapy for lupus and the beginnings of roentgen therapy for skin conditions in 1896, the discovery of *Spirochaeta pallida* in 1905, the Wassermann reaction in 1906, and the development of Salvarsan in 1910.[96]

Numerous factors thus explain the widespread perception that Germany had become the world leader in clinical specialties. The large number of academic specialists active in those few fields accepted in virtually every medical school in the German-speaking world, the impressive resources invested in the specialist clinics that were established, and the existence of numerous private clinics and dispensaries where new specialties could make their mark (at a time when French private teaching was being severely curtailed[97]) all contributed to propagating this view. But I would like to emphasize one final factor that strikes me as both critical and insufficiently appreciated by historians: the sheer unprecedented size of the German-language scientific domain. Just as Paris medicine represented research and teaching on a uniquely large scale at the beginning of the nineteenth century, so the German network of universities at the end of the century functioned on a vast new scale that transformed the very nature of scientific communities.

Although politicians might make much of the difference between the Kaiserreich and the German parts of the Austro-Hungarian Empire, universities were part of a large network of German-speaking universities and scientific institutions that transcended political boundaries. This scientific and medical linguistic space (*Sprachgebiet*) included a network of twenty-seven German-language institutions, among them those in Vienna, Zurich, and Prague as well as Berlin.[98] Each had different strengths: experimental science in Prussia, clinical specialties in Vienna. Such variation made the whole network appear stronger, richer, and more versatile than any of its constituent parts. The number of researchers working in this network dwarfed numbers elsewhere.[99] The amount of scientific work coming out of the numerous institutions of the German-speaking world was equally prodigious. The demographically challenged French, no matter how much they built up their Parisian institutions as international showcases, were in no position to compete because of fundamental population inequalities; nor was anyone else, at least until the twentieth century, when American institutions came to occupy an even more vast and varied scientific space.

Perceptive readers will note here that I am providing an alternative explanation to the one offered in the classic study by Joseph Ben-David, which emphasizes free competition among institutions as the key variable in the strength of German (and later American) science during the nineteenth and twentieth centuries.[100] I believe that Ben-David's thesis is generally valid and explains a great deal, but only if one takes account of the size and economic resources of the various national players in the international scientific arena. Thus France in the early nineteenth century, Germany at the end of that century, and the United States in the twentieth, each in its time and its unique way, represented an unprecedented expansion of the scope and resources of the scientific enterprise.

Specialist Practice

The distinction between specialties as university disciplines and specialties as forms of medical practice remained especially pertinent in Germany. As late as 1890, the dermatologist-venereologist Albert Neisser wrote that academic specialization could in fact serve to protect against specialization of practice:

> *The more the university offers every individual the opportunity to be trained adequately in all the specialty disciplines, the more every* general *practitioner [praktischer Arzt], if I can speak thus, is trained as a specialist, that much less would be the necessity to become pure specialists; a rupture* [of the profession] *would not only not be advanced by the establishment of specialist clinics in the universities,* I believe rather that directly through these and only through these, it would be prevented.[101] (Italics in original)

Despite such arguments, academic specialization was becoming closely connected with specialist medical practice. Medical research and teaching for specialists took place in clinics. Early specialists tilling virgin territory made significant advances that attracted referrals and patients. As early as 1852, the Berlin ophthalmologist Graefe reported to his colleague Donders that he saw from 100 to 120 patients a day.[102] The success of leading specialists encouraged many others with little or no academic credentials, or even training, to claim specialty status. As a result, specialist practice became increasingly widespread during the last decades of the century. A few leading academic specialists, such as the medical dentist Moritz Heider, even played a central role in creating professional specialist associations.[103]

Furthermore, for some specialties, humanitarian and public health considerations rather than academic concerns were paramount. In fields such as psychiatry, orthopedics, and obstetrics, hospital institutions grew out of efforts to help or to control certain classes of needy poor and, in the case of obstetrics, to do something about high infant and maternal mortality rates. The institutions that resulted nonetheless provided the basis for developing specialist knowledge. The lack of certain institutions also had scientific implications. It has been argued, for instance, that the weakness of pediatrics in Germany owes something to the fact that there was no widespread movement—as in other countries—to establish foundling hospitals where medical knowledge of children could be cultivated.[104] Public health concerns, we shall see, increased in influence as a result of growing state involvement in all aspects of health care.

Specialized practice expanded rather slowly until 1880. Predictably, it encountered criticism. As early as 1862, specialists were denounced for greed and medical incompetence, and specialization was likened to assembly-line work in factories.[105] Both the number of specialists and debates around them multiplied rapidly during the 1880s. There are no national statistics, and a major government survey of medical personnel in the Empire published in 1889 completely ignored specialties as a relevant professional category.[106] But another survey found that among large cities in 1886, Hamburg had the highest density of specialists, with 14.2 percent of the medical population, while Hannover, with 3.7 percent, had the lowest.[107] German medical directories, we shall see in chapter 5, were inconsistent at this time about listing specialty designations, a reflection of differences among local medical associations on this matter. In an early edition of Börner's famous *Reichs-Medizinal-Kalender* published in 1884,[108] most city lists of doctors did not include specialty information; a few, however, did. One of these was Hamburg, where 13 percent of those listed as doctors identified themselves as specialists, with about half (fourteen of thirty) claiming diseases of the eye as their sphere of activity. While Berlin's doctors lacked specialty designations next to their name in this particular publication, the city's professional directory did include a specialists list. In 1883, fifty-two individuals were listed as dentists (*Zahnärzte*), forty-two as specialists of the nose, thirty-nine as gynecologists, twenty-four as specialists of the eye, and twenty-three as specialists of the throat and larynx.[109] In Württemberg, the proportion of specialists among all doctors rose from 9.5 percent in 1885 to nearly 20 percent in 1900, with the largest group being psychiatrists, followed less surprisingly by gynecologists and ophthalmologists.[110] About one-eighth (N=3,431) of all German doctors listed in the *Reichs-Medizinal-Kalender* for 1901 described themselves as specialists. And it was cities such as Stuttgart, Dresden, and Frankfurt—rather than Berlin—that had the highest proportions of specialists.[111]

The *British Medical Journal* commented in 1906: "Cultured Germany appears to be the land where medical specialism most runs riot."[112] Such judgments, however, must be evaluated with care. The German figures are pretty much comparable with those in Paris, where specialization was equally rampant. The major difference is that specialization in French provincial cities appears to have been considerably less widespread than it was in similar-sized German cities. If this difference is not an effect of source bias, the most likely explanation for it is that the large number of specialists in mid-sized and small German cities reflects the relatively large number of medical faculties in such cities, as well the better representation of specialties in these schools than in the handful of French provincial institutions. This meant that the academic prestige of specialties could be directly transferred to local medical practitioners who were provided with both professional models and opportunities for specialist training. The creation of a health insurance system in 1883 also supported the growth of specialty practice because the major health insurance boards recognized most specialties in matters of payment.[113]

Conclusion

From the 1860s to the 1880s, specialization became closely identified with university research, and in consequence became fully established in the German Empire and the German-speaking world more generally. During these same decades, another process unfolded simultaneously: national bodies emerged to represent the interests of the medical profession in Germany. Although it was largely unrelated to the specialization process that I have described in this chapter, this development was to have a determining influence on the subsequent history of German specialties.

As was also the case in the United States, difficult conditions provoked the German medical profession to create well-organized, if not always effective, national representative bodies that set out to tackle a wide variety of issues. Professional associations were initially slow to get started in the politically divided German states. But once they began to be established in the second half of the nineteenth century, they spread widely.[114] In 1873 the Deutsche Ärztevereinsbund (DÄV) was established as an association of regional medical societies. This institution, which at the end of the century represented about 65 percent of all physicians in private practice,[115] spoke for about 95 percent in 1927. Although it initially aspired also to become active as a scientific society and to deliberate on public health issues, it soon came to focus on professional matters. The DÄV provided German doctors with a national political voice as well as an important national forum for discussion, its annual meeting, the *Ärztetag.*[116] Its success in bringing together the German medical profession reflected the larger processes of unification going on in German society during the same period.

The activism of the German medical profession reflected as well certain unique problems. The profession perceived itself to be under onerous state tutelage; perhaps the single most disturbing symbol of this inferior position was the legal obligation to provide medical care (the *Kurierzwang*). One of the results was to prompt doctors to join together in a movement to free the profession from state supervision and introduce freedom of practice. The movement was successful, and in 1869 *Kurierfreiheit* was introduced in the North German Federation, and extended to the entire empire in 1872.[117] Henceforth, anyone could practice medicine so long as he did not claim the title of doctor. While freeing doctors to some extent from certain forms of state intervention, *Kurierfreiheit* also presented them with unprecedented competition that exacerbated their other economic problems. Before long, the profession was demanding new legal controls on medical practice as well as the suppression of unlicensed practitioners, termed *Kurpfuscherei.*[118] This struggle served as a further incentive to organize in order to pursue the profession's collective aims. The creation of medical disciplinary "chambers," *Ärztekammer,* including all doctors in a given area, began in the 1860s and culminated in the royal decree of 1887 creating such chambers throughout Prussia; these provided yet another venue for professional discussion and debate.[119]

New political conditions also made issues of professional self-regulation more critical for the well-being of the profession. The early introduction of state health insurance in 1883 was by far the most urgent and controversial problem that had to be faced. This program covered 10 percent of the population at its inception and 20 percent by 1911; these figures do not include separate insurance funds for specific categories of workers such as civil servants and miners. The effects of insurance programs on doctors came to dominate medical journals and professional meetings.[120] Associations created to deal with the issue at the political level and to negotiate with sickness insurance funds, notably the Leipziger Verband (Hartmannbund) added to debate within the profession. Also critical to medical practitioners were growing fears of professional overcrowding, demands for the reform of medical education, and the claimed proliferation of "polyclinics," private dispensaries that provided free care to patients. Many of these issues were closely identified with specialization. Polyclinics were particularly characteristic of specialists seeking clinical material in order to pursue academic careers.[121] And the numerous discussions about reforming medical studies, while primarily concerned with increasing the amount of practical training for doctors, inevitably raised the issue of specialty clinics in the education and examination of doctors.[122] This professional concern with a broad range of professional issues led to relatively early debate about ways of controlling the consequences of specialization. We shall argue in chapter 6 that the profession's preoccupation with organizational reform of every sort would make Germany the first of the four countries under discussion to resolve the issue of specialist certification and training.

Chapter 4

The Rise of American Specialties

There are many similarities between the development of specialties in the United States and in Germany. In both countries, a decentralized political system combined with fierce professional competition to provoke medical elites to identify themselves closely with science and specialization. National professional associations responded to these conditions by taking on a central role in the reform of medical education and practice. The American Medical Association (AMA) was established, and became involved in issues of training, research, and specialization, well in advance of the comparable German medical association. Like its German counterpart, the AMA would show a marked proclivity for solutions based on professional self-regulation rather than state intervention. Other parallels were consequences of the direct influence of German medical science on members of the American medical elite.

There were, however, critical differences between the two nations. Whereas in Germany early specialization was closely identified with state-controlled academic medicine, in the United States freedom to establish private hospitals and medical schools left considerably less social distance between the medical elite and rank-and-file practitioners and created more fluid social conditions. The introduction of specialties into elite American institutions was thus facilitated substantially by the competitive environment fostered by large numbers of private institutions. This environment also fostered a more practical, utilitarian approach to specialties than was the case in continental Europe. Consequently, specialist practice and debates around it loomed earlier and larger in American perceptions of specialties than they did in Germany. Market pressures and economic incentives behind the spread of specialties also seem to have been, if not more potent, then more visible and transparent in the United States. Finally, while European academic specialists largely ignored issues of practice, and left rank-and-file generalist and private specialist practitioners to battle things out, American academics were directly involved in practical professional issues.

The Early History of
American Specialties

Few of the conditions that produced specialization in early nineteenth-century Paris existed in the American states of this era. Neither hospitals nor the few medical schools in existence at the time were publicly controlled or very large. Consequently they faced few of the pressures for administrative rationalization that promoted specialization on the European continent. Nor was there much incentive to create research communities on the Paris model. As Tocqueville famously perceived, Americans valued practice over theory, and this applied as much to doctors as anyone else. John Harley Warner describes the negative response of Dr. James Jackson, Sr., to his son's desire to spend several years in Paris pursuing clinical research, and explains: "for an American physician scientific investigation was not a legitimate substitute for practice."[1] It is thus hardly surprising that we have few indications of significant specialty development during the first half of the nineteenth century. What *is* perhaps more astonishing is the swift spread of specialization in the years that followed.

There is no evidence for the significant development of specialties in the United States before 1855. Historical studies of pre–Civil War American medicine are almost completely silent on the subject. For reasons to be discussed in chapter 5, no national medical directories existed at this time, but several collections of medical biographies,[2] while not representative of the profession as a whole, suggest how little specialized elite American medicine was at midcentury and how speedily this situation changed in the following two decades.

Stephen W. Williams's collection of medical biographies appeared in 1845.[3] His 104 subjects were all deceased, which meant that many had pursued their careers in the eighteenth or early nineteenth century. As one would thus expect, there is little mention of specialist interests. Only two traditional domains are occasionally described in peripheral ways: surgery and obstetrics. John Bartham was a general practitioner who "obtained some celebrity in the practice of surgery,"[4] and Andrew Harris was the most distinguished surgeon in eastern Connecticut.[5] Thomas James was "a distinguished obstetrician"[6]; William Potts Dewees was "[f]avorably introduced to the citizens of Philadelphia as a practitioner, and to the professional public as a teacher of, the science of obstetrics, his practice became extensive."[7] Several individuals directed asylums, but only Eli Todd "devoted his life to the subject of insanity" and to "diseases of the brain and nervous system."[8]

In the context of American medicine, the desire to limit practice along European professional lines can look to historians like an early precursor of specialization. In contrast with the situation in Britain, where the medical elite was sharply divided institutionally between physicians and surgeons, with *accoucheurs* becoming increasingly distinctive, the norm in the sparsely populated United States was to combine all three branches (often with drug-dispensing as well). But as cities developed, the separation of activities became more feasible. In 1765, after spending five years studying medicine abroad, John Morgan publicly announced that he would limit his practice to physic and renounced surgery and drug-dispensing.[9] His action, like his stated justification that each of these activities required distinct skills, can be seen either as an attempt to import the professional divisions of eighteenth-century Europe into the colonies or as a foreshadowing of the logic that would drive specialization a century later.[10] There is, however, no question that surgeons became an increasingly visible and distinctive category of practitioners in the nineteenth century and that the process of segmentation continued in major cities.

A half-century after Morgan's declaration, the Boston physician James Jackson, having already renounced the practice of surgery, felt called upon in 1818 to send a letter to his patients to explain why he was also renouncing the practice of obstetrics.[11] While such a limitation was not unknown in other cities, he wrote, "[i]t has not been the custom here." The reasons he offered for his action were not dissimilar to those that would apply to later specialists: the unpleasantness and physical difficulty of certain activities; the greater perfection that could be achieved by concentrating on a single field; the need to adapt his practice to the teaching and research duties associated with his university professorship in medicine. Such motives would be invoked for the ever narrower forms of specialization that gradually made their appearance. But until much later in the century, the most common form of specialist practice involved emphasis on a particular field within a predominantly general practice. Thus Jackson's younger colleague Walter Channing received special training in obstetrics in Scotland and Britain and set himself up as one of the leading obstetricians of Boston. All the while he maintained a general practice and served as first assistant physician and then physician at the Massachusetts General Hospital.[12]

There is also a dearth of specialists in Samuel David Gross's edited volume, *Lives of Eminent Physicians and Surgeons*, published in 1861.[13] Here there are essays on thirty-two deceased American medical men. Among these are a considerable number of surgeons, but only five individuals presented as having some specialist interest. Thomas C. James, who held the first chair in midwifery in Philadelphia, was described as an obstetrician.[14] Jacob C. Randolph was characterized as "devoting himself to the treatment of stone in the bladder."[15] Daniel Drake was presented as an all-round physician but especially as a distinguished oculist who had "acquired no little skill as an ophthalmic surgeon."[16] In the case of Charles Frick, "urinary pathology had become a favorite subject with him."[17] Amariah Brigham was not described as having any special interests, but the career discussed was nonetheless centered on asylum posts and psychiatric publications.[18] Gross's collection suggests only a modest development of specialization during the first half of the century.

The impression that this was indeed the case is confirmed by William Atkinson's 1878 work briefly describing a large number of *living* practitioners, the "real workers in the profession," who "by their work had brought themselves more or less prominently to notice."[19] A little less than 20 percent of those profiled were described as having some sort of specialty interest. (If we add those whose careers consisted of an unbroken series of specialist posts even if a specialty was not specifically invoked, the figure is slightly higher.) These figures include surgery, treated by now pretty much like any other specialty interest. Atkinson's essays suggest clearly that certain forms of specialization had become widespread by the 1870s, but they also confirm that this was new. Most of those described as specialists obtained their MD diploma after 1850 and did not necessarily begin practicing as specialists until after 1860. Very few obtained their medical diploma before 1840.

Atkinson's list is fragmentary and cannot be taken as a representative sample of American doctors during this period. Nonetheless, it suggests a number of general observations.

As was the case almost everywhere else, surgery was a pivotal category because it existed long before specialization as one of the two basic divisions of medicine. Once it became possible to think of medicine as divided into specialties, surgery eventually became the largest, and in many ways prototypical, specialty. Similarly, obstetrics loomed very large in the development of specialist self-consciousness because it had been established as a distinctive medical activity since the eighteenth century. By the nineteenth century, in the United States as elsewhere, it was represented by lying-in hospitals and professorships in medical schools.[20] When the American Medical Association was founded in 1847, it immediately treated midwifery as a distinct professional category.[21]

Obstetrics traditionally included diseases of women and young children within its boundaries. But by midcentury, gynecology was on its way to becoming an autonomous medical category and was becoming very visible among the budding specialties in America. Among Atkinson's subjects who took their MD after 1845, more than one-third included "diseases of women" or "gynecology" among their specialty interests. In many cases this was combined with midwifery, but in many others it was not. Similarly, in a *Philadelphia Medical Directory* of 1885, nearly 30 percent of those who identified themselves with a specialty used one or both of these terms.[22]

Gynecology, like other specialties in the United States, based its claims to acceptance on the need to advance medical science and invent new procedures. But there also existed a strong utilitarian orientation among specialists that was less strongly developed in countries where hospitals were public institutions. The fact that American hospitals were philanthropic establishments appealing to patrons for support meant that they had to be seen to offer medical procedures that provided significant practical benefits to the deserving poor. One model for specialty development was for an early specialist to develop a procedure, build a hospital or dispensary around that procedure, and then pursue further clinical research. This is the pattern followed by the pioneering gynecologist Marion Simms. As is well known, Simms spent several years in the late 1840s experimenting on women slaves in order to develop surgery to repair vesico-vaginal fistula. Several years later he moved to New York City, where in 1855 he convinced prominent citizens to fund the Woman's Hospital, which was largely devoted to fistula surgery. This hospital was presented, Deborah Kuhn McGregor has suggested, as a philanthropic effort to alleviate the suffering resulting from childbirth. It went on to become a place for both charitable care and further clinical study and research.[23]

Although this was not reflected in Atkinson's book, ophthalmology also seems to have constituted an important early specialist category in the United States, due to the capacity of its practitioners to combine scientific and philanthropic impulses. George Frick of Baltimore is generally considered the first American practitioner to study in Vienna and to then restrict himself to ophthalmology (from 1819).[24] By the 1820s several American cities had infirmaries, dispensaries, or hospital wards devoted to eye diseases.[25] This early activity almost certainly reflected widespread familiarity with medicine in Britain, where a large number of eye hospitals were founded during the same period.[26] A small number of difficult but frequently successful procedures—notably removal of cataracts, therapy for lachrymal fistula, and removal of objects embedded in the eyes—provided specialists with activities requiring considerable skill, alongside more routine treatments for inflammations and infections utilizing topical and systemic medications. This allowed founders of eye hospitals to present their activities as immediately beneficial means to combat blindness.

Thus the appeal to the public in 1823 of George McClellan's unsuccessful Hospital for Diseases of the Eye and Ear in Philadelphia argued that in London and Vienna, "[t]housands have been annually relieved and cured of diseases of the eye and ear, who otherwise would have lost the use of these all important organs and proved a burden to themselves and to society."[27] Similar sentiments were expressed by Henry Noyes in publicizing his New York Eye and Ear Infirmary, founded in 1820.[28] Such utilitarian motivations did not, of course, preclude the advancement of knowledge. On the contrary, Isaac Hays published regular reports on Philadelphia's Wills Hospital (where he had an appointment) in his *American Journal of Medical Science.* "It is unquestionably in such institutions that these diseases can be studied with most advantage, and we hope in these reports, especially should our colleagues unite in the plan, that most of the forms of the disease to which the eye is subject will eventually be illustrated."[29] Following the invention of the ophthalmoscope in 1851 and the publication of Donders's work on refraction, ophthalmic clinics in Vienna began attracting many American doctors and the field took on especially high intellectual stature.[30] In 1864 its practitioners organized one of the first specialist societies in the United States.

Finally, it is worth noting that in the United States, as elsewhere, the spread of lunatic asylums provided the institutional foundations for the relatively early visibility of psychiatry. However, the fact that we identify so many of these practitioners from institutional appointments and publications, rather than specific references to special interest in the diseases of the insane, suggests that many early practitioners defined themselves primarily as administrators of special institutions rather than as specialists producing new knowledge. Whatever its basis, their sense of identity was real and was bolstered by the early foundation (in 1844) of a professional society, the Association of Medical Superintendents. As we shall see below, they kept their distance from the AMA and the medical profession more generally.[31]

Atkinson's listings suggest that doctors in the major American cities of the Northeast embraced specialization in significant numbers about two decades after those of Paris and about a decade after those in Vienna. From 1860 on, this process unfolded with dizzying speed. Doctors looked back at this early period and remembered the animosity felt by the regular profession toward the specialist.[32] Specialties entered the general hospitals first in the form of outpatient departments. Boston City Hospital, for instance, established such departments in dermatology (1868), otology (1869), gynecology (1873), and neurology and laryngology (both 1877). Much the same occurred at Massachusetts General Hospital. Higher-status inpatient specialty wards, however, were more difficult to obtain, and hospital specialists in Boston seem to have been restricted to the outpatient staff until the end of the century, when the situation changed dramatically.[33] This exclusion undoubtedly explains the development of specialist hospitals in that city. Boston, in 1860, had one general and two special hospitals. The latter had forty-three beds. Thirty years later, there were five general and fourteen special hospitals in the city; and by 1910 there were no fewer than twenty-one specialist hospitals with almost as many beds as the city's eight general hospitals.[34]

Philadelphia doctors appear to have accepted specialties with less ambivalence than their colleagues in Boston. As late as 1868, there were relatively few signs of specialist activity in the city of brotherly love. *The Philadelphia Medical Register and Directory*[35] of that year lists the recently established Obstetrical Society of Philadelphia among local medical societies. (A similar society had been established in New York City four years earlier.) The major distinctions among hospital wards involved separation of the surgical from the medical, and male from female.[36] On the other hand, the Hospital of the Protestant Episcopal Church reflected the growing tendency to express philanthropic impulses in highly focused ways. "One ward founded by bequest of Miss Grasby and called the 'Hannah Ward' is for the reception of patients with diseases of the chest; the receipts from the fund maintain at present ten patients."[37] Other hospitals, such as the Pennsylvania Almshouse Hospital, the Municipal Hospital, St. Mary's Hospital, and St. Joseph's Hospital, included one or more obstetricians among their medical staffs; and the latter institution also offered special clinics for diseases of the eye on Wednesday and Saturday mornings.

A number of specialized hospitals were also in existence; the Pennsylvania Hospital for the Insane was one of several institutions for this class of patients. The Pennsylvania Infirmary for Diseases of the Eye and Ear was founded in 1822. It appears to have been replaced by the Wills Hospital for the Relief of the Indigent Blind and Lame, established in 1833[38]; set up as a fairly standard charitable institution, the Wills began to offer clinical lectures in 1839 and by 1868 advertised formal lectures as well as private courses "by different members of the staff, who seek to make this a practical school of ophthalmic medicine and surgery."[39] There were also a children's hospital founded in 1855, the Woman's Hospital (founded in 1861), and several lying-in charities. The Philadelphia Orthopaedic Hospital was incorporated in 1867 and included such Philadelphia luminaries as Samuel D. Gross, Thomas

Morton, and David Hays Agnew on its staff. It would eventually add a service for nervous diseases directed by Silas Weir Mitchell.[40] But the institution that most reflected the growing development of specialization was the Howard Hospital and Infirmary for Incurables, founded in 1853. The hospital was in fact not functioning due to lack of funds, but its infirmary was active. "The distinctive feature of the charity is that each physician confines his attention to a specific class of affections."[41] There were eight specialists, each responsible for biweekly clinics in such fields as diseases of the eye and ear, digestive organs, and nervous system. There was as well a daily morning clinic for infants and small children.

Specialization thus existed on limited scale in late-1860s Philadelphia. This was acknowledged in 1874 by a leading medical periodical in that city, which disputed an assertion by the *New York Tribune* to the effect that New York had overtaken Philadelphia as a center of medical science: "New York is, however, decidedly ahead of this city in the cultivation as well as the literature of specialties; this we freely acknowledge; and it seems to us the only danger, so far as New York is concerned, of our city's losing its medical preeminence."[42]

Less than twenty years later, the institutional landscape of Philadelphia had been transformed. The most striking changes were connected to medical education. At the University of Pennsylvania in 1885, there were now six professorships in clinical specialties.[43] The one in obstetrics and diseases of women and children had been in existence for some time. Most of the others had been more recently upgraded to full university status from clinical professorships and lectureships at the Pennsylvania Hospital following reforms of the medical school in 1877. These professorships included clinical gynecology, diseases of the eye, diseases of the ear, nervous diseases, and skin diseases. There were also six demonstrators or lecturers in clinical specialties, and nine assistants or instructors. Jefferson Medical College was less well endowed with specialist staff—only obstetrics, gynecology, and ophthalmic and aural surgery were formally represented. But the school offered two-month spring and fall courses in seven specialized areas including electrotherapeutics, venereal and genito-urinary diseases, and anal and rectal diseases. Ten postgraduate courses were also offered.[44] Woman's Medical College and the Medico-Chirurgical College also had small numbers of specialist teaching staff.

The Howard Hospital continued to exist as a dispensary, but the institution that now most clearly represented the new specialties was the Philadelphia Polyclinic and College for Graduates of Medicine, which had been established in 1884. This institution was the local manifestation of a new type of institution sprouting up in the major cities of the United States in order to offer practical training in the specialties and general medicine.[45] In Philadelphia, the Polyclinic dispensary was divided into special departments under the direction of a professor. These offered short postgraduate courses usually lasting six weeks. Although many of these professors were relatively young, with few holding senior posts in the city's most prestigious institutions,[46] and many were foreign-born or Jewish as well, they were in most cases well-known figures with affiliations in one or another of the major medical institutions of Philadelphia.[47] The Polyclinic's charter described its tasks as offering free care to the sick poor and providing facilities for physicians to study the special branches. By 1909 it had thirty medical staff, all specialists, and many more junior personnel.[48]

What is striking about these developments in Philadelphia is not just the rapid spread of specialties but also the rapid integration of specialists into established institutions. Multiple affiliations were common. The dermatologist Louis Duhring held appointments at the University of Pennsylvania and the Philadelphia Hospital, and was a lecturer at Woman's Medical College and consultant in charge of skin diseases at Howard Dispensary. The laryngologist Jacob Solis-Cohen was honorary professor at Jefferson, physician at the German Hospital, and professor at the Polyclinic. Solis-Cohen's entire career illustrates the remarkable fluidity and openness of the numerous private and public institutions of the city. Having received his MD degree in 1860 from the University of Pennsylvania, he opened a private practice in 1866. A year later he performed the first successful laryngotomy to remove a cancerous growth. One year after that, he was named professor of electrotherapy at Jefferson Medical College, and in 1869, lecturer in laryngoscopy and diseases of the chest. In 1871 he became a fellow of the College of Physicians and would later be among the founders of the Polyclinic.[49]

Little wonder that claiming a specialty was beginning to carry considerable cachet. Philadelphia was one of the first, if not the first, American city to produce a medical directory (in the early 1880s) that included specialty designations, in spite of the strictures of the AMA against this practice. Approximately 13 percent of those listed mentioned specialty interests.[50] Even the venerable College of Physicians of Philadelphia could not resist the pressure, and in 1892 overcame substantial opposition in order to establish specialty sections.[51]

Philadelphia was not unique. Specialties had an imposing presence in the medical schools and hospitals of many cities. Harvard Medical School in 1884 had fewer professors in specialties but large numbers of junior staff; most of the standard specialties were included on the examination given at the end of the fourth year.[52] This being said, it is important to note that, as George Rosen emphasized, there were still relatively few specialists in much of the United States; most of these had acquired what special knowledge they had in general practice, and relatively few gave up general practice in order to become exclusive specialists.[53] Nonetheless, the change effected in large eastern cities (and a few in the West)[54] within a period of two decades is remarkable. Many of the procedures and instruments developed by specialists were incorporated into the practice of more ambitious generalists.[55]

Explaining the Spread of American Specialties

Medical specialization in the mid-nineteenth century developed in the great cities of Europe. It was based on dense networks of medical researchers, teachers, and institutions that had emerged in these cities and on population size that made specialist practice increasingly viable. No American city during the first half of the century had the kind of medical infrastructure that could produce internationally recognized medical knowledge and, in the process, stimulate something more substantial than isolated instances of specialization. The small, often competing medical schools had at best eight to ten professors and hardly constituted environments conducive to such development. At least some of this was clearly recognized by reformers who wished to transform American doctors into producers of significant medical knowledge. It was suggested in 1850 that a serious medical literature could come only "from those in charge of public hospitals and other medical charities. . . . Our country, however, possesses as yet, but few of these institutions sufficiently extensive to afford materials for any extended series of clinical observations; consequently the physicians of the United States are as yet shut out from one of the most important means of becoming able and distinguished medical writers."[56]

Others, however, suggested that it was not so much lack of institutions as habits of mind that were the chief problem. Samuel D. Gross argued that hospitals and other charities did in fact exist in sufficient numbers in larger cities; no one, however, was utilizing them for purposes of clinical research.[57] Some attributed the situation to more general conditions of professional life.

> The advantages for the investigation, on the largest scale, and in the most thorough manner, of the profounder problems of life and death, health and disease, which have surrounded for centuries past, the favored and gifted men of Europe, as found in vast hospitals, in the aggregation of men, in the encouragement given to scientific pursuits, in the immediate rewards of success, and in incentives of every kind to avail themselves of the opportunities almost thrust upon them— these advantages have not always prevailed here, nor do they now, to as great an extent as abroad.[58]

Given such inauspicious conditions, how can one explain the extremely rapid development of specialization among urban medical elites? The growth of American cities and their medical professions clearly provides a part of the answer, as does the related and remarkable spread of hospitals in the latter decades of the century.[59] Bonnie Blustein has argued that the unprecedented number of cases treated in hospitals during the Civil War allowed doctors to focus on specific conditions and problems, and thus facilitated the emergence of clinical specialties in the years that followed.[60] Most significant, I would suggest, was a profound change in attitudes among elite doctors in the United States that is expressed in the long passage quoted above. Many American doctors were quite simply determined to enter the world of international medical research, which had by now become synonymous with specialization.

It is widely acknowledged among historians that American doctors in the second half of the century faced what was perceived as a desperate crisis. The repeal of licensing laws, the proliferation of proprietary medical schools that lowered professional standards and produced a glut of inferior physicians, the popularity of medical sects calling into question orthodox medicine, and a general sense of scientific inferiority with respect to European medicine all seemed to demand major institutional reforms. Significant segments of the urban medical elite responded to this call. In 1847, the American Medical Association was founded to unify the profession and coordinate reform activities. This resulted in an effort to reform medical education that would last many decades.[61] Simultaneously, American medical elites identified themselves closely with European "science."

John Warner has argued that aspirations to elevate the profession drove leading American physicians to adopt the clinical empiricism associated with Paris medicine.[62] More generally, they began to claim the advancement of medical science as a central function; during the 1840s and 1850s, a profusion of new medical journals appeared. In its early years, the AMA decided that improving the quality of American medical literature was a vital task and entrusted it to a special committee. In 1850 this committee's report concluded with the following statement: "*Resolved,* That the Association regards the cultivation of medical literature as essential to professional improvement, and as adapted to form one of the broadest lines of distinction between physicians and all pretenders to the name."[63] This concern continued well into the second half of the century. A selection of papers published in 1876 to celebrate the history of American medicine during the preceding century included a long essay by John Shaw Billings, of the National Medical Library, on the "literature and institutions" of American medicine; this erudite survey displayed, along with some national pride, considerable awareness of the relatively low quality of American medical writing.[64]

To improve medical writing, it was sometimes suggested, American doctors needed to rely less on general medical periodicals and more on journals devoted to special branches of medical science. By "special branches" reformers referred primarily to traditional academic subjects such as physiology, pathology, surgery, and midwifery.[65] But this notion of special branches could easily be expanded as new clinical subjects gained acceptance. The advantages of specialization for mastering a body of knowledge, keeping up with the literature, and producing original results based on numerous cases would certainly have come into play for aspiring producers of knowledge in the United States, as they had in Europe. But the rapidity of this shift in the United States suggests something more. Particularly ambitious young American doctors had for some time gone to Europe to complete their training, and this trend accelerated after midcentury. Already in the Paris of the 1840s and 1850s, they followed private courses in the specialties and frequently went on to specialist careers. According to Warner, "students who took such private specialty courses in Paris were the first large cohort of Americans to embrace and proselytize for specialism as an appropriate professional model for medicine in the United States."[66]

In subsequent decades, those most serious about postdoctoral training increasingly went to Vienna and other German-language universities, instead of or in addition to Paris, largely because of the perceived excellence of practical clinical instruction in the specialties.[67] Many, if not most, returned home with some specialist knowledge and the belief that specialization provided the means to advance both medical knowledge and careers devoted to "science."[68] These set the tone for other aspirants to elite status who could not afford travel to Europe.[69] But this explanation still begs the question. Why was specialized knowledge perceived in this way, and why did it, as opposed to pathological anatomy, experimental physiology, or more general medical and surgical education, become the most common badge of foreign training? Why, in other words, did young American doctors in many cases go to Europe with the idea of obtaining specialist training?[70] And why was this training not perceived, as in the past, as just one component in a well-rounded medical education?

To some degree Americans were merely reflecting European attitudes and developments. Specialists still constituted a small minority of urban practitioners in Europe, but specialties constituted the most dynamic and fastest-growing areas of medical science. Since French and German medical graduates were increasingly making such career choices, it is not surprising that Americans did so as well. The budding otologist Clarence Blake wrote to his parents from Vienna: "The general feeling among the men studying abroad is that a revolution in medical practice which has already commenced here is to be extended to America, viz. the splitting up of the profession into specialties."[71] Such choices became more socially acceptable than they had been in the past. The mistrust of specialized professional knowledge that characterized American society during the first half of the century seems to have given way to a new "culture of professionalism" that increasingly valorized specialized knowledge in all domains.[72]

A more banal but equally pertinent factor had to do with the constraints of travel and the relative brevity of even the most ambitious trips abroad. There was simply not enough time for anything but the acquisition of particular specialist skills, which might require a relatively long period of training. Clarence Blake wrote from Vienna: "[i]f a fellow has studied abroad he is expected at home to be most perfectly fitted in *everything*, rather a mistake because the very thoroughness of study here obliges him to give his whole attention to one thing in order to grasp it fully, and so the Vienna school breeds American specialists. . . . "[73] A few individuals, such as Henry P. Bowditch, became proficient in general pathology or physiology, but this was a relatively rare occurrence because training in experimental science led to a very narrow range of careers. Most travelers were seeking more conventionally to combine "research" with lucrative medical practice, an association that was identified with specialists.

Clarence Blake's letters to his parents from Vienna and Munich wonderfully illustrate these dual motives. They are full of phrases emphasizing the research component of his chosen field, otology: it is described as "a specialty where one is continually treading new ground"; those building it up must "be not merely givers of other men's prescriptions but above that, be observers and experimenters"; professional success could be achieved at the price of "hard work, experiment and observation in an extending field of labor. . . . "[74] Even more ambitiously, Blake wrote from Munich: "I hope, however, that in due course of time and through the efforts of the American specialists who have had the advantages of an European education and the broader thought resulting therefrom, we may stand at home on a par with our Continental brethren in the devotedness to and thoroughness in, scientific research."[75] Such ambitions did not, however, preclude more practical professional and material considerations. Blake desired a post at the Boston Eye and Ear Infirmary not only because "such a position will give me material for study" but also because it would be "the best possible opening to practice as an aural surgeon." And, perhaps attempting to assuage anxious parents, he stressed that "considered also in the light of expediency, I cannot but feel that there is more promise of a speedy reward in this than in a general practice. The number of general practitioners is very large, the number of specialists comparatively few. . . . "[76] Blake himself railed at those doctors who thought, mistakenly, that they could master a specialty in six months.[77] But brief courses were, in all probability, one of the chief attractions of specialist training abroad, which frequently involved learning to use instruments such as the ophthalmoscope and laryngoscope.[78] To some observers, "obtaining more complete knowledge of some special branch of medical science" was the *only* reason to study abroad, the only kind of medical experience not readily available in the United States.[79]

Specialist knowledge did not just allow young doctors to return to a relatively less crowded form of medical practice; it also provided advantages in carving out elite careers. In the United States, as elsewhere, professors and hospital clinicians initially resisted sharing prerogatives and powers with newly minted specialists.[80] As in Britain, special hospitals were established because specialists could not at first obtain proper facilities in general hospitals.[81] However, private hospitals, dispensaries, and polyclinics were relatively easy to set up in the American context and were not, as was the case in Britain, repudiated by medical elites centered in general hospitals. On the contrary, the fluidity of social relations in the United States, and the absence of a long-standing medical aristocracy with a deeply ingrained sense of group identity and entitlement, allowed specialist institutions to become integrated more or less easily (depending on local conditions) into municipal medical networks.[82]

The three-way relationship between specialization, clinical research, and career success was summed up with a wonderful combination of lucidity and cynicism by John Shaw Billings in 1876. There were, he wrote, "very few" men who were totally devoted to research, and the products of their efforts had been until then "for the most part fragmentary. . . . Of the highest grade of this class we have thus far produced no specimens." There was a much larger class of individuals whose education was often defective and who took no interest in medical science. In between these two, there was a third large class of physicians, mainly in cities, whose principal object is to obtain money, or rather the social position, pleasures, and power, which money only can bestow. They are clear-headed, shrewd, practical men, well educated because "it pays," and for the same reason they take good care to be supplied with the best instruments, and the latest literature. *Many of them take up specialties* because the work is easier, and hours of labor are more under their control than in general practice. They strive to become connected with hospitals and medical schools, not for the love of mental exertion, or of science for its own sake, but as a respectable means of advertising, and of obtaining consultations. They write and lecture to keep their names before the public, and they must do both well, or fall behind in the race. They have the greater part of the valuable practice, *and their writings, which constitute the greater part of our medical literature, are respectable in quality and eminently useful.* [83] (Emphasis added)

In the long run, resistance to specialties in even the most conservative medical schools and hospitals was overcome comparatively quickly for several reasons. First, intense competition and local control of medical institutions made it both necessary and quite easy to create junior posts for specialists of every sort (putting them in charge of outpatient clinics, for instance) and eventually reward with beds and senior posts those who had gained sufficient stature. Second, there was among American medical elites relatively little *collective* principled opposition to specialization of the sort found in Britain. On the contrary the American elite at the national level was preoccupied with the need to reform medical training, a task that included, among other things, admitting to the curriculum the latest in specialist knowledge.[84] As part of its permanent effort to improve the quality of medical education, the AMA regularly called for expanding the teaching of emerging specialties "so completely ignored as to leave these branches almost outside the profession and either in the hands of pretenders, or to be cultivated solely by experts."[85] Third, from about 1865 on, the desire to reform medical training became associated with the larger movement to create research universities in the United States. As universities took increasing control of their medical schools, which had until then enjoyed almost complete autonomy, the desire of medical reformers to transform medical schools became a critical component of the movement for university reform that in turn reinforced the momentum to bring about change in medical schools.[86]

The American educational context thus combined profound dissatisfaction with existing medical teaching, deference to European (increasingly German) academic models of both medical and higher education, and decentralized management of competing institutions that were still small enough to expand with relative ease. Furthermore, new courses and hospital posts in specialties allowed young doctors to enter elite institutions without competing directly against their elders who held the more general clinical posts. It is in this context that some specialties, such as neurology, gynecology, and dermatology, found a place in at least a few American elite medical institutions considerably earlier than in much of Europe. By 1870, virtually all of New York City's medical schools had professorships in neurology.[87]

Even the relatively small and recently developed specialty of pediatrics was being taught in medical schools during the 1860s and 1870s by figures such as Abraham Jacobi in New York City.[88] Historians may disagree about whether Harvard's famous reforms of 1871 reflected the emerging attitudes to laboratory research that would dominate educational reform in the last decades of the nineteenth century or the more traditional desire of the AMA to make medical training more rigorous and effective,[89] but it is indisputable that one result of these reforms was the addition of professorships of ophthalmology, dermatology, and mental diseases; an instructorship in otology; and a special course on syphilis.[90] Similarly, the creation of specialty posts at the University of Pennsylvania, described above, followed closely on the reform of medical training at that institution in 1877. However one defined the medical science that needed to be added to the curriculum, the development of medical specialties constituted an essential component of the task at hand. By 1890, elite medical schools in the United States had a complement of specialty chairs and courses that could rival, in quantity if not necessarily quality, those of all but the largest European medical schools.[91] Hospitals, dispensaries, and clinics devoted to specialties, as well as specialist inpatient and outpatient departments in general hospitals, proliferated in major northeastern cities during the latter decades of the century.[92]

Advance and Resistance

Although the institutional acceptance of specialties was justified chiefly by the need to provide future general practitioners with necessary knowledge, it went hand in hand with increasing specialist practice. For the academic elite, specialty research and teaching were, as Billings observed, the basis of lucrative private practice. With the growing stature of specialties, physicians outside elite circles were stirred to make their own claims to specialist expertise. By the 1860s, public declarations of specialist expertise were sufficiently visible to provoke considerable debate within the AMA. This situation was to some degree unique to the United States. In France there was no national representative body capable of dealing with this issue, and the same would be true in Germany for another decade; in Britain the hostility to specialization was so general and vigorous that one-sided attack rather than debate was the rule. The American situation was considerably more convoluted. The AMA actively supported the development of specialization in medical schools. When it came to specialist practice, urban medical elites tended to be positively inclined toward at least partial specialization[93] while rank-and-file general practitioners tended to oppose it as a threat to their status. As a representative association dependent on local member societies, the AMA had to reconcile both sets of interests without provoking a schism in the profession. The focus of the American controversy was also singular. During the 1860s, French doctors were preoccupied with acceptance of specialties in the Paris Medical Faculty, while in

Britain competition between general and specialist hospitals dominated the agenda. In the United States, the AMA's intense concern with issues of medical ethics made specialist self-advertising the central focus of debate.

In 1864 Julius Homberger, an ophthalmologist in New York City, was suspended by the state medical society for publishing an advertisement stating his specialty and making great claims for his abilities.[94] At its annual meeting, Homberger asked the AMA "to go into committee of the whole to define the position of specialists and the duties of the profession toward specialists, as well as the duties of the specialist toward the profession."[95] Instead, it was decided to appoint a committee of five members, chaired by Homberger, to report at the annual meeting the following year. At that meeting, however, the New York State Medical Society was allowed to precede Homberger in presenting a resolution that termed any references to a specialty in advertisements "an extra inducement to patronage" that should be "deemed a violation of the code of medical ethics."[96] Homberger tabled a report favorable to specialization signed by no other members of the committee; one other committee member, the Boston gynecologist Horatio Storer, tabled a separate minority report also favorable to specialties.[97] The issue was then referred to the Association's Committee on Medical Ethics.

At the annual meeting the following year, this latter committee presented majority and minority reports. The former, signed by Worthington Hooker, professor at Yale, and James Kennedy, a practitioner and member of the state legislature of Ohio, went well beyond the issue of advertising to discuss the advantages and disadvantages of specialization; the chief disadvantage was a narrowness of perspective and inability to take account of complex interconnections within the body. The authors admitted the usefulness of specialization only if specialist knowledge was based on a foundation of general medical knowledge and if it emerged gradually from years of experience in general practice. But they went considerably farther by also suggesting that *any* exclusive specialization, even if it grew from general practice, was necessarily harmful. Hence *partial* specialization—a combination of general practice with emphasis on a particular field—was to be encouraged. Advertising by specialists was of course characterized as illegitimate. What is notable about the majority report is that it referred almost exclusively to specialist practice; not a word was said about specialism as form of research and teaching.[98]

The brief minority report was presented by Henry I. Bowditch, a quintessential member of that part of the urban medical elite committed to research. Bowditch was at this time professor of clinical medicine at Harvard and was known for his work on lung disease. His report treated specialism largely from the perspective of research, and was thus favorable to a development that he saw as characteristic of all modern sciences.[99] Nor was the advertising of an individual's specialty shocking to Bowditch. Such advertisements "may be a grave question of *taste* . . . but on the question of *right* the undersigned protests that no association of physicians can have any reason for expressing an opinion, unless the advertisement is evidently of the mountback character. . . . "[100] The author concluded by presenting a resolution to the effect that "the consideration of the subject of specialties in medical practice be indefinitely postponed."[101]

These reports "elicited much discussion," and in the end *both* were adopted.[102] The AMA also adopted another resolution: the subject of specialization should be treated as a specific order of business at the meeting of 1867, and meanwhile local societies should discuss the issue.[103] However, the presidential address of 1866 by David Humphreys Storer,[104] professor of obstetrics and medical jurisprudence at Harvard (and father of Horatio Storer, mentioned above), essentially articulated the position that the AMA would eventually adopt. Despite links to quackery and "disloyal competition," specialization had become a necessity of medicine because no individual could grasp or investigate all knowledge. Proper behavior toward colleagues, however, was expected of the specialist.

> We would not then discountenance the specialist as such: we would not speak disparagingly of him; we would neither ridicule nor condemn him. . . . Every atom he can add to our stock of knowledge, every grain he can place upon the mound already raised, shall be appreciated and rejoiced in; and as long as his conduct shall prove him worthy of our esteem, so long may he claim to possess it.[105]

The presidential address the following year was presented by a nonacademic surgeon, Henry Askew, and was even more positively disposed toward specialization, characterized as the inevitable consequence of scientific advance as well as the prerequisite for further progress.[106] Nonetheless, Askew added, where medical practice was concerned, specialists in many cases had little more to offer than did GPs:

> He who announces publicly that he claims superior practical skill in diseases of the lungs, the stomach, or the bowels, proclaims either his ignorance or his venality, and should be declared "hors de profession" at once and without reserve.
>
> But the case is very different with diseases of the eye, ear and skin; . . . there is often requisite an extent of observation on the changes of structure in the organ . . . and a practical adroitness in the employment of delicate and peculiar instruments . . . very seldom attainable by the general practitioner. . . . [107]

In 1868, Homberger was finally expelled from the AMA.[108] A year later, another report on specialization was presented.[109] Written by E. Lloyd Howard, professor of anatomy at the Baltimore College of Dental Surgery, and Christopher Johnston, professor of surgery at the University of Maryland, this was, if anything, even more supportive of specialization than earlier reports:

> As to the advantages of specialties to the *science* of medicine there can be but one opinion; that "division of labor," that has accomplished so much in the history of all other sciences, must give like results in the broad field of medicine; and indeed it has already been demonstrated in ophthalmology, in uterine surgery, in the researches of Dr. Brown-Séquard, and others in neuropathy, that the cultivation of

these branches can best be accomplished by a special devotion to one of them, by such as have become proficient in general medicine.[110]

If the advantages of specialism in science were clear, the report continued, there was "great diversity of opinion as to its benefits to the *profession.*" The main objection was the implication that GPs were incompetent. But the authors felt that eventually an adjustment in practice would occur that would benefit GPs and "elevate and improve the profession." In the meantime, some specialists "have shown a tendency to exceed their natural boundaries within the code of ethical obligations" by advertising to the public "for that support which only a faithful apprenticeship and work should bring." The authors proposed that the AMA recognize the legitimacy of specialties in medical practice but prohibit specialists from advertising themselves as such or assuming "any title not granted by a regularly chartered college."[111] The Assembly of the AMA adopted the resolution and added the proviso that handbills and cards in medical journals that called attention to specialties also be declared a violation of the Code of Ethics.[112]

Protests were raised against this latter limitation on the grounds that cards, especially, constituted communication among doctors and not advertising.[113] But the AMA, having found a way to live with specialization, reaffirmed its position in 1874 and unveiled a formula that allowed specialists to make known their field of practice. Instead of specialist titles it permitted only

> a simple honest notice appended to the ordinary card of the general practitioner, saying "Practice limited to diseases of the eye and ear" or "to diseases peculiar to women". . . . Such a simple notice of limitation, if truthfully made, would involve no other principle than the notice of the general practitioner that he limits his attention to professional business within certain hours of the day."[114]

Any more positive claim to specialist status, it was explained a decade later, "would be to invest him with special advantages inconsistent with the equality of rights and duties pertaining to the profession."[115]

This limitation was not universally accepted, and one of its chief practical effects was to prevent the many local medical directories that sprang up after 1875 from including the specialties of the doctors listed. Among dozens of directories published before 1902 that I have examined, only one consistently included specialty designations.[116] On the other hand, medical biographies, such as the one by Atkinson, had no compunctions about mentioning specialties. The prohibition on advertising was not a defeat for specialization,[117] but rather one of those compromises at which the AMA excelled; it fully accepted specialization but satisfied both GPs and many specialists who viewed advertising as a form of quackery; it elaborated a definition of specialization that, although widely ignored in reality, insisted formally on equality within the profession. GPs would continue to criticize specialists for the next three decades; but neither this criticism nor the prohibition on advertising significantly hindered the spread of specialization in the United States.

Specialists, however, posed a different, more serious problem for the AMA. Its officers saw the Association as the single, unifying body representing the medical profession and as the central locus of medical knowledge in America. In 1860, as part of its drive to introduce more scientific discussions at meetings, it created six sections devoted to specialized disciplines.[118] While morning sessions were given over to general business and medical education, afternoons and evenings were taken up by the "scientific" work of the sections.[119] Nonetheless, the scientific status of the AMA was not high. John Shaw Billings wrote in 1876 that the Association offered little to physicians interested in scientific work since there was little oversight of papers presented and published in the AMA's *Transactions* and because meetings were dominated by professional and ethical issues.[120]

The scientific role of the AMA was directly called into question by the rapid proliferation of specialty societies. In 1864 the American Ophthalmological Society was formed, joining the Association of Superintendents of Asylums, which had been in existence for close to two decades and had already spurned a number of overtures from the AMA requesting closer ties.[121] In 1865, the AMA decided to appoint a delegate to the annual meeting of the Association of Superintendents with the aim of once again seeking closer ties between, if not the actual integration of, the two bodies. Simultaneously the AMA established a new section in psychological medicine "intended more particularly for the reception of superintendents."[122] It also set up several committees to report on issues relevant to the psychiatrists.[123] The AMA's delegate, the gynecologist Horatio Storer of Boston, reported that superintendents expressed little interest in closer ties, and went on to expound on the dangers posed by independent associations:

> However decided one's sympathy with efforts to advance all legitimate specialties, still the good of the general practitioner must rise superior to all other considerations. For this reason, every attempt to directly separate any class of specialists from the mass of their fellows is to be deprecated. . . . Through your so-called [AMA] Sections, wisely and, if thought necessary, permanently organized, all the work of special organizations can be effected as thoroughly as by any other method, and with infinitely more advantage to the mass of the profession.[124]

Superintendents and ophthalmologists were soon joined by many other specialties in organizing societies, which characteristically restricted membership to individuals perceived as having contributed to medical knowledge.

Leaders of the AMA bemoaned the proliferation of these societies[125] but nonetheless continued seeking the support of specialists. The Association increasingly chose as presidents of annual meetings, specialists and surgeons rather than general practitioners.[126] More significantly, the AMA's system of sections gradually evolved into a parallel form of representation for specialists. As specialties grew, sections divided and subdivided. In 1885 there were seven sections, and fifteen years later there were thirteen.[127] Before 1885, an associationwide committee of nomination chose the officers of the sections, but thereafter sections elected their own officers. In this way the AMA came to provide an alternative form of representation for specialties that, as AMA representatives never tired of pointing out, was not exclusive and restrictive in membership, as specialist societies were, but was instead open to nonelite specialists and general practitioners.[128] Indeed, many of the papers read in these sections during the latter decades of the nineteenth century seem to have been aimed chiefly at educating GPs in specific skills and teaching them when to consult a specialist.

A brief controversy was created by the coming together in 1888 of twelve national specialty societies in an annual Congress of American Physicians and Surgeons. This followed on the heels of several unpleasant conflicts between the AMA leadership and the notables of academic medicine, many of whom were specialists. During the early 1880s there was much disagreement about the clause in the AMA's Code of Ethics that prohibited doctors from consulting with homeopaths. Many elite physicians opposed this prohibition on the grounds that scientific expertise rather than professional codes should determine proper practice. A serious dispute broke out when the Medical Society of New York State enacted a code of ethics without a consultation clause; this caused a split in the society, and for the next decades two medical societies coexisted in New York State. Many members of the AMA saw the campaign for freedom of consultation as a self-interested attempt by predominantly urban specialists to increase their fees. This provoked hostility toward specialization as well as a famous warning against it by Austin Flint.[129] In 1885 another dispute erupted over the organization of the International Medical Congress in Philadelphia. The original organizing committee, made up of leading academics and specialists, was dismissed and replaced by a committee more closely identified with the AMA and its support for the Code of Ethics.

In response, those most associated with the fight against the Code of Ethics organized in 1886 the Association of American Physicians, an exclusive body representing the scientific elite of medicine.[130] Two years later the annual Congress of American Physicians and Surgeons met for the first time. This was a restricted event controlled by equally restrictive specialty societies that claimed to be devoted to medical knowledge rather than to medical politics or medical ethics.[131] Both the Association and the Congress were perceived as direct attacks on the AMA. One editorial in the *Journal of the AMA* condemned specialist societies for their "disintegrating influence" that was "antagonistic to any general and harmonious organization of the whole profession"; it went on to attack the new Congress for seeking "to ultimately displace and supersede" the AMA.[132] In contrast to specialist societies, which encouraged "class differences" and their attendant bickering and rivalries, the sections of the AMA were presented as a means of accommodating specialists while also maintaining unity and homogeneity within the profession.[133] But the Congress, which never became more than an annual meeting of the member societies, limited itself to scientific issues; its members also feared the excessive proliferation of specialties, and its rules stipulated that the admission of any new specialist societies required the unanimous agreement of all member societies.[134] The Congress's existence in fact encouraged efforts to increase the number of specialty sections within the AMA, to improve the way these functioned, to make them more autonomous, and, increasingly, to transform them into the dominant units within the organization.[135]

After 1890, relations between elite specialists and the AMA were not without conflict. It could hardly have been otherwise, Rosemary Stevens has argued, given that the AMA was seeking to unify the profession and to bring uniformity to medical training while the activity of specialists tended toward fragmentation.[136] The specialty societies and the Congress of American Physicians and Surgeons offered specialist leaders an attractive alternative to the sections of the AMA as well as the opportunity to express hostility to the AMA's attempts to prohibit contacts with irregular practitioners.[137] But by 1896 an editorial in the *JAMA* proclaimed: "The American Medical Association has become what the Congress of American Physicians and Surgeons sought to be, a veritable confederation of medical bodies devoted to independent lines of thought and practice. . . . "[138] The specialty sections of the AMA continued into the twentieth century to be characterized as the true associations of specialists precisely because they were inclusive.[139] The AMA's claim to represent specialists would continue to have serious consequences as the twentieth century advanced.

Viewed from another angle, however, the AMA complemented the specialty societies. Both promoted many common goals at very different levels. While the scientific work of the sections may have been of low quality, they presented to general practitioners newly developed specialist knowledge and contributed to the growing acceptance of specialization within the profession. Presentations by specialists to their generalist confreres frequently emphasized the need to consult specialists in complicated situations; they thus contributed to the carving up of the medical market in a manner that everyone could live with. The AMA never ceased to call for more teaching of specialties. By resisting pressure to grant more marginal specialties their own sections, the AMA irritated some groups but helped control the unbridled proliferation of specialties, a goal supported by most academic specialists.[140]

Becoming a fully autonomous section of the AMA became a status symbol for specialties and something to strive for in the case of emerging or marginal groups.[141] Voices within the AMA and the profession more generally continued to attack "Specialism on the Rampage," to quote one medical editorial of 1881.[142] Another physician called specialization a "monstrous incubus which casts a shadow over every department of medicine."[143] More moderately, another recognized that medical schools needed expert specialists as teachers. However, "[t]he interdependence of each part of the animal economy upon the state of the general nutrition, forbids exclusive specialism in practice."[144] These were hardly isolated voices, but neither were they particularly influential. During the 1890s professional unity was imperative in order to achieve such goals as reforming medical education. This resulted in various measures to recognize and satisfy specialists. By 1894 the AMA was considering a revision of the Code of Ethics that emphasized the necessity of specialization and allowed the advertising of specialty interests.[145] This was not implemented, but in 1903 the AMA decided that a revised Code of Ethics was no longer to be binding, but only "advisory."[146] This finally defused the issue of prohibiting consultations with irregulars and, at the same time, made possible the widespread advertising of specialty interests in medical directories.

Conclusion

Despite conditions that did not initially appear very congenial, specialization developed in the United States for much the same reasons as in other nations: the identification of specialties with medical research and innovation proved too powerful to resist, despite considerable opposition and the more visible role of profitable specialist practice. It is worth noting that with the exception of the debate about the validity of specialization that broke out in the 1860s and that proved to be self-limiting, the major conflicts of the second half of the nineteenth century were not about specialization per se, but rather about positions that leading specialists took on more general medical issues (such as consultation and codes of ethics) or about how specialists related to the major institutions of the profession such as the AMA. It is a moot point whether the AMA represented the interests of general practitioners, specialists, or both. In a context within which the medical elite was firmly committed to specialization as a necessity of medical science and teaching, while the national medical association viewed the avoidance of conflict and schism within the profession as a vital professional necessity, there was little choice but to accommodate specialism within limits that were in the last analysis mainly symbolic.

Part II

REGULATING AND STANDARDIZING
SPECIALIST PRACTICE, 1890–1950

Chapter 5

Regulating Specialists in National Medical Directories

For much of the nineteenth century, I have argued, specialization was primarily about research and teaching. Sometime during the 1880s, specialist medical practice began to expand at a vertiginous rate, generating numerous problems in its wake. The medical history of the next half-century was in large measure about coming to terms with and exerting regulatory control over this relatively new form of practice. I begin this chapter by examining briefly the expansion of specialist practice from the 1880s to the mid-1930s. I then move on to medical directories, a genre of medical publication that has been used by historians as a source of data but that has never been fully analyzed as a genre of medical publication. After presenting a historical survey of the development of directories in the four countries under discussion, I examine the measures introduced by different national directories in order to cope with the rapid spread of specialties. I will suggest that these differences—predetermined definitions of acceptable categories in Germany and the United States, benign neglect in France, and blanket prohibition in Britain—prefigured the strategies that national medical professions would eventually pursue in dealing with the issue of specialist certification.

The Rapid Expansion of Specialty Practice

By the mid-1880s, in most large cities for which we have data, from 10 to 15 percent of doctors announced themselves as specialists in one medical directory or another. In the years that followed, the number of those claiming to be specialists increased at a spectacular rate. In 1905 something like 30 percent of all doctors in Berlin identified themselves in directories as specialists; in many other large German cities the proportion was even higher. In Paris, where the most important directory made little attempt to control use of specialist designations, the figure was 35 percent. Although criteria of inclusion are very different, the figures are roughly comparable in major American cities such as New York and Boston.[1]

By the mid-1930s, the figures everywhere were substantially higher: 52 percent in Paris and 46 percent in the major French provincial cities; approximately 40 percent in both New York and Boston; and over 50 percent in Berlin, where fairly rigorous criteria governed mention of specialties in a directory. Only in Great Britain does the number of specialists appear to have been somewhat smaller; but even here, in the one directory that appeared during the 1920s that allowed individuals to mention specialty interests without imposing the usual restrictions, the proportion of those with specialty designations was over 40 percent nationally and more than 50 percent in London.[2]

Behind these increases lay the massive influx of nonacademic, nonhospital physicians into specialties. Certainly, as the number of hospitals multiplied everywhere during this period, the absolute number of specialists with hospital posts climbed significantly while their proportion among all specialists remained stable or, in some cases, even rose slightly.[3] (The same is undoubtedly true on a smaller scale for teachers in medical schools, the number of whom also expanded very rapidly during this period.) But except in Britain, where the growth of specialties is impossible to chart and where specialists were frequently defined by hospital posts exclusively, it was the increasingly routine turn of private practice physicians to specialties after 1880 that accounts for the largest increases in the numbers of specialists.

The fact that so many doctors described themselves or were described as specialists in directories was the result of many factors. Demographic pressures certainly played a major role. From 1876 to 1909, the number of doctors in the German Empire rose from 13,728 to 30,558. The number of American doctors increased from 64,500 in 1870 to 132,000 in 1900, rising more slowly thereafter as the number of medical schools gradually declined. Less dramatically, the medical population in Britain rose from 15,061 in 1876 to 25,553 in 1911, and that of France from 14,000 in 1886 to over 21,000 in 1911.[4] Competitive pressures, especially in the largest urban areas, encouraged many to specialize in order to find more comfortable and lucrative professional niches. Governments, moreover, were investing in specialized medical domains, such as child health and venereal disease services, that provided jobs for doctors desperately in need of supplementary income.

The rise of academic specialties eventually produced enormous amounts of new medical knowledge difficult for generalists to master and for educators to teach. The popularity of specialist practice was also a consequence of working conditions that were perceived as less onerous than those in general practice, where home visits (often at night) were the rule.[5] As specialism became indissolubly associated with science and expertise, it offered prospects of substantially higher incomes and greater social status.[6] That life generally was better for specialists is suggested by American statistics that indicate that by 1940, mortality rates were substantially lower for full-time specialists than for nonspecialists. (The rate for the former was about 70 percent that of the latter.) Even radiologists and dermatologists suffering relatively high rates of mortality due to exposure to radiation enjoyed lower rates than nonspecialists.[7]

If the reasons for specialist self-identification in directories are understandable, the practice is nonetheless problematic for historians, as it was for the early statisticians who tried to determine exactly what it meant.[8] Among other difficulties, no one can know exactly what relationship specialist self-descriptions in directories or on doorplates had to actual medical practice. Charlotte Borst, for instance, found that doctors in Milwaukee who identified themselves as obstetricians often attended fewer childbirths than did certain general practitioners. And doctors complained continually about unfair competition from individuals who called themselves specialists while continuing to engage in general practice. No one knows just how many practitioners of this sort there were, but it is fairly clear that many, if not most, "specialists" in the late nineteenth century were "partial" specialists who spent more or less time in general practice. As late as 1913, the number of full-time specialists among Harvard medical graduates was only slightly higher than the number of GP-specialists. At a time when formal specialty training did not yet exist, general practice often provided the experience that led to expertise in a specialty. In George Rosen's words, partial specialization "was a way station for physicians who eventually became full-time specialists."[9] The ambiguity of the term "specialist" is one facet of the problem that historians, like the historical actors themselves, have had in fully grasping the meaning of specialization a century ago. The imposition of widely accepted definitions of specialist practice is the subject of chapters 6 through 9.

A second sort of ambiguity has to do with the shifting nature of specialist categories. The widest assortment of fields could bring doctors together in a common enterprise and identity: an organ or organ system; a particular group of patients who were targets of government programs of intervention (children, the insane, sufferers from venereal disease or tuberculosis) as well as groups who were not ("nervous" women); a therapeutic or diagnostic modality or technology (electricity, radiology, surgery); administrative or legal institutions (public health, legal medicine); an industry such as the railroads (whose medical employees had specialist aspirations); or a cultural activity (sports medicine). Groups emerged, joined together in various permutations and combinations, split apart, and sometimes disappeared. Judgments about which fields were or were not specialties were made constantly, in multiple arenas and contexts.

With benefit of hindsight, the historian can distinguish between two distinct sorts of logic to specialty claims. The first involved aspirations to elite status. For specialists, this meant acceptance of their field as a recognized category in medical schools, hospitals, national associations, and international congresses. Such aspirations kept the number of specialty categories relatively small, since in this context, specialty categories had to be more or less conventional and their practitioners had to make a case for themselves in predictable academic ways. They had to demonstrate that substantial numbers of individuals were creating a significant body of knowledge or technical procedures that all doctors needed to be taught and that specialists alone could manipulate in particularly difficult cases. They typically did so by creating specialist societies and by infiltrating general medical associations and congresses that established specialty sections in the latter decades of the nineteenth century. If they were excluded from official clinical settings, they might set up private hospitals or dispensaries where they could teach and pursue some form of clinical research.

By the 1860s, there existed a core of ten or so specialties that were pretty much recognized internationally and that were beginning to organize and make knowledge claims. These included obstetrics, diseases of the eyes, diseases of women, psychiatry and neurology (sometimes separated and sometimes combined), diseases of the skin (usually including venereal disease), diseases of the nose and ears, and diseases of the throat. A few others, including diseases of children, urology, and orthopedics, were visible in some countries but not in others. As time went on, new fields appeared: in the 1880s, electricity; at the turn of the century, radiology, endocrinology, tuberculosis, and various fields devoted to internal organs. By the early years of the twentieth century, fifteen to eighteen fields were generally recognized; these either had succeeded in achieving recognition in elite institutions or were making respectable efforts to do so. For some of these, the extent to which they were discrete specialist categories or part of some larger entity was still being worked out.

As academic specialties emerged, they were subject to contradictory pressures. On one hand, the mark of a scientifically respectable field was narrowness—restriction, for instance, to a single organ or organ system. This was the model of ophthalmology, which enjoyed especially high status. But not all organs or fields provided sufficiently broad scope for teaching, since costs of maintaining permanent teaching staffs were high and clinical material in large quantities was not easy to find; and in private practice there were not enough patients to provide practitioners with adequate income. Consequently, individual specialists and entire specialties frequently laid claim to other fields that were related by either anatomical or functional proximity. Sometimes such pressures led merely to boundary disputes over lucrative practices. Medical journals everywhere were rife with debates about who could best perform abdominal surgery, tonsillectomies, and birthing. Occasionally they generated conflicts about whether a field should be divided into several narrow specialties or combined into a single comprehensive category. The relationship of diseases of the ear to those of the throat was one of the most striking examples of this tension, but there were others, as we shall see in chapter 11.

There was, however, a second and very different kind of logic to specialist development in which practitioners eschewed aspirations to elite medical institutions; instead, they focused exclusively on private medical practice and appealed directly to potential patients. Such appeals were of course unregulated, allowing for the widest (and wildest) sorts of claims. Many fields that were not part of the elite academic consensus might thus appear in directories or on doorplates: actinology, gout, diseases of old age and even of middle age. And they could be combined in the most creative ways. Such appeals could be cast in very narrow terms indeed. In 1921, for instance, a general directory of Parisian occupations included a medical section listing the city's physicians divided according to specialties; the list was split into no fewer than 120 specialist categories.[10] Among those categories represented by only a single practitioner were acne, anemia, autointoxication, chronic bronchitis, and something called nasal centrotherapy, to cite only those at the beginning of the list.

Specialists at this second level frequently appealed to the public by claiming to treat widespread health problems with huge numbers of potential patients. And in fact the majority of specialists, we shall see in chapter 10, were concentrated in such fields as diseases of women, diseases of the ear and throat, and, in some countries, diseases of children. The extent of practice in such fields could vary from one nation to another because government programs might transform the national landscape of practice and because certain categories of doctors, whether specialists or not, might effectively monopolize certain clienteles, leaving little room for specialists who appealed directly to the public.

Many of the specialties with a large client base were also part of the academic consensus; these fields in which many self-proclaimed specialists coexisted with academic specialists posed especially acute problems for medical professions in all four countries under examination. In such cases, discrepancies in specialist training were particularly visible. Practitioners who had received elaborate professional education deeply resented the claims to specialist status by those who had not. Full-time specialists and GPs took exception to specialists who also practiced as generalists. Working out solutions to these problems took more than half a century and required the establishment of elaborate regulatory frameworks in each national context.

Practitioners who made narrow but wild specialty claims constituted a different problem entirely; they seemed to devalue all specialties by making them look ridiculous. They placed specialists in the same category as the much-maligned charlatans. In some cases it was not so much the specialty category as the principle behind it that appeared threatening. "Natural therapeutics," for instance, hardly constituted an overcrowded field, nor was there anything shocking to most doctors about the principles upon which it was based. But claims to expertise in it were deeply resented because of the implication that each therapeutic modality needed its own specialists rather than being part of the complete arsenal of general medicine.[11] It is true that academic models had a trickle-down effect that gradually inculcated professional norms about which specialties were legitimate and which were not. And it is likely that those who did not adhere to such accepted categories declined in number in the twentieth century. But as the Parisian professional directory cited above suggests, the possibility of appealing directly to the public allowed such practitioners to continue to exist and sometimes to flourish.

Achieving a measure of regulatory control over definitions of acceptable specialties was no simple task. One option available to national medical associations was to try to prevent advertising by doctors. Although such rules of professional etiquette had much broader implications—seeking, for instance, to shape both the public image of the profession and its moral values—they could be used to prohibit doctors from advertising *any* specialist interest. In three of the four countries we are examining—France is the single exception—this was the strategy that professional associations initially followed. It had several shortcomings, however.

First and foremost, it was difficult to enforce. One could do little about the local medical groups that refused to abide by it or commercial publications that allowed maverick doctors to advertise their specialty and much else besides. Second, such a blanket prohibition did not discriminate between those specialists and specialty categories that were achieving academic and professional legitimacy and those that were not. And as the system of health-care provision became increasingly large, complex, and segmented, it seemed necessary to provide adequate descriptions of this domain to doctors, if not the public. As we saw, the issue of advertising provoked serious conflicts within the American medical profession during the 1860s. Elsewhere, controversy emerged somewhat later. For all these reasons, in the first decade of the twentieth century both the American and the German medical professions abandoned all such blanket prohibitions. Instead, they sought to predefine the categories that specialists could utilize to describe themselves. One of the key arenas for this attempt at control was the medical directory.

The Natural History of Medical Directories

The medical directory is a curious genre with a complex literary pedigree. One early precursor was the astrological almanac, itself a successor to the medieval *computus* manuscript, which might contain all sorts of practical information, including lists of professionals.[12] As directories developed, they frequently retained the most characteristic feature of the almanac, the calendar. Until the 1870s, the British *Medical Directory* contained an elaborate calendar including information about the phases of the moon, times of sunrise and sunset, days of meetings of scientific societies, historical anniversaries, days of religious significance, and days for renewing fire insurance, paying taxes, and voting in county elections.

Long before they abandoned calendars, directories had become primarily devoted to the representation not of time but of social space. As social life became increasingly complex from the seventeenth century on, individuals required practical guides to the intricate patchwork of institutions, groups, and persons that constituted their society. By the late seventeenth century there existed several different sorts of directories appearing at more or less regular intervals. One important category described the major elite institutions and corporations of the nation, ranging from the royal family and state officials to members of occupational groups; the *Almanach royal*, which appeared in France from 1699 until the twentieth century, and Debrett's *Royal Kalendar* (1765–1893) in Britain were among the most successful examples of this genre. A second category of works, whose origins in Britain go back to lists of guild merchants of the fourteenth century, was trade and business directories, which proliferated especially in Britain. A German variant of this sort of publication was the *Berliner Adreßbuch,* which began to appear in 1704 and was regularly published under various titles and imprimaturs for two centuries.[13]

In the late eighteenth century, directories devoted to specific professional groups began appearing sporadically. The first medical directory in France appeared in 1776, and in Britain in 1779.[14] Almanac-agendas (*Taschenbücher*) for doctors began to appear in Germany in the 1780s; although not quite directories, they contained, in addition to scientific articles, information about well-known doctors and medical institutions.[15] It was not until the nineteenth century that the growth of medical professions and the emergence of large-scale publishing enterprises allowed medical directories to truly proliferate.

In France, two directories began appearing on something like an annual basis during the 1820s. One of these, the *Almanach général de médecine* (founded in 1827), managed to survive in various forms until World War I.[16] It was joined in the next decades by a variety of other publications, including the *Annuaire Roubaud,* founded in 1849.[17] Competition for what was undoubtedly a restricted market was already brutal in the 1840s, and intensified thereafter as new directories were launched.[18] The *Annuaire Roubaud* and *Almanach général* merged in 1886[19]; the unified publication was printing 4,000 hefty copies (over 1,000 pages in length) annually before World War I.[20] It was one of a half-dozen publications struggling for a share of the admittedly growing medical market. Even in the 1930s, there were at least three serious Parisian directories in operation, as well as a host of more specialized or local directories, in spite of the growing dominance of one publication, the *Guide Rosenwald.*[21]

This plethora of medical directories undoubtedly reflects the general fragmentation of the French medical profession, the absence of a dominating medical association, and the lack of powerful publishing houses specializing in this domain. In Britain, a single publication, *The Medical Directory,* dominated the market, though it always faced sporadic competition. Founded in 1845 as *The London Medical Directory,* it was taken over a year later by the medical publisher John Churchill and continued to appear annually while expanding in scope. In 1847 it incorporated *The Provincial Medical Directory,* and a few years after that, the medical directories of Scotland and Ireland. The catalog of the British Library is full of short-lived competitors to this publication, whose success is all the more remarkable in view of the fact that it managed during its early years to antagonize an influential segment of the medical profession due to the tolerant way it treated homeopaths in its pages.[22] As a result of this policy, Thomas Wakley briefly produced a rival directory more in keeping, on this issue at least, with the wishes of the organized medical profession.[23]

That directories could be central to the reformist and exclusionary aspirations of segments of the medical profession is confirmed by the case of the United States. From the first meetings to set up the American Medical Association, that organization showed an interest in creating a directory or registry of physicians legally entitled to practice medicine.[24] In 1856 an effort was made "to enlist some enterprising publisher" who could help put together such a directory.[25] In 1868 a committee was actually set up. Such a directory, said AMA President Samuel Gross, "would be of incalculable benefit to our profession in preventing mistakes in regard to consultations with irregular practitioners, at the same time it would serve to bind its members into a firmer and closer union."[26] Despite such hopes the effort had to be abandoned, so great were the logistical difficulties.[27]

Nor was the private sector in the United States any more successful in publishing directories. For much of the nineteenth century, American medical almanacs were regularly published, but they seldom attempted to list medical practitioners. The difficulties of compiling national lists of practitioners in a land of huge distances and few state licensing laws were nearly insurmountable. One directory that did appear in 1874 nicely illustrates these difficulties. The preface to *The Medical Register and Directory of the United States* indicated that work on the publication had begun fifteen years before (the author, Dr. Samuel Butler, had in fact died just before publication):

> When we consider that there are between 70,000 and 80,000 members of all shades and grades scattered throughout such vast tracts of country, where only semi-civilization ofttimes exists, and the postal arrangements, if there be any, are often of very primitive character—where also education has been in the past so sadly neglected, and diplomas easily obtained, even by those unable to read and write—the difficulties . . . were sufficient to deter the most enterprising.[28]

Complaints about the difficulty of collecting information in the American medical context were echoed by the editors of the first permanent national American directory, *The Medical and Surgical Register of the United States*, published from 1886 by R.L. Polk and Company of Detroit. This enterprise could overcome such barriers because of the scale of its operations and, as it explicitly stated, "the great facilities and long experience of the publishers in Directory work."[29] The company, founded in 1870, produced state gazetteers and business directories in about thirty states and Canadian provinces, city directories for nearly fifty urban centers, and *The Architects and Business Directory* of the United States.[30] A publishing house of a rather new kind, it had, in 1890, branch offices in thirteen North American cities. All physicians were asked to submit information through the mails, and the replies were checked against official college records; as a result, about one-third of the names in the register in 1890 appeared without educational information because the diplomas claimed could not be confirmed.

During the next decade many state and interstate directories appeared. A second national directory, *The Standard Medical Directory of North America*, surfaced in 1902. Clearly, the development of administrative structures and of recordkeeping within state agencies and medical associations was making it feasible (if still not easy) to identify medical practitioners. Furthermore, as the medical profession struggled to organize itself, the desire to identify and distinguish fully trained and licensed practitioners gained intensity.

By the early twentieth century the AMA was finally prepared to step in. There was a widespread feeling that existing directories were unreliable, and if there was money to be made, it should be the AMA that profited.[31] In 1901 the issue of a directory was first raised. Initially the various administrative organs of the Association hoped to produce a "Blue Book" of AMA members. In 1905, however, the proprietors of *The Standard Medical Directory* offered to sell their directory to the AMA, which agreed to the nominal price of $6,000. This provided the AMA with a list of names on which to base a more comprehensive work.[32] Soon after, the Committee on Reports and Officers decided to produce a directory of all American physicians: this would "be of great aid in effecting more complete organization of the profession" and would provide a new source of income; but it was "only incidental to the other work," that of preparing a biographical card index of all American physicians from information submitted by state and county medical societies and state licensing boards. This would provide the Association, as well as insurance and railway companies, with accurate information about properly licensed physicians and with a means of verifying practitioners' educational claims.[33] It was perceived as a "first step in purging our ranks of the dishonorable and criminal classes."[34] *The American Medical Directory* (*AMD*) first appeared in 1906. Although it regularly lost money due to the labor and expense of maintaining the records on which it was based,[35] it gradually assumed a monopolistic position nationally.

The early difficulties of producing a national directory in the United States were not dissimilar to those encountered in a decentralized setting such as Germany, which did not become a unified nation until the eighth decade of the nineteenth century. I have located few real medical directories during the first half of the nineteenth century. Doctors and patients seem to have relied for their medical information on city directories (*Adreßbücher*). However, a few years before Polk brought out the first American national directory, Paul Börner launched the first national German directory, the *Reichs-Medizinal-Kalender* (*RMK*), in 1880. Börner was an extraordinary presence on the German medical stage. He was an important figure in the public health movement, a mover in the national medical association, the Deutsche Ärztevereinsbund (the DÄV), and he created a publishing empire. In 1875 he began publishing the *Deutsche medizinische Wochenschrift*, arguably the most prestigious medical journal in imperial Germany (and that is still published today). Three years later he began putting out an annual handbook of practical medicine, and two years after that, came out with his medical directory. His successors continued to edit these varied annual publication; the most important was Julius Schwalbe, who ran this publishing empire from 1894 to his death in 1930.[36]

In the absence of any real competition, the *RMK* quickly became the semi-official directory for the German medical profession. Börner, who had been active in the DÄV, was eulogized on his death in that organization's journal, the *Ärztliches Vereinsblatt für Deutschland*,[37] which regularly published positive reviews of the annual volumes of the directory. (The word "indispensable" [*unentbehrlich*] was an invariable adjective in these reviews.) Börner's successors maintained these close links with the national organizations of medicine, links that became increasingly official.[38] In 1937 the *RMK* was designated by the Nazi regime as the official organ and directory of German medicine.[39]

Lists of practitioners were the primary but not exclusive component of the medical directory. Most directories included information about major medical institutions, societies, administrative organs, and establishments (ranging from prisons to theaters) employing physicians. Reprinting of major legislation that regulated medical practice was also common. Directories closely linked to professional associations often printed fee schedules, and Börner's *RMK* sometimes reprinted the resolutions of the annual congress of the DÄV. Some included practical indications and optimum dosages for medications, scientific articles, and medical statistics. As medical life became increasingly complex, one might find lists of ambulance services, home nurses, laboratories, instrument makers, and masseurs. A directory for New York City contained a detailed list of conveyances for moving around the metropolis and of routes to leave it.[40]

With the exception of *The American Medical Directory*, run by a representative medical association, directories were ordinarily commercial ventures. From the mid-nineteenth century on, the advertising of pharmaceuticals, rest homes, instruments, and practitioners became increasingly ubiquitous and, most likely, a growing source of profits. But the direct sale of directories to readers remained economically significant. Who in fact were these readers? It is impossible to say for certain, but it seems that in the vast majority of cases they were physicians rather than laypersons. The statements in editorial introductions, the sheer bulk of the more successful publications, the copious professional information, and the fact that advertisements were directed at a medical audience suggest that physicians themselves were the targeted market group. For the general public, different sorts of publications—popular health guides, general city or commercial directories—could provide appropriate guidance.

Physicians contributed to profits both as purchasers of the directories and as an attraction for advertisers seeking to sell medical products. During the 1850s, the high "monopoly" price of *The London and Provincial Medical Directory* was one of the major criticisms leveled against it.[41] Despite intense competition in Paris at the end of the nineteenth century, most directories cost 3 to 4 francs—not expensive, to be sure, but not a giveaway either. British and American directories faced less competition and could be more costly. *The Medical Directory* before World War I cost almost 12 shillings for those who paid early and 14 shillings for those paying later; at the same time, a six-month subscription to *The Lancet* cost less than 13 shillings.[42] In 1900 Polk's annual *Register* cost a whopping $10, twice as much as an annual subscription to the *Journal of the AMA* and far more than any of the medical textbooks advertised in its pages.[43] The German RMK, by now virtually an official publication of the DÄV, cost 14.50 marks in 1929—quite a substantial sum, considering the terrible economic climate.[44] Judging from protests issued by the British Medical Association in the 1920s, some more marginal directories attempted to tie the appearance of physicians' names in the directory to purchase of the publication.[45]

Still, the ability to reach large numbers of physicians constituted the major appeal of directories to advertisers. Some advertisers even took matters a step farther by establishing their own directories. It has been said that one of Lucien Rosenwald's motives for founding the phenomenally successful *Guide Rosenwald* was his desire to create a platform for advertising certain proprietary remedies that he owned.[46] In 1901 a mineral water enterprise, the Source de Paradis, published a directory that does not seem to have taken root, since no further volumes appeared.[47] The giant Vichy mineral water concern had better luck when it published a Belgian national medical directory, which appeared from 1898 until after World War II.[48]

By the 1930s, Britain's *Medical Directory* remained (at 36 shillings) quite expensive.[49] But for other publications, the revenue from advertising was looming increasingly large and making the actual purchase of directories less important. The always innovative *Guide Rosenwald* responded accordingly by offering copies free to physicians.[50]

By the twentieth century, substantial differences existed among national medical directories. In France, the competition among directories was fierce. *The Medical Directory* largely dominated the market in Britain. In the United States and Germany, directories appeared only late in the nineteenth century. In the former the *AMD* took on a fully official role as a publication of the AMA. In the latter the *RMK* assumed a quasi-official position. Curiously, market domination did not preclude constant innovation. It is true that struggling French publications had to make more of an effort. Editors tried to make their publications stand out by constantly adding new features that would make them more useful: alphabetical listings of practitioners were supplemented by street and neighborhood listings; provincial listings were added to those for Paris. But even in those countries where one publication dominated the market, editors felt compelled to regularly add new features. One could, after all, hold on to a volume for quite a few years before it became truly out of date. In 1902, for instance, the *RMK* added the most significant annual decisions of the medical honors courts and a section on postgraduate courses.[51] The rather staid *Medical Directory* also added new features from time to time. Finding ways to present the growing group of medical specialists might, in some contexts at least, constitute one such publishing innovation.

Medical Directories Confront the Specialties

For many decades, we saw, calling oneself a specialist was as valid a criterion as any for determining specialty status. Medical directories constituted one potential and particularly visible location for making specialty claims. Editorial strategies for handling such claims thus represent a key manifestation of the way struggles over the definition of specialization were being worked out in different nations. To the extent that a directory was recognized as an authoritative representation of the medical profession, its method of labeling individuals helped shape the way in which specialty categories were perceived.

Directories could identify physicians as specialists in several ways. The most traditional was to add information about specialty practice (within parentheses or in italic type) to other data in an alphabetical listing of physicians. In both medical and general directories in France, this was the standard practice from the early nineteenth century on. It is not entirely clear whether such information was obtained from administrative lists that circulated widely or from personal communications. But there was never any significant opposition in France to such self-advertising by specialists. It does not seem to have been perceived any differently from announcing oneself as a hospital physician or former intern of the Paris hospitals (both prestigious titles).

In contrast to the French situation, mention of a specialty in any publication was considered a form of advertising, and thus unethical behavior, in Germany, the United States, and Britain. The taboo was especially strong in Britain. *The London and Provincial Medical Directory* initially allowed practitioners to specify their area of practice but, as we saw in chapter 2, abandoned this policy in 1849. In subsequent years, it became rare, though not impossible, for individuals to specify that they were specialists. (One gets the feeling it was considered infra dig rather than formally prohibited.) Instead, specialists made themselves known to readers by listing their specialist hospital and teaching posts, publications, memberships in specialist societies, and (later) diplomas. This would remain the pattern in this publication (called *The Medical Directory* from 1870) in the twentieth century.

In the United States, conditions of practice made it difficult to determine who was legally authorized to practice, let alone who was a specialist. Here, too, any public identification of specialists was widely viewed as unethical advertising.[52] Most state and regional directories followed the guidelines of the AMA and state medical societies to the effect that "all references to special branches of medical practice, as extra inducements to patronage should be deemed a violation of the Code of Medical Ethics."[53] Even in the last years of the century, Polk's *Register* identified sectarian practitioners such as homeopaths and eclectics, but not specialists. By the early twentieth century, however (and in contrast to the British situation), such opposition had been overcome and American directories were identifying specialists.

Much the same was true in Germany, once national directories began to appear. Börner's *RMK* was close enough to the medical associations not to ignore their ban on specialist identification. In an early volume published in 1884,[54] lists of doctors for most cities did not include specialty information; a few, however, did. The most likely explanation is that this reflected variations among local medical societies in rules governing the advertisement of specialty status. It is worth noting, however, that Berlin specialists who could not identify their specialty in the *RMK* did not hesitate to do so in the local trade directory of that city.[55]

The rapid spread of specialties at the end of the nineteenth century produced new methods of identification. Alphabetical lists that included specialty information were not a very effective way for physicians in large cities to attract clients or referrals; only readers who took the trouble to look up the names of specific individuals would know that they were specialists. Far more effective as a means of calling attention to one's practice were specialty lists, which brought together the names of all specialists in a given locale.

Distinct specialty lists were relatively rare in the early and mid-nineteenth century. The *Guide médical* published in Paris in the 1820s included such a list but did not survive for long, and the initiative was not followed. The earliest specialist lists were not in fact published in directories aimed at medical practitioners, but in publications targeting clients. Popular almanacs and guides frequently contained health-care advice, and some were devoted completely to it. While many emphasized self-help, others provided counsel about appropriate specialists to consult for specific complaints. Such lists did not have to be comprehensive: they could be presented as selections of the best specialists available. The categories tended to be based on types of health problems, and thus were rather more numerous than those found in professional directories. One of the earliest I have located is the *Annuaire des familles*, published in 1859.[56]

By the end of the nineteenth century, some popular guides were devoted exclusively to helping people find the right specialist for their needs. *London Medical Specialists*, published in 1890, was intended, according to its preface, "for the guidance of those who require to consult an eminent authority on any malady to which special attention has been paid by various members of the medical profession."[57] A similar publication devoted to specialist practitioners in New York City, published nine years later, was intended "as much for the use of general practitioners as for patients."[58] Both editors claimed to be presenting only the most eminent practitioners in each field and emphasized that the selection resulted from the best judgments of the medical profession. Specialty practice in New York City clearly was widely accepted, but the American editor nonetheless spoke of the "embarrassment" of omitting the names of "men of great eminence . . . who have not consented to be classed as specialists."[59] And the editor of the London volume reflected the prevalent hostility of the British doctors to specialization by emphasizing that a majority of those listed "are in no sense 'specialists' though distinguished by their knowledge of certain subjects."[60] Another British publication that appeared at the same time, and that apparently made less modest claims, was violently attacked by the *British Medical Journal* (*BMJ*) as an "impudent attempt to increase the demand for the supernumeraries and camp followers of medicine. . . . It may be taken for granted that respectable specialists will do all they can to keep their names out of a book in which they are likely to find themselves in company with a good deal which will be very distasteful to them; it might be worth the while of the better set of specialists to write to the publisher, forbidding the inclusion of their names on any such list."[61]

The fact that the editor of *New York Medical Practitioners* sought to appeal to general practitioners indicates that complete specialty lists could be useful to physicians needing advice or referrals. They could also provide knowledge about the number of specialists in a city or town, information helpful in making career decisions. It is thus not surprising that specialist directories aimed directly at the medical professional eventually made their appearance.

A specialty directory published in London in 1889 sought to provide practitioners with comprehensive listings of all specialists on staff at recognized hospitals; this publication did not survive beyond its first volume.[62] It had been preceded by a slightly more successful and quite bizarre French annual publication, the *Annuaire des spécialités médicales et pharmaceutiques,* which began appearing in 1880 under the editorship of the orthopedist P. Bouland and was something like a general almanac for medical practitioners.[63] The word *spécialités* in the title had a double meaning. In French, as in German, this word referred to the proprietary remedies that were beginning to be produced industrially during this period. Bouland provided practitioners with a practical guide to the bewildering variety of existing pharmaceutical products through an inventory that filled nineteen pages in the first volume. He added to this a twelve-page listing of medico-surgical materials, ranging from batteries to instruments to manuals. He also attempted to deal with a second, more recently accepted meaning of *spécialités:* specialized medical practice. He began his volume with an alphabetical listing of specialist practitioners according to name. This did not identify specialties, but rather included the major publications of each individual. Bouland also added a short one-and-a-half-page listing of specialist practitioners, without any descriptive information whatsoever; it was organized according to specialties and included names of foreigners as well as Frenchmen.

This brief specialist listing was a major French publishing innovation, although Bouland's *Annuaire* survived only until 1886. The following year, a somewhat more conventional medical directory, the *Guide Rosenwald,* made its debut. Like other publications of this type, the new directory contained an alphabetical listing of Parisian practitioners that included specialist self-descriptions; but in its second year of publication, it added a separate list of Parisian specialists divided according to specialty categories. In 1892 the venerable *Annuaire Roubaud,* already in existence for sixty-five years, broke with tradition by adding its own Parisian specialist listing. Henceforth lists of Parisian specialists became a feature of all major French directories.[64]

It is not clear just how these lists were compiled. Although they were supposed to be comprehensive, most Parisian directories exhibited a substantial discrepancy between specialty identifications in the alphabetical listing and the specialist lists. In many cases, specialist lists omitted individuals who were identified as specialists in the alphabetical list; in others, individuals without such identifications were included. While this certainly reflected the growing pains of a new and complex publishing practice, as well as the extreme fluidity and uncertainty of specialist status at the turn of the century, editorial decisions certainly played a role.[65] Editorial choice functioned in other ways as well. Someone had to determine the specialist categories under which names were presented, and this inevitably excluded many of the less conventional descriptions that individuals used in the alphabetical listing. But overall, French editors tended to be quite liberal. By 1935, the *Guide Rosenwald* included thirty-six specialties on its list.

Outside France, specialist lists did not become established, I suspect, because they visually highlighted divisions within the medical profession. An exception occurred in 1902, when a new American publication, *The Standard Medical Directory of North America,* came into existence; in its second annual edition it added to its alphabetical directory (arranged by state and city) a specialist directory. The editor felt compelled to explain: "The compilation of these lists being the first of the kind, we believe, in any publication, either of local or national scope, has met with some professional scepticism as to its feasibility."[66] Shortly thereafter, this directory was purchased and put out of business by the American Medical Association, which began producing *The American Medical Directory.* From that point onward, only directories in France, among the countries being examined, included self-standing specialty lists.

Instead, the major directory of Germany, the *RMK,* introduced in 1901 a significant innovation to the traditional form of specialty identification. Like more traditional publications, it contained an alphabetical list of doctors in each city that included space for specialists to identify their special interest. But this publication was the first, to my knowledge, to restrict the way specialists could do this. This part of the directory began with a list of official pictograms that could be placed next to names in the alphabetical listing. A rudimentary scalpel represented surgery; a brain, psychiatry; and so on. The motivation for this innovation, the editor declared, was to provide useful information to readers.[67] But it was also a response to intensifying discussions about the regulation of specialties and to ongoing administrative efforts to determine exact numbers of specialists that we will discuss in chapter 6. In contrast to specialist lists that sent the message that the medical profession was divided into separate and distinct parts, this visual format presented the image of a united profession with very discrete differences among practitioners. Specialist pictograms were not much different from those representing other identifying features, ranging from state honors to hospital posts. Many would have been incomprehensible to the casual reader who could not find the pictogram key. At the same time, and more important for our purposes, the list of pictograms rigidly defined the domain of acceptable specialist categories and excluded marginal specialty groups.

Although he regularly requested that doctors submit information to supplement and correct the official data used to determine initial listings, the directory's editor, Julius Schwalbe, was in fact picky about what information he accepted. He refused to apologize for not providing symbols for infrequently mentioned specialties such as gout and rheumatism. Furthermore, he counted as specialists only those in established practice and refused specialty markers to hospital assistants (akin to residents) or volunteers in specialty clinics, even though he realized that many would eventually become specialists.[68] Several years later, a new French medical directory, *Medicus*, took a similar approach to specialty identification, specifying through use of abbreviations rather than pictograms the specialties that could be represented.

But the most far-reaching application of this principle was certainly implemented by *The American Medical Directory*, backed by the authority of a well-organized and increasingly activist American Medical Association. The second volume, which appeared three years after the first, began the daunting task of representing specialty practice; the editors started with only a handful of specialist categories and added new ones in subsequent volumes. The *AMD* also utilized a list of abbreviations inserted into alphabetical listings to define the domain of legitimate specialties. It went even farther by beginning to introduce criteria for defining individuals as specialists and distinguishing different types of practice. By 1914, the *AMD* was indicating with an asterisk those specialists who claimed to practice their specialty exclusively. In keeping with the policy of not being satisfied with the claims and statements of individuals, the directory from 1921 stated clearly that practitioners requesting mention of their specialty status had to satisfy a number of conditions: membership in a state association or specialty society listed in the *AMD*, or a professorship in a specialty in a medical school with an "A" or "B" rating from the Council on Medical Education.[69] The directory of 1914 specifically stated that the individuals listed could mention only one of the recognized specialty categories (several of which were in fact combinations), thus further limiting self-expression.

In contrast to the efforts made in Germany and the United States to redefine the domain of specialties, the British medical profession continued to fight efforts to make specialties more visible. The dominant *Medical Directory* was regionally and alphabetically organized, with individual entries containing a wide range of information—but there were no specialist lists, and very few entries in the alphabetical lists specifically mentioned specialties. However, discerning readers could find rather opaque abbreviations referring to specialist diplomas, hospital posts, and membership in specialty societies. Recognizing these abbreviations required considerable professional knowledge. Any effort to make such information more visible to the public was vigorously combated. In 1923 the British Medical Association responded with some alarm to a circular from the publisher Grafton announcing the imminent publication of a new medical directory, *London Doctors and Dental Surgeons*. The wording of the circular seemed to suggest that the appearance of names in the directory would be contingent on purchasing the volume. Even more serious was the announcement that it would contain a "particularly full and comprehensive" specialty list. The BMA reiterated a position it had taken in the past: the best person to advise patients about specialists was "a patient's ordinary medical attendant. The grouping of practitioners under various specialties in a directory intended for public use is to be deprecated."[70] Practitioners were advised not to allow their names to be included in the volume.

Grafton immediately contacted the BMA's Ethics Committee, stating his willingness to defer to its wishes, and thus gained its official approval.[71] He wrote in the preface, with some ill humor: "In deference to the views of the British Medical Association, the publisher has abandoned a proposed classified list of Consultants and Specialists . . . although no objection to this practical feature, which had been strongly urged and was desired by many leading practitioners, was raised in other quarters." Instead, each page of the alphabetical directory was divided into columns into which information about individuals was fitted; under the heading "Nature of Work" (suggested by the BMA), specialty information sent in by physicians was presented. "The Ethical Committee of the British Medical Association, after deliberations took no exception to this arrangement."[72]

London Doctors and Dental Surgeons did not reappear. But in 1925 Grafton resuscitated, after a hiatus of seven years, another, more conventional-looking directory, *The Medical Who's Who*, which had appeared from 1912 to 1918 from a different publisher. The editor announced in the preface that he had "been inundated with requests for a classified list of consultants and specialists"; he had nevertheless decided "that the time has not yet come when this would be approved by the whole profession and he has preferred to defer to the views of such a representative body as the British Medical Association."[73] Practitioners were, however, given "the ethical opportunity . . . to state precisely the nature of their work" among the other information contained in their listing.[74] Grafton was no more successful in this new venture than in his previous one, and only one further volume followed (in 1927). It is worth noting that even though the BMA grudgingly accepted the principle that physicians could include specialist interests within the context of alphabetical professional directories, it continued to object strenuously to such specialty designations in telephone directories or other publications directed at the general public.[75]

Conclusion

The major national medical directories thus treated specialties in quite different ways. Most of the competing French publications allowed practitioners total freedom to identify specialty interests in alphabetical directories and granted specialists further visibility (with some modest limitation of category choice) in separate lists of specialists. No one thought to define what specialist identification actually meant for practice in the French context. By the twentieth century, opposition to specialist self-advertising had been overcome in the United States, Germany, and, at least officially, Britain. The first two, in contrast to most (though not all) French publications, predefined acceptable specialties, and the *AMD* even went so far as to define criteria for claiming a specialist designation. In Britain, simple opposition to specialization had been transformed into the more complex referral system. *The Medical*

Directory included information relevant to the identification of specialists, but kept it obscure and refused to highlight specialization as a significant feature of medicine. The BMA eventually and grudgingly acquiesced to clear identification of specialists in medical directories, but it is telling that none of the publications that followed this practice survived for long.

The strategies of medical directories presage national efforts to regulate medical specialists. The fact that directories in both Germany and the United States undertook to define acceptable specialist categories after the turn of the century reflected intensifying medical concern with the larger problems of specialization. In both countries, the organized profession would seek an early resolution of this issue by creating mechanisms to define and regulate competent specialists. This would prove to be a lengthy and complex process.

Chapter 6
Regulating Specialists in Germany

German was the first of the four nations under discussion to organize a national system of specialist certification. It was preceded by Sweden and Denmark, whose medical associations introduced specialty regulation in 1911 and 1918, respectively.[1] The grave problems facing the German medical profession, the existence of an active national medical association, and uniquely difficult political conditions made a relatively early resolution of the issue both desirable and possible. But it was above all the tactics chosen that allowed the profession to overcome massive differences of opinion and conflicts of interest. These tactics were based on the avoidance of legal and state machinery in favor of professional self-reliance; the national association provided general guidelines while local medical associations applied them with maximum discretion. Widespread desire to preserve general practice, lack of interest in professional issues on the part of the academic specialist elite, and the magnitude of the political and economic crisis that forced doctors to make painful concessions in order to remain unified, produced a system of certification that attempted to satisfy some of the major concerns of general practitioners. The agreement that was finally reached in 1924 was by no means unproblematic. But it would exhibit remarkable longevity, surviving even the Nazi reorganization of medicine and the postwar reconstruction of Germany.

From Academic to Professional Concerns

In the twentieth century, medical education continued to be central for German specialists. As in other nations, finding room in the curriculum for the ever-expanding accumulation of knowledge and techniques proved to be difficult. In the state-controlled German education system, acceptance in curricula and examinations, notably the final *Prüfung*, constituted the most significant form of official recognition for developing specialties. Struggles for academic acceptance were intensified by the fact that German universities remained, on the whole, conservative in acknowledging specialist disciplines. In 1919, for instance, there were no chairs in German universities in orthopedics, otorhinolaryngology, urology, and neurology (independent of psychiatry), all of which existed in a number of French medical schools.[2] And the situation was little changed at the beginning of the 1930s. Some medical schools, such as the one in Halle, tenaciously resisted the introduction of professorships in the specialties.[3] In 1931–32, only eight clinical specialties, *including* internal medicine and surgery, were represented in all or nearly all of the twenty-three German medical faculties.[4] Nor were these limitations completely mitigated by junior personnel (*Privatdozenten*), who became surprisingly scarce in the twentieth century and who tended to be concentrated in disciplines with already existing chairs.[5] General hospitals without university affiliation also provided few career alternatives for specialists. In the 1920s, those in Berlin did not have specialty wards, and the situation was only slightly better in the general hospitals of other German cities.[6]

Both before and after World War I, intense preoccupation with the reform of medical education kept medical schools at the center of specialist concerns.[7] Increasing state intervention in medicine in the early twentieth century further promoted traditional professional strategies for academic recognition. A plea for the introduction of new methods for dealing with infectious diseases published in 1919 culminated almost reflexively in the demand that universities establish a separate teaching and clinical division in this field; this would result in serious research, the transmission of research results to medical practitioners, and an improvement in the nation's health.[8] Much the same logic was used to argue for the acceptance of the newly emerging field of insurance medicine as an academic subject.[9]

Such tactics seemed entirely appropriate in view of the rapid spread of both pediatrics and dermatology-venereology throughout medical schools in the early twentieth century; this occurred because training in these fields for GPs was thought necessary for the successful implementation of state campaigns to lower infant mortality and eradicate syphilis.[10] The government did not always get its way, however. In 1908, pressure from the Prussian administration to create chairs of "social medicine" provoked intense and successful opposition from medical schools. Political pressures were not necessarily based on practical public health needs. While colonial medicine shrank as a real medical activity during the years following the loss of Germany's colonial empire, a chair of tropical hygiene was established in 1919 at least in part because Germany's attempt to reclaim her colonies and revise foreign accounts of German colonialism seemed to require such a symbolic gesture.[11] Less successfully, representatives of sports medicine tried to exploit growing interest in physical fitness to establish themselves academically. As the number of specialties increased, the clamor by specialty disciplines for a place in curricula and examinations became deafening. Some individuals realized that choices boiled down to reducing time devoted to the basic sciences, extending the length of medical studies, or curbing the academic claims of specialties.[12]

In spite of the continuing relevance of such academic concerns, Germany was the first of our four countries to begin serious debate about specialist practice and ways to regulate it. The academic elite, preoccupied as it was, did not participate actively in this debate, but medical practitioners filled the breach. There were several reasons for this early concern with the *Spezialistenfrage,* as was suggested in an earlier chapter. First, specialization seems to have been somewhat more widespread in middle-sized and even smaller cities than in other countries, where it was usually concentrated in the largest urban centers.[13] A second factor was the continued attachment in Germany to ideas of intellectual and educational "wholeness." While such views were not powerful enough to prevent the growing fragmentation of disciplines in German institutions, they did produce unease with excessive specialization. The fact that specialization was so closely identified with academic teaching and research may also have contributed to the disquiet over widespread specialist practice that frequently lacked all academic legitimacy. Third, the multiplicity of state regulatory codes organizing medicine, and the very late reform of most of these, meant that in many states, before 1860 or so, special degrees had in fact existed for such specialists as oculists and obstetricians.[14] The direct precedent for specialty certification was thus more immediate than in the other countries under discussion.

Most significant, I have suggested, was the mobilization of the profession in order to deal with a variety of professional issues, notably the repercussions of *Kurierfreiheit*—the freedom to practice for irregular and alternative practitioners— and campaigning to extend to all doctors the right to work in the health insurance system set up in imperial Germany. German doctors thus created national professional associations, notably the Deutsche Ärztevereinsbund (DÄV), to deal with all these issues. By 1927 the DÄV represented about 95 percent of all doctors in the country.[15] For the most part, it and other professional associations and institutions were only moderately effective in forcing the hand of local and national governments and in winning satisfactory concessions. But the one thing their members *could* do was talk, and they did so incessantly, vigorously, and at a national level. As a result, systematic professional debates of various sorts occurred nationally from the 1880s on. Specialization was one of many issues discussed in this way.[16]

Early Debates

Specialization was not the most serious problem facing the medical profession; it popped up sporadically, provoking intense discussion for brief periods of time. The first such outbreak occurred from 1888 to 1893 before being displaced by seemingly endless discussion about professional regulation, reform of medical studies, and, above all, the new health insurance system. A second period of intense debate erupted in 1904 and lasted until 1909 before petering out. The tone of discussion differed substantially during the two periods.

In late nineteenth-century Germany, no one questioned that specialization in teaching and research was fundamental to the advancement of medicine.[17] Specialist practice, however, remained controversial. It was still common to defend the introduction of a subject into medical schools on the grounds that providing specialist knowledge to GPs was the best way to *prevent* specialist practice. A leader in his field, Albert Neisser, denied repeatedly that dermatology-venereology was a field of specialty practice.[18] Such views were to some degree a result of the logic of academic recognition; a place in curricula and examinations was justified by claims of relevance to the training of generalists. But they went deeper, and in some cases reflected profound hostility to expanding specialist private practice. Balancing the usual metaphors of "division of labor" and "industrial modes of production," utilized to characterize specialization, were themes of "wholeness" of knowledge and of the individual that remained powerful in Germany even as they were being ignored by the expanding universities. This allowed more sophisticated GPs to cast themselves as healers of the individual in all his or her complexity and to portray specialties as exclusively technical and even mechanical forms of practice.[19] Some wished for nothing less than the disappearance of specialties. But even at this relatively early date, the majority of critics usually admitted that specialty practice was an inescapable reality of modern medicine; rather than abolishing it, they hoped to correct or moderate its numerous abuses.[20]

By far the most common approach was to distinguish between "true specialists" and "pseudo specialists." The former were well trained in general medicine as well as in their specialty and sought to benefit patients and science; medical peers recognized their competence. Pseudo specialists, in contrast, were poorly trained, to the point of posing a danger to patients, to whom they appealed directly through advertising; they simultaneously refused to renounce general practice. Self-advertising was critical to this process because it fostered false claims of specialist competence and popular belief in the superiority of specialists over general practitioners.[21] The worst of the *Schwindler,* the "most vulgar species" of specialist, it was said, were those specializing in women's diseases, a field that attracted huge numbers of practitioners, many seeking to insinuate themselves as family physicians. Like the watchmaker or roofer, said one critic, the specialist in this field seldom had his work carefully scrutinized.[22] Equally pernicious were the numerous specialists of the larynx who, it was charged, would over a long period putter around the esophagus and larynx, claiming to improve the digestion of credulous patients.[23]

The critical question was what to do about these "pseudo specialists" or "six-week specialists" (referring to their brief training). The Brunswick *Ärztetag* of 1889 was unable to come to a decision about a course of action, but did pass a resolution prohibiting self-identification as a specialist; this prohibition was enforced by some local societies.[24] If it was fully enforced, the logic went, pseudo specialists would be unable to survive by appealing to the public. However, there were two weaknesses associated with this approach. It was, in the first instance, impossible to enforce; in the second instance, it displeased "true specialists," who could no longer make themselves known to their peers or the public. Preventing information from circulating, it was argued, might actually constitute a danger to public health in large cities.[25] It was noted that in the United States, medical societies enforced this kind of rule against specialist advertising, but this hardly constituted a ringing endorsement. In America, it was said dismissively (and in French, yet), "les extrêmes se touchent."[26] A number of alternative solutions were thus proposed for Germany.

The Prussian commission that planned the reform of medical examinations in 1891 suggested the establishment of a special examination to accredit specialists.[27] The issue was placed on the agenda of the Leipzig *Ärztetag* of 1892 in the form of a question: Should doctors be forced to pass a special state examination in order to call themselves specialists? The response was overwhelmingly negative.[28] Some speakers criticized the meeting organizers for giving this option credibility by even putting it on the agenda.[29] Many arguments justified the unequivocal dismissal of this proposal. No one was happy about the prospect of further state incursion into the medical domain.[30] Establishing a postgraduate degree would create two categories of doctors, it was argued, turning generalists into second-class practitioners and destroying the fragile professional unity that had recently been established. The public's belief that specialists were superior practitioners would be reinforced. Such examinations, it was predicted, would lead the courts to consider as malpractice all specialist procedures performed by those without certification. Specialists feared, in addition, that any form of licensing would be administered by local medical societies, frequently hostile to specialists, that would impose draconian conditions on specialist practice.

One of the draconian conditions that specialists feared most was a requirement that they renounce all forms of general practice. However, for many this was precisely the solution to the "pseudo specialist" problem that would render special state examinations unnecessary; it was recommended in the commission report that served as a reference for the meeting.[31] This measure, it was thought, would eliminate the incentive for announcing oneself as a specialist because one would no longer be able to advance a general practice in this way; nor would unqualified practitioners be capable of competing as exclusive specialists against the truly qualified. This solution was attractive to at least some general practitioners but was hugely unpopular among specialists and attracted little support at the *Ärztetag*. It was argued that few doctors, even among well-trained specialists in big cities, could as yet survive economically in exclusive specialist practice. Furthermore, such exclusiveness would harden divisions between specialists and general practitioners, ensuring that the former would not receive adequate general training and the broad perspective thought desirable, while making it impossible for generalists to gradually transform themselves through practical experience into specialists.[32]

Yet a third solution proposed that individuals be allowed to practice as specialists only after having spent at least three years in general practice. This recommendation inverted the reasoning behind the plan for specialist examinations. Rather than dividing the profession, the goal was to create stronger links between specialists and general practice. Experience in general practice would avert the "one-sidedness" that specialists were regularly accused of. The specialist familiar with general practice would fully understand just how tiny the domain of medicine that he or she cultivated was. [33] Unfortunately, this solution did not address the fundamental criticisms against "pseudo specialists": that they were incompetent in their specialty and competed unfairly against GPs. It simply assumed that this would not be the case.

Not surprisingly, the Leipzig *Ärztetag* of 1892 rejected all these solutions. Nor did it consider seriously a variety of more limited proposals, including one prohibiting doctors from calling themselves *Spezialarzt*, which to many implied superiority over GPs, in favor of more descriptive and neutral terms such as *Augenarzt* or *Chirurg.* [34] (This hostility to the term *Spezial,* we shall see, did not dissipate.) The only positive resolution that emerged from discussion was a vague statement to the effect that the abuses of specialism could be dealt with only through the advance of professional consciousness (*Standesbewußtsein*) and the gradual elaboration of comprehensive legal regulation of medical practice. [35] If there was general agreement about the need to combat the abuses of specialization, there was clearly no consensus about solutions.

Criticisms of pseudo specialists continued to appear regularly and gradually had some effect on what doctors admitted publicly; in 1909 only about one-third of the Prussian specialists inventoried, admitted to engaging in some form of general practice. Nonetheless, pressure to do something about the specialist problem continued to mount for several reasons.

First, the rapidity with which specialists and specialty categories were spreading proved deeply shocking to German medical leaders. The proportion of those identifying themselves as specialists in most large cities rose from 10 percent or less in the 1880s to anywhere from 30 to 45 percent by 1906. Only 11 percent of all specialists were older than fifty, and almost 35 percent declared they had had two years or less of specialist training. [36] Just as shocking was the growing number of specialist categories, most of which were not represented in universities, as more and more fields split off from internal medicine and surgery. [37] In the early twentieth century the *Reichs-Medizinal-Kalender* (RMK), we saw in the previous chapter, began allowing doctors to identify themselves as specialists, largely as a way of monitoring the spread of specialization. Since the editor of the *RMK,* Julius Schwalbe, was also editor of the *Deutsche medizinische Wochenschrift* (DMW), the leading medical periodical of the era, that journal was able to publish annual quantitative surveys of the medical profession. These frequently highlighted the growing number of specialists and culminated in calls for "an urgently needed" mechanism to regulate specialists.

Second, a consequence of the spread of specialists was intensification of conflict within the profession. Generalists' diffuse hostility to specialists turned into focused animosity when directed against pediatricians. Pediatrics was a relatively new and untested field in the first years of the twentieth century. GPs saw it as a direct form of competition different in kind from that of other specialties. The problem with many specialties was that practitioners *combined* them with general practice. Pediatrics *was* general practice, and provoked distinctive hostility.[39] Its position among specialties, moreover, was relatively weak: it could claim neither difficult technical procedures nor special skills nor specific organs. It was simply a form of general practice directed at children—older children who, moreover, did not appear all that different from adults. (Unlike pediatrics in France, which grew out of obstetrics and focused on newborns and infants, German pediatrics grew out of internal medicine and centered on older children.) If faculty positions in the field could be justified by the educational needs of medical students, the oft-repeated question "Is pediatrics a specialty?" was frequently answered in the negative. At most, more tolerant GPs and many specialists were willing to concede that pediatrics might be a consulting specialty based in hospitals. But there was no justification for home visits that impinged on the prerogatives of the family physician (*Hausarzt*). As time went on, such criticisms were increasingly directed at the expanding field of internal medicine as well.

Third, the conflict between GPs and specialists at the core of the *Spezialistenfrage* was being raised in another idiom by the intensified debate over reforms of the health insurance system. The organized profession overwhelmingly supported the idea of allowing members of insurance plans the freedom to choose from among all physicians in a locality, and fought bitterly against the widespread practice of appointing only small numbers of panel physicians to treat members. Bringing about this change was at the core of the profession's political strategy to mold the insurance system into something it could live with. Not only did this struggle require unity among practitioners, and thus a resolution of the specialist question, but it also raised the thorny issue of differential honoraria. An influential segment of the profession argued that the insurance funds (*Krankenkassen*) could afford to allow all doctors to participate in the insurance system only if specialists renounced the higher reimbursement rates now received by the few specialists with insurance practices. Free choice of physicians could become very expensive indeed if patients chose to visit specialists paid at existing rates. Many specialists were willing to accept equality of fees in order to obtain the right to participate in the insurance system, while others hotly contested this reasoning.[40]

For GPs, of course, the issue was simpler. Formal fee differentials, it was argued, pretty much served as a public declaration that general practice was worth less than specialist practice. Specialists responded that no issues of value were involved; that such differences merely rewarded specialists for renouncing general practice and seeing fewer patients. But to this traditional argument in favor of differential fees were sometimes added other, more controversial claims: that the work of specialists was harder and more time-consuming, and required greater concentration and skill than general practice. These arguments provoked vigorous protests from GPs and confirmed their fears that generalist work was devalued.[41] Specialists, for their part, felt that their interests in insurance matters were being neglected by existing medical associations.[42]

The final and probably most significant factor behind the increasing urgency of the specialist question was the fact that governments, in the absence of collective action by the profession, were beginning to take initiatives on their own. By 1904 the Prussian government was widely considered to be preparing its own solution to this problem, possibly through the introduction of state examinations.[43] There were several forces pushing it in this direction. The most critical had to do with the significant number of specialists now working in health insurance plans.[44] Defining competence was becoming a practical administrative necessity. In 1901, the Prussian government allowed the creation of private asylums to care for the insane. As part of the package, the administration was given responsibility over determining whether doctors working in these institutions had the requisite training in psychiatry.[45] It was, in other words, directly evaluating specialist competence. In subsequent years, the Prussian government's increasing role in health care created a demand for trained personnel to work in new programs being introduced. The next logical step would be to seek to ensure that those staffing these programs had the necessary competence.

We saw above that in 1891 the Prussian Commission to Reform Medical Examinations had proposed to establish examinations for specialists. Doctors raised a collective howl, and the idea was abandoned. However, at the turn of the century, Friedrich Althoff, the powerful and autocratic director of the Department of Higher Education in Prussia, developed a special interest in continuing and postgraduate medical training.[46] In 1901, he established a Prussian committee for postgraduate education; a year later a state collection of medical training aids was set up and located at the University of Berlin. And in 1903, a privately funded but state-supported foundation, the Kaiserin-Friedrich-Stiftung für das Ärztliche Fortbildungswesen, was set up with the idea that it would provide space for all the various activities being developed in this domain. None of this seemed particularly threatening until it was announced a year later that two academies of practical medicine were being set up, one in Cologne and the other in Düsseldorf. These academies were organized by municipal authorities in each city but were under the formal jurisdiction of the Prussian Ministry of Education, which, no one doubted, was the real power behind these initiatives. The goal was to use city hospitals (Düsseldorf had just built a new 1,000-bed institution) and other municipal clinical facilities for purposes of postgraduate training. This meant, first of all, the year of practical training demanded of all graduates wishing to become eligible for medical licensure; in the second instance, it meant specialist training. The academies were meant to be models for other cities, and there was talk of another one being planned for Frankfurt.

The response of the profession to these announcements and rumors was deafening.[47] Although the Cologne institution opened as scheduled in 1904, the opening of the one in Düsseldorf was delayed until 1907. The outcry forced Althoff's supporters to deny that his various initiatives in this domain were acts of centralization; far from being an intervention by the state, they constituted an innovation "von Kollegen für Kollegen. . . . "[48] And Althoff himself conceded that no more academies would be created until the experience in Cologne could be properly evaluated. (The Düsseldorf Academy was exempted from this promise because planning was already advanced.[49]) The Cologne academy was denounced in a presidential address at the thirty-second *Ärztetag* in Rostock and was a major subject of discussion a year later at the *Ärztetag* in Strasbourg, where it was the target of mostly negative comments. Among the numerous criticisms—that the new institution was too big, that it would destroy small hospitals and medical faculties, that military physicians and surgeons had been allotted too many places, that the staff would compete unfairly against local medical practitioners—one essential point stood out: that its founders had without appropriate consultation meddled in issues reserved for the organized profession; and one of the most critical of these issues was the training of specialists. After much discussion, the *Ärztetag* affirmed that the organized medical profession, independently of the political process, should resolve the problem of specialization. It was also resolved that specialists should practice their specialty exclusively.[50]

There were other troubling indications that the Prussian government intended to intervene. In 1904, it requested a report on specialists that eventually appeared in 1906. Based on doctors' answers to a questionnaire, the report identified 2,779 specialists in Prussia, excluding all university teachers; most of these specialists were inadequately trained for their specialty, with a third having had less than two years of appropriate training. The report repeated the usual criticisms that had been directed at such specialists in earlier decades. It also recommended that a comprehensive system of specialist regulation and training be introduced.[51] In 1907, the scientific delegation of the Prussian Ministry of Education made a similar recommendation, although the specific details of the report were not released until the following year.[52] This year of silence led many doctors to expect the worst. It is worth noting that the Prussian report of 1906 represents the first government-sponsored survey of specialists undertaken in any of the four nations examined in this book; for many years, Germany was the only one of these countries that collected official government statistics on this subject.

Other German states or provinces were doing more than making recommendations. An ordinance issued in 1902 by the government of Anhalt made the right to publicize specialty status dependent on passing an examination following two years of specialty training in a hospital or medical school.[53] By 1907, authorities in the states of Hamburg, Schleswig-Holstein, and Saxony were demanding some evidence of appropriate training from anyone wishing to call himself or herself a specialist.[54] Such pressures were not restricted to imperial Germany but extended as well to Austria.[55]

As in the United States, the German medical profession was viscerally hostile to all forms of state dirigisme in this domain; most doctors thus continued to reject the notion of state examinations for specialists and looked instead to professional organizations to introduce and administer the regulations that seemed to be required.[56] Some local medical groups came up with internal regulations that applied to their members. Thus in 1902, the Medical Chamber of the Rhineland decided that specialists were required to renounce all general practice; many other local medical societies and chambers announced similar rules.[57] But if state action was to be averted, the profession would have to come up with a national plan. During the next few years, many such plans were proposed and discussed.[58]

In reality, the Prussian government abandoned any effort to impose a political solution, if indeed it had ever had such a plan. In 1908, the Prussian Ministry of Religion and Medicine finally made public the recommendations of the scientific delegation that had been completed the previous year and that were based (though with major deviations) on a lengthy report by Professor H. Löbker, a major figure in the DÄV.[59] The plan called for seven recognized specialties; one could call oneself a specialist by producing documentary proof of at least three years of practical postgraduate training in the field. Much was left out, including the agency that would administer this plan and whether it was necessary to practice specialties exclusively. However, a commentary by the editor of the *Ärztliches Vereinsblatt für Deutschland* (*ÄVD*) claimed that the majority of the scientific delegation was of the opinion that "the *Spezialistenfrage* should be handled as a question for the medical profession (*eine ärztliche Standesfrage*)" and that the next step was for the issue to be taken up by professional organizations.[60]

The plan of the scientific delegation served as the basis for medical debate in local medical associations and chambers, which prepared numerous recommendations over the next few years. But Althoff's death late in 1908 may well have eliminated much of the urgency to resolve the issue; and, in any event, it became clear that little consensus existed within the profession. Many medical chambers and local associations rejected the delegation's proposals.[61] If nearly all doctors opposed formal examinations to judge specialist competence, the alternative was not clear. Many thought that even the simple evaluation of training credentials that had been proposed would, like a formal examination, divide doctors into two classes. Substantial numbers felt that any such measure was unnecessary because the number of unskilled specialists was in fact low and could be dealt with either by allowing the public to judge competence or by utilizing the normal disciplinary powers of medical associations.[62] And while most specialists wanted free access to patients in primary care situations, many GPs wanted most specialties to become forms of consultant or hospital practice exclusively.[63]

Although support for demanding the renunciation of general practice by specialists was clearly gaining momentum,[64] opposition to this measure continued to be fierce. Nor was there agreement about which specialties should be included in any certification process. Almost everyone wanted to keep numbers small, but deciding which categories qualified and on the basis of what principle was not easy.[65] The essential features defining a legitimate specialty—focus on specific organs, special technology or skill, a specific disease, therapy, or social need—became a common topic of medical debate. Some, such as Heinrich Quinke, took the liberal view that all these principles might define legitimate specialties[66]; most others picked one or two. For many, organ systems and technology were key.[67] Others saw "completeness" as the essential requirement of true specialties. Completeness might mean that both medical and surgical procedures had to be included within the boundaries of a specialty or that both diagnostic and therapeutic activities were required.[68] Given the actual heterogeneity characteristic of specialties, any effort to develop a classification based on abstract principles was doomed to failure. In the face of so many fundamental disagreements, and the absence of any imminent threat of government action to spur doctors on, debate over this issue gradually petered out.

Nonetheless, the general principles enunciated by the scientific delegation would gradually attract more and more support. It would take another fifteen years or so for a consensus to finally emerge around these principles. The debates of this period were also notable for planting another seed, this one semantic. During this entire period, we have seen, the specialist was called *Spezialist* or *Spezialarzt*, and the problem of specialties was the *Spezialistenfrage* or, increasingly, *Spezialarztfrage*. In 1909, two anonymous articles by Dr. W. from Brunswick on the debates of the day suggested a new nomenclature: *Facharzt* should replace *Spezialarzt* and the problem of specialists, the *Spezialarztfrage*, should become the *Facharztfrage*.[69] This suggestion was justified as part of a package of measures to diminish distinctions between specialists and generalists, which included equality of insurance fees.

Dr. W's objection to *Spezialarzt* was that it was a foreign word, "half Latin, half German," that should be replaced by a German word. *Facharzt*, which had been proposed by a dictionary of contemporary German usage,[70] seemed to him the best translation. But this was not merely a matter of linguistic purity or clarity. "The designation '*Spezial*' contains a critique of remaining doctors and represents . . . an advertisement [*Reklame*]"[71]; furthermore, the prototypical specialists, university professors, did not call themselves "Special Professors for . . .," so why should practitioners call themselves special doctors? *Facharzt*, in contrast, described a doctor practicing a particular division of medicine and not only implied absolute equality with general practitioners but even suggested that the specialist had mastered only a small part of medicine, while the generalist "treats the organism as a harmonious whole."[72] Dr. W's suggestion did not receive much attention at this time, but in the postwar years his nomenclature would be widely adopted as the proper designation for specialists.

The Bremen Guidelines

The early years of the Weimar Republic were intensely difficult for the German medical profession.[73] Postwar political instability and economic hardship added to the long-standing troubles of the profession. The number of practitioners nationally continued to increase, from 5 doctors per 10,000 population in 1911 to 6.67

in 1925; in Berlin it grew from 11 to 13.5 per 10,000 population; and in Munich, from 16.5 to 22.[74] Competition from unofficial healers also intensified.[75] With the worsening economic situation and a climate of limited resources, already intense conflicts with health insurance funds deteriorated further. The ability of doctors to stay independent of the insurance system shrank considerably in the face of consumers' lessened ability to pay for private medical care and the extension of insurance to those earning higher wages. Medical strikes become a fact of life in Weimar Germany. One response to what was perceived as the "crisis" of medicine was to blame others. Traditional medical hostility to Jewish colleagues assumed new and disturbing proportions.[76] Alternative and holistic forms of medicine, while increasingly popular everywhere, proliferated more widely in Germany than anywhere else in the Western world.[77]

But the democratic Weimar regime also offered new political opportunities to special interest groups. This, in combination with harsh economic realities, resulted in a plethora of reform proposals affecting all areas of medical practice. The health insurance system remained the most intensely disputed issue. The medical profession won a significant victory in 1931 when a right-wing government revamped the insurance system by establishing associations of insurance doctors to negotiate payment rates with insurance funds and distribute payments to doctors. This greatly strengthened the medical profession and weakened the insurance funds.[78] But this measure was only the tip of the iceberg. Many domains, ranging from public health to medical training, were the subjects of intense reform agitation.

The issue of specialization (now referred to the *Facharztfrage* because the word *Facharzt* had completely displaced *Spezialist* and *Spezialarzt* in the lexicon of professional associations)[79] was frequently implicated indirectly in these proposals. For instance, the active promotion of public health programs targeted specific diseases (tuberculosis, syphilis) or singled out segments of the population (children, pregnant women, "cripples," the insane) at the center of specific kinds of specialty practice.[80] Political pressures led to the spread of chairs of pediatrics in medical schools and the introduction of this subject as the third section of the *Prüfung* in internal medicine. This gave pediatricians considerable leverage against both internists and general practitioners who insisted that children were an integral part of their own domains of practice. Consequently, the proportion of pediatricians among all specialists rose from 4 to 8 percent between 1903 and 1937.[81] Campaigns against venereal disease led to the introduction of dermatology-venereology as the fourth section of the *Prüfung* in internal medicine.[82]

Some of the proposals being hotly debated during the immediate postwar years—notably the reform of medical training and the reorganization of state medical boards and honor courts—also touched on the issue of specialization. If irregular practitioners without diplomas and growing numbers of doctors were perceived as the chief causes of economic distress, the existence of so many competing specialists was nonetheless viewed as a serious problem. Medical anti-Semitism was also directly relevant to many specialties within which Jews were highly visible. The overspecialization of German medicine, it was argued, was a direct result of the excessive numbers of Jews within the profession.[83]

Discussion of reform in so many different domains had several major consequences for specialty certification. First, specialization emerged at regular intervals as a secondary issue and gradually become a primary focus of attention. Second, in the atmosphere of crisis that characterized this period, divisions within the profession came to be seen as a serious handicap that reduced the ability of doctors to intervene effectively in their many ongoing battles. Finding an acceptable solution to the specialist problem thus came to be viewed as an indispensable step toward achieving professional unity. Third, much of the profession's reform activity quickly became stalled in the complex political process and, later, by the crippling budgetary problems faced by the Weimar government[84]; this confirmed the profession's traditional determination to keep the issue of specialties outside the bounds of politics and state regulation. In fact, specialty certification appeared to be one of those rare reforms that might be implemented quickly and successfully by the profession itself.

In the years following the war, postgraduate courses directed at GPs and budding specialists proliferated.[85] In some cities, all categories of specialists came together in local associations. The association of specialists in Hamburg justified its foundation on the grounds that the coming battles against the health insurance funds required an "unbroken Phalanx of all German medical specialists as a particular group."[86] In 1921 several local medical chambers or associations undertook to elaborate their own regulations for determining specialist status.[87] A year later, specialist associations joined together to form a national specialist federation.[88] Not everyone was happy with this development. One writer argued that it divided specialists from generalists at a time when the profession needed to stand together against the "external enemy [äusseren Feind]."[89] But the creation of this new organization succeeded in bringing specialists' views to the forefront and was followed almost immediately by widespread debate about a comprehensive national system of regulation. The specialists' association published a draft plan and requested its widest possible discussion.[90] Two years later a comprehensive proposal was introduced at the Bremen Ärztetag of 1924. This was one of many controversial points of discussion—number 7, in fact—on a highly charged agenda of nine points that included the proposed unification of the DÄV with another association, the Hartmannbund, and the reform of the health insurance system. Several months before the meeting, the head of the specialists' association and a prominent general practitioner together prepared a comprehensive proposal for certifying specialties, under the banner of compromise and professional unity. It was then widely precirculated. One medical writer was pessimistic about its chances because too many controversial issues remained unresolved.[91] As it turned out, he was wildly wrong. The profession was by now prepared for compromise.

During the next months some opposition to the reform proposal emerged; it was argued that it set rules that were excessively detailed, formalistic, and dependent on paper credentials, and that the interests of generalists were not sufficiently protected.[92] Despite such misgivings, the profession was moving decisively toward an agreement. An article by a general practitioner published in the *Deutsche medizinische Wochenschrift* a month before the Bremen *Ärztetag* clearly expressed this emerging trend. Despite a highly critical tone that blamed misbehavior by specialists for most of the hardships faced by GPs, the article by the Königsberg physician O. Schellong[93] proposed a solution in the name of professional compromise and solidarity; this was based on the acceptance of formal training and certification for specialists, something that generalists had long opposed. In exchange for this concession, according to Schellong, three foundational requirements needed to be met: (1) Specialists had to restrict their practice exclusively to their specialty. (2) The number of specialties should include only those large fields recognized by and largely based in faculty and hospital clinics, and a few smaller, more recently established fields that were highly technological (orthopedics and radiology, for example). His list of recognized fields included thirteen specialist categories. Pediatrics, a traditional target of GP hostility, could continue to exist so long as it limited itself to children younger than six years of age. (3) Specialists were to receive serious training; this meant inevitably that the number of specialists was to decline substantially.

The proposal presented to the Bremen *Ärztetag* went some way toward satisfying these demands, in principle if not in all details. It was based on the guidelines proposed by the Prussian scientific delegation sixteen years earlier. The 313 delegates representing 298 medical associations passed the measure with minimal controversy, agreeing to introduce a system of specialty regulation that would become known as the Bremen *Richtlinien* (Guidelines).[94] Certification was to be introduced and controlled by professional institutions representing both specialists and generalists. Certification thus had no legal validity and depended for its application on purely professional sanctions. The *Ärztetag* also refused to make formal examinations the basis of specialist status. Such status would depend, rather, on the evaluation of an individual's qualifications by local medical societies. This gave general practitioners an influential voice in the certification process, to a degree that would not be duplicated in the United States. Although the two authors of the Bremen Guidelines had markedly different views about internal medicine (the generalist, Kustermann, saw the existence of a specialty devoted to this field as a "calamity [*Unheil*]," both agreed that it was to be restricted to consultant practice and not compete against general practice.[95] The entire process was considered part of the larger effort to achieve professional unity. A separate resolution that passed by an overwhelming majority stated: "The *Ärztetag* recommends the coming together of specialists and generalists, in the interests of establishing the unity [*Einigkeit*] of German doctors."[96] The gradual working out of these guidelines resulted in the following system of certification.

A candidate for specialty status had fourteen recognized specialties to choose from.[97] The exact content of the list was the subject of much controversy in the months preceding and following the *Ärztetag*.[98] Individual candidates for specialist status would apply to the local medical society, which decided, on the basis of documentary evidence presented, whether recognition in a particular specialty would be granted in *that locality*. Characteristically, the examining committees in Germany were divided evenly between GPs and specialists, with the addition of specialists in fields being examined who had a deliberative voice but no vote. The major requirement was evidence of adequate training: four years in surgery, obstetrics-gynecology, and internal medicine, and three years in the other specialties. This training would take place in university clinics, academies, specialist departments of larger hospitals, sanatoriums, and suitable private clinics. Proof of training was in the form of certificates signed by directors of clinics and detailing services performed. The candidate could appeal a negative decision to a regional council.

Once recognized, specialists had to confine themselves "essentially" (*im wesentlichen*) to the specialty and limit practice to office consultations and hospital services, leaving house calls to GPs. In order to further protect general practice, the boundaries of certain fields were established. Pediatrics, for instance, was defined as the care of children up to the age of thirteen. In an early edition of the draft proposal, faculty or hospital appointments in internal medicine defined internists, but this restrictive formulation disappeared from the final working paper discussed by the *Ärztetag*.[99] The terms used to describe specialties were codified and many common appellations disallowed. The claim to be a specialist in more than one field was not generally permitted except where combinations were common. And in some of these—surgery and orthopedics, surgery and gynecology—preliminary training was at least six years. In any case, such combinations were seen as a transitional option that would eventually be terminated. Local societies were granted leeway to determine many details; among these was the possibility of allowing individuals in exceptional circumstances to become recognized in fields not on the approved list of specialties. Although the Bremen Guidelines lacked legal force and anyone could continue to call himself or herself a specialist, the local association could exclude from membership anyone who did so without proper authorization.

Specialist regulation was clearly in the air throughout central Europe. In Czechoslovakia a system very similar to the one in Germany was set up almost simultaneously.[100] And several years later a comparable system was created in Austria.[101] In Hungary, a rather different kind of state system of regulation was established. Here the Ministry of Public Welfare, after consulting with medical associations, passed regulations having the force of law.[102] In North America, we shall see in the next chapter, American doctors were already in the process of setting up their own version of professionally controlled certification.

Implementation of the Bremen Guidelines occurred quickly; by late 1925, most large medical associations and physician chambers had accepted and implemented them. A survey by Friedrich Prinzing in 1926 estimated that only 10 to 15 percent of those claiming to be specialists did not yet have the proper credentials, with the incidence especially high in midsize cities.[103] The DÄV followed up on the regulation of specialties by introducing detailed guidelines on medical advertising, and on information that could be placed on doorplates and in directories.[104] Crucially for the success of this voluntary system, the health insurance funds accepted these criteria in determining which physicians were eligible to participate in their plans as specialists; their policy became formalized in the *Zulassungsordnung* of 1928.[105] Professional regulations also began insinuating themselves into the legal sphere, mainly through existing laws against false advertising that were used to prosecute individuals making public claims to specialty status.[106] Nonetheless, the lack of legal status for the Bremen Guidelines troubled some legal experts who questioned the legality of the profession's efforts to enforce compliance through internal professional discipline.[107] There were sporadic demands for a formal state approbation of specialties, and the move by Czechoslovakia in 1932 from profession-controlled to state-sanctioned specialist regulation was observed with great interest in the German medical press.[108] Nonetheless, the idea of placing certification under state control did not win the approval of many German doctors.

Working Out the Details

The Bremen Guidelines provoked a variety of practical problems that needed to be worked out; in the years just after their passage, Otto Stuelp (co-author of the guidelines) himself frequently judged disputes and problematic questions in the pages of the *ÄVD*. Later a special committee of the DÄV took up the task. The thorniest and most frequently recurring problems revolved around the compromise between specialists and generalists.

The latter became increasingly disillusioned with the Guidelines, arguing that they had done little to curtail the spread of specialties, improve the status of general practice, or end conflict.[109] A continuing source of friction was the prohibition of home visits by specialists, in one writer's words the "Conditio sine qua non for a tolerable state of affairs between specialists and generalists [*Praktikern*]."[110] GPs argued that the prohibition was being interpreted so liberally that it lacked all meaning.[111]

Specialists had their own complaints. According to Stuelp, GPs in some local societies imposed excessive restrictions on specialist qualification. In one case, he disputed decisions made by local professional bodies that allowed only lung specialists holding posts in hospitals and sanatoriums to become qualified.[112] Those in such fields as orthopedics, not recognized as fully autonomous categories, were disgruntled and continued to agitate for greater recognition.[113] Overall, however, specialists did not have a lot to complain about and recognized the sizable gains they had made. In conformity with the Bremen Guidelines they dissolved their specialist association in 1928.[114] This was to some degree a symbolic act since they were allowed to maintain associations of specialists on the local level, where most of the action was. They also went on to establish new associations dedicated to promoting their economic interests. Nonetheless, the symbolism was powerful and expressed general satisfaction with the new situation. Generalists, in contrast, pointedly refused to dissolve their association, which they perceived as vital to protecting their interests.

In 1928 the leadership of the DÄV moved to resolve the issue of home visits by specialists. A new set of guidelines was widely circulated and discussed before being presented at the forty-seventh *Ärztetag* in Danzig.[115] The new regulations sought to define relations among three groups with overlapping clienteles: generalists, internists, and pediatricians. Internists and pediatricians with hospital posts were to limit themselves to consultative and office practice. Those in private practice could make house calls, but only in cases directly relevant to their specialty and where patients were not capable of making office visits; they were expected to end such visits as soon as the patient was ambulatory. The plan stated clearly that the *Ärztetag* "considers it its obligation to declare explicitly that the German people must perceive the well and generally trained *Hausarzt* as its qualified adviser." At the same time, the reform sought to situate pediatrics more closely within internal medicine, requiring that at least one year of the four-year training program in pediatrics should be devoted to internal medicine. (The organ specialties associated with internal medicine were also linked more closely to the mother discipline by requiring that at least two years of the four-year training be devoted to internal medicine.) The age limit of children to be treated by pediatricians was left to the *Ärztetag* to decide.

Generalists were not satisfied with this tinkering along the edges of the Bremen Guidelines and demanded a much more radical revision. An alternative proposal was circulated before the meeting in Danzig. This version prohibited all house visits by specialists and restricted them to their field exclusively.[116] Training programs, it was argued, had to become more restrictive in order to reduce the influx of doctors into specialties.[117] But this alternative proposal was defeated at the Danzig *Ärztetag* of 1928, while the official submission was successfully passed.[118] The regulations resulting from the Danzig *Ärztetag* went some way toward satisfying generalists by tightening up use of specialist titles[119]; it was also decided that public positions for physicians in schools, welfare institutions, and inoculation programs were to be reserved for general practitioners and could be held by pediatricians only if GPs were not available.[120] (This latter provision, vehemently opposed by pediatricians, was eventually qualified somewhat.) The *Ärztetag* of 1933 passed a resolution forbidding any practice of general medicine by a specialist.[121]

Another issue that emerged from time to time was what to do about generalists who performed highly technical specialist procedures. Legally, any licensed physician was permitted to perform any medical act. But the intent of specialist regulation was to ensure specialized competence, especially where surgery was involved.[122] The DÄV and other professional bodies and associations had considerable influence in determining the solutions to these issues. But sometimes they were outflanked by the health insurance system, which could make unilateral decisions with major implications. In 1931–32, for instance, the insurance administration decided that only those specialists who had completed three years of training as "assistants" in a hospital (akin to residents) could be eligible for insurance practice. (GPs were required to have had a two-year assistantship.) This requirement was in some ways more stringent and specific than the regulations for normal specialty practice that gave practitioners a wide degree of latitude in obtaining specialist training, because hospital assistantships were relatively rare. As a result of this measure, the number of foreigners in such posts was reduced so that German specialists might fulfill their obligations.[123] But in other ways, the measure was less severe than official practices because certain specialties (surgery, among others) required *four* years of training. Some commentators worried that these new regulations would lead to a significant increase in the number of specialists.[124] Whether professional rules needed to be revised in the wake of the new insurance regulations was a subject of intense discussion in the medical press until National Socialism consigned it to insignificance.[125]

Local professional bodies wielded enormous influence. Sometimes this was perceived as unjust. Someone certified as a specialist in one locality might be refused certification if he or she moved to another. But local bodies also played a major role in working out the many ambiguities in the Bremen Guidelines. Resolution of boundary disputes among specialties often occurred at this local level. Could surgeons treat the pneumonia of patients on whom they had operated, or did they have to call in an internist? Who was responsible for treating pleurisy?[126] Where, exactly, was the boundary between gynecologists and surgeons?[127] Was sciatica the province of the internist or the neurologist?[128]

Specialist certification thus imposed a new logic on specialist relations. Nonetheless, the old logic centered on acceptance within medical education remained central, especially for newly emerging fields.[129] As in the past, nonmedical social groups might exert significant pressure to introduce into curricula relevant new fields, such as "accident" medicine.[130] On occasion the old logic of medical education clashed with the new logic of controlling specific domains of practice. In 1932, the central committee of the DÄV rejected a proposal by the National Association of Radiologists that any specialist who wished to utilize X-rays in his practice needed an extra two years of training in radiology. One reason advanced for this decision was the assumption that competence in the specialist uses of radiology could be obtained in the context of normal specialty training. But the judgment went farther; given the growing importance of radiological training in medical education (largely as a result of radiologists' insistence that these skills were necessary for all doctors), it suggested that there was no reason why X-rays should not become a generalized diagnostic procedure used by all doctors.[131] As a consequence, local medical authorities set up short courses in radiology for GPs rather than requiring two full years of extra training.[132]

It was thus impossible to abandon the logic that specialties were forms of knowledge that had to be taught to all doctors.[133] An intermediate position that was frequently proposed was that specialist practice should be consultative. GPs would perform diagnosis and routine therapeutic procedures while referring complex and difficult cases to specialists. The professor of ophthalmology in Berlin, in his inaugural lecture of 1935, justified this view at some length.[134] Specialists without elite posts, however, were loath to give up primary care, which constituted a significant part of their practice.

Battles over jurisdiction frequently combined issues of medical education with matters of practice. In the 1930s, a battle erupted between surgeons and orthopedists in which competition worked at many levels. While surgeons insisted that orthopedics was a branch of surgery limited to chronic problems of joints and limbs, orthopedists insisted that they constituted an autonomous specialty that should have sole responsibility over all the modalities of care given to "cripples" and all matters relating to the organs of support and locomotion, whether chronic or the result of injury; their proposals seemed to leave only internal organs to surgeons. But while these were crucial matters of practice to the extent that the health insurance system accepted one or another of these conflicting claims, more traditional issues were not ignored. Orthopedists claiming to be excluded from senior positions in medical schools argued for, while surgeons argued against, the introduction of obligatory lectures in orthopedics in the medical curriculum and the creation of a special examination in the field.[135] Given the inequalities of size and power between the two groups, the surgeons emerged victorious. In 1934, an agreement left orthopedics as an addition to surgery in academic courses and examinations. As far as practice was concerned, surgery was given responsibility over all relevant surgical procedures, while orthopedics was left with "bloodless actions and the utilization of orthopedic apparatuses. . . . "[136]

It was frequently noted and deplored that the combined efforts of GPs and specialists in private practice successfully restricted specialist practice. Leaders of the national DÄV regularly reminded local medical committees that using specialty certification to prevent practitioners from settling in the region was not the way to garner public support for the right of the medical profession to regulate itself.[137] But things were not much better at the national level; the fact that the national Ärztetage determined the list of recognized specialties had a profoundly negative impact on the emergence of new domains. By 1930, the widespread consensus that bacteriology and pathology required some form of certification was not being acted on, leading to suggestions that the Administrative Committee of the DÄV take over responsibility for deciding such matters.[138] Reluctance to recognize new specialties would continue to be a feature of German medicine throughout the twentieth century.[139]

By the end of 1932, the problems associated with the certification of specialists had accumulated to substantial levels. Among the worst were fluid boundaries between related specialties, professional associations' loss of power to the insurance funds and their inability to impose or enforce regulations on doctors who were not members, and inequalities caused by the local nature of certification. Convinced that the Bremen Guidelines needed revision and clarification, the DÄV began planning for another discussion of the subject at a forthcoming Ärztetag.[140] Discussion in the professional press again became very lively. In this context, it was finally decided in 1933 to do something about a transitional feature in the Bremen Guidelines that allowed certain specialties to be combined. Two common combinations—surgery with gynecology and dermatology with urology—were eliminated from the list of acceptable combinations.[141] And a year later the Prussian Medical Chamber prohibited all combinations of distinct specialties.[142] The Nazi seizure of power cut short all plans to reform the Bremen Guidelines.

Specialization Under the Nazis

The Nazi takeover of Germany transformed medicine in that country deeply and in ways that have shocked and perplexed historians, ethicists, and psychiatrists for more than half a century. Specialties were not immune to these developments. The persecution and elimination of Jewish physicians transformed many specialties that lost their leading figures.[143] Racial ideologies became prominent. The significance of congenital and hereditary diseases for Nazi ideology had a decisive influence on the practice of certain specialties. The Berlin professor of ophthalmology dwelt on this topic in his inaugural lecture of 1935, insisting that, second only to neurological and psychiatric illnesses, the most numerous congenital illnesses were those of the eyes. In view of what was eventually done in the name of eliminating hereditary illness, there is something blandly chilling in his claim that the family doctor who could discover congenital illnesses of the eyes within a family "in this way, prevents further, grave harm among descendants."[144]

I am not competent to enter into the difficult and painful issues raised by Nazi medicine and will limit myself narrowly to the regulation of specialties. Here change occurred in the midst of surprising stability. The organizations representing and holding power over the profession were transformed. And yet, the essential features of the system of specialties created by the Bremen Guidelines remained unchanged. Many Nazi medical leaders were deeply hostile to specialists and wished to reduce their number, redistribute some of them to rural areas, and encourage more young doctors to enter general practice. General practitioners, in the words of the head of the Berlin Medical Chamber, provided the foundation of the nation's health:

> Population policy, also military policy and the nation's health, are represented by the well-trained, selfless, consciously responsible general physician, especially the country doctor [*Landarzt*], dependent on himself alone, who masters all pains and illnesses of the countrymen entrusted to him, a personage who is so significant and irreplaceable that comparing his value to that of specialists is senseless and therefore impossible.[145]

But initial success in this respect (the proportion of specialists declined from one-third to one-quarter of the medical population in the first years of the regime) was temporary and due primarily to the exclusion of Jews from medicine.

The essential features of the Bremen Guidelines remained largely and surprisingly intact during the Nazi era, with only minor changes introduced as a result of other reforms. The relationship between the medical profession and insurance funds, already altered by the reforms of 1931, was permanently transformed by the Nazi in 1935, when they destroyed the leadership of the insurance funds and subjected the funds to state control; this left power effectively in the hands of the associations of insurance doctors, now organized nationally. (This was accompanied by the promulgation of a national physicians' regulatory code, long a goal of the organized profession.[146]) The creation of a new organization representing the medical profession, the Kassenärztliche Vereinigung Deutschlands (KVD) led to some modifications of the specialty system.[147] However, these changes deliberately stayed close to the existing regulations, which, it was admitted, represented the will of the medical profession and had essentially resolved the problem of specialties.

Most elements remained unchanged. The training time of several specialties was raised from three to four years. Leading hospital physicians were expressly forbidden to make house calls and were enjoined to hold all consultations in hospitals or clinics. The most significant change was to extend certification as a specialist to the entire country, so that it applied if a doctor moved to a new locality. In fact, the evaluating commissions in small localities were eliminated altogether. Judgment of credentials was now to take place in the provincial branches of the KVD.[148] At the same time, the rules now applied to every doctor in the country and not just to members of medical associations or those in insurance practice. These regulations reaffirmed that specialists—except for academics and heads of hospital departments, who were prohibited from this—might make home visits, but were on no account to act as *Hausärzte.*

Several months later, the grandfather clause that allowed specialists in fields not recognized by the Bremen Guidelines to continue to use these specialist titles was brought to an end.[149] Another reform introduced mandatory continuing education for doctors, in the form of a course in a hospital every five years.[150] This applied to everyone, and its goal was as much to inculcate National Socialist ideals as to provide practical training. Specialists were especially encouraged to study general medicine. In part, this reflected the desire to raise the status of general practice, but it had a practical dimension as well. As war loomed on the horizon, one justification for training in general medicine was its usefulness for the future military physician, who would then be versatile enough to function in a variety of positions and contexts.[151]

Continuing structural reforms also forced authorities to reconsider aspects of specialist governance. Regulations determining participation by doctors in the insurance system (*Zulassungsordnung*) appearing in 1934 and a new code of medical practice (*Reichsärzteordnung*) introduced in 1935 and 1936 changed some of the rules of the medical game. The 1934 regulations, for instance, introduced a quota—1 doctor per 600 inhabitants—and limited the proportion of specialists in any jurisdiction to 40 percent. Above these limits, permission to participate in the insurance system might be denied. Under such conditions, formal certification of specialists might become a rather moot point.[152] The *Reichsärzteordnung* of 1936 created a new national medical chamber, the Reichsärztekammer, with responsibility over all postgraduate training. This measure finally (though not definitively) gave professionally controlled certification of specialists the force of law.[153]

Other minor revisions of the regulations governing specialists were introduced in the following years.[154] More important, the prohibition on combining a specialty with general practice was strengthened. "The specializing physician is now as a matter of fundamental principle excluded from general practice: he must virtually limit his activities to his own particular discipline and never permit his work to develop into a general family practice."[155] In response to the new interest in various forms of alternative medicine, naturopathy (*Naturheilverfahren*) and homeopathy were recognized as specialist categories under the Nazis, as was tropical medicine (for rather different political reasons).[156]

World War II raised the status of specialists, as acute shortages of competent physicians forced military and civilian authorities to compete for their services.[157] Income rose substantially for all doctors during the Third Reich. But as was the case in other countries, specialists benefited especially. Michael Kater cites the following figures from the city of Brunswick: in 1943 generalists earned RM 12,350 while specialists earned 19,300. Not surprisingly, surgeons received the highest fees.[158]

Conclusion

In spite of the close identification of specialties with academic medicine in that country, Germany was the first of the four countries under discussion to develop a comprehensive system of specialist regulation. This was largely due to a unique set of political circumstances that encouraged early discussion of the subject and pushed the national professional association to seek wide-ranging reforms in a variety of domains. The severity of the crisis they faced after the Great War encouraged German doctors to overcome deep divisions and achieve consensus on this issue. The relative speed with which this was implemented reflected the tactics chosen. The German medical profession chose the path of least resistance; certification was professionally controlled, avoiding the pitfalls and delays inherent in the political process. National guidelines tended to be general, leaving details and interpretation to be worked out by local professional bodies. This strategy permitted quick implementation of specialist regulation and also left considerable power in the hands of local professional associations—including general practitioners—rather than specialist societies. The significance of this latter choice becomes clearer when we examine the American case.

Chapter 7
Regulating Specialists the American Way

Interest in specialty training and certification emerged in the United States a few years after its appearance in Germany. Unlike the system of regulation that emerged in the latter nation after many years of debate and that was associated with a single national set of guidelines introduced in 1924, American doctors began almost immediately to implement certification in a piecemeal way. Consequently, a comprehensive system of specialist certification was gradually introduced over a period of two decades. As was the case in Germany, a national medical association preoccupied with all aspects of medical practice played a central role in these developments. The organized American profession was acting from a position of increasing political strength that allowed it to move from success to success. Furthermore, the interventions of the American Medical Association (AMA) into the affairs of individual specialties went significantly beyond the actions of other national medical associations. Nonetheless, for all its power and accomplishments, the AMA, unlike the Deutsche Ärztevereinsbund (DÄV) in Germany, did not fully dominate the issue of specialist certification. It was only one of several forces and organizations that sought to shape specialist certification in the United States. The AMA's efforts were in large measure reactions to initiatives taken by specialist associations led by academic elites.

Despite the fact that both systems were set up by medical professions acting independently of the state, the American system of regulation was quite different from the one set up in Germany. While the German profession rejected examinations as a requirement for specialist status and preferred instead the evaluation of training credentials, the American system was based on examinations. While uncertified German doctors found it difficult to identify themselves publicly as specialists, American doctors faced no such restrictions. Finally, in Germany the entire medical profession, organized locally and nationally, administered specialist regulation; in the United States, national specialist organizations played a predominant role, with the result that much less was conceded to GPs.

Disciplines to Specialties

Specialist practice provoked substantial criticism in the United States during the second half of the nineteenth century, as we saw in chapter 4. Nonetheless, specialization here, as elsewhere, was justified primarily as a requirement of medical science and education for general practitioners.[1] Certainly boundary conflicts emerged, and numerous speeches and papers addressed the issue of when a patient should be referred by the GP to a specialist. Nonetheless, specialist societies, as well as the AMA, had as their declared goal the development of specialist science. During the first decade of the twentieth century, the specialist sections of the AMA remained preoccupied with improving the quality of presented papers and ensuing discussions at annual meetings.[2] However, the rapid expansion of the specialist population provoked the same concerns with regulating practice that had emerged a decade earlier in Germany.

Detailed statistics did not become widely publicized until after the First World War, when information in the *American Medical Directory* and a series of studies about recent American medical graduates documented the extent of specialty practice.[3] But overall trends were clear well before then. The reorganization of the AMA in 1901 created a much more effective, unified, and representative professional association with greatly expanded membership and increasing capacity to tackle difficult issues.[4] Its chief activity during this period, reforming medical education and licensing, was producing more standardized medical practitioners who took longer and spent more money to complete their training than had their predecessors. Having made such investments in their education, they were understandably attracted to the most prestigious and lucrative forms of practice—increasingly, specialist practice.[5] Reforms of medical education also encouraged the emergence of larger, more all-inclusive medical schools containing all the resources, disciplines, and personnel now thought to be imperative; this further intensified pressures for increasing disciplinary specialization. Growing numbers of specialist academics served as professional models to more and more students. Once these developments were well under way, the place of specialist practitioners within this reconstituted profession emerged as the next order of business.

The older question "What counts as an academic specialty?" remained central. It was asked by curriculum committees, editors of medical directories, and, increasingly, medical associations. Some specialties continued to define themselves in traditional terms, emphasizing their role in developing new medical knowledge and diffusing this knowledge in medical schools: "The idea of investigation, therefore, is fundamental in the conception of the real specialist, whether he be a specialist in medicine or in another subject. The problems in clinical medicine which more often attract the practicing physician differ only in kind from the problems which the distinctly laboratory worker sets out to solve." The true specialist, the author continued, "must identify himself with scientific medicine and win his spurs by making some real contribution to medical science."[6] This required substantial training in research, preferably in a university department; in the absence of such training, "the nearest approach to a scientific contribution, from so many who share this advantage of working in restricted fields, is the more or less garbled case report."[7]

Pediatrics provides a notable example of a specialty in which many leading practitioners identified themselves in such terms until well into the twentieth century. The first generation of American pediatricians, led by Abraham Jacobi of New York City, viewed pediatrics not as an autonomous specialty but as part of general medicine, with the pediatrician acting as a partial specialist outside the academic milieu. To some degree, this was a result of the same forces that made the specialty so controversial in Germany (and also encouraged there the definition of the field as an academic discipline); it dealt with a particular age group and borrowed most of its procedures from other branches of medicine. (However, it seems not to have aroused the same degree of animosity in the United States as it did in Germany.) A second generation of specialists around the turn of century was, according to Sidney Halpern, preoccupied with enlarging and consolidating its place as an autonomous discipline within reforming medical schools.[8] The academic status and achievements of the field thus assumed primacy in professional rhetoric.[9] But the application of this pediatric knowledge was the task of general medicine. "[A]lthough often referred to and practiced as a specialty, pediatrics belongs, not to the few, but essentially to all practitioners of medicine, for they [general practitioners], rather than the specialist, are called on to apply its teachings in family practice to the vast majority of infants and children."[10] Internal medicine provoked very similar kinds of professional rhetoric.[11]

Pediatrics and internal medicine were in many respects unique. But in the context of the educational reforms stirring the American medical profession, leading figures in almost every specialty cast their claims to status in similar terms. Neurologists maintained that the various fields in which they worked should not be seen as "highly specialized branches," but as fundamental to clinical medicine and necessitating a more central role in the education of medical students.[12] One of the dominant figures in the newly emerging field of neurosurgery, Harvey Cushing, advanced a particularly dynamic view of his subject and of surgical specialties more generally. Not only were they not domains of practice, they were not even stable academic disciplines. In his view, each arose around a new discovery or technology, then enjoyed a period of creative development, after which both the field and its achievements would be reabsorbed into general surgery.[13] Psychiatry, too, became increasingly preoccupied with its potential contributions to medical education. Widespread interest during the 1930s in curing "maladaptation," and new interest in "psychosomatic" factors in disease, provided psychiatrists with effective arguments for ending their traditional isolation from medicine and increasing their role in general hospitals and medical schools.[14]

Emerging technical specialties such as radiology frequently insisted on their potential role in training doctors and on the imperative that they become recognized academic departments.[15] Institutional acknowledgment of this sort was especially critical in a field that was highly technical and in which lay practitioners continued to function. But the rationale given for efforts to integrate medical schools was sometimes less the needs of generalists than "educating the profession and the public to the fact that a real radiologist has to be more than a photographer. He should be a very versatile general practitioner specializing in radiology. All of us know that no specialty in medicine requires a greater knowledge of general practice than does radiology. . . . "[16]

Anesthetists made claims of this sort based on the increasing use among general practitioners of medications for the relief of pain and the "management of depressed states," traditionally areas of anesthetic expertise, it was claimed:

> By anesthesiology is meant not only the science of the administration of drugs for the comfort of patients during operations but also the management of patients in depression from other causes. Pneumotherapy, intravenous therapy, therapeutic and diagnostic procedures involving the use of anesthetic drugs, and other efforts based on similar scientific knowledge, logically fall within the scope of anesthesiology. Clinical instruction in this subject is sound educational policy in the broad training of every physician.[17]

A study of obstetrics published in 1912 adopted this traditional perspective and focused on the inadequacies—indeed, the incompetence—of most of those who taught the subject in medical schools (many of whom were general practitioners), as well as the general lack of resources and facilities in obstetrical departments; consequently "the average practitioner, through his lack of preparation for the practice of obstetrics, may do his patients as much harm as the much-maligned midwife."[18] One of the most powerful arguments against midwives was not that they took work away from doctors but that proper obstetrical training for medical students was impossible so long as so much of the clinical material (75 percent was a figure commonly cited, and this predominantly among the poor) that might be used for training of medical students was monopolized by midwives who contributed nothing to the advancement of obstetrical knowledge.[19]

Academic arguments of this sort were presented in Germany as well, but since there was great distance between the elite preoccupied with medical schools and specialist private practitioners, there was a sharp distinction between such academic discourses and those focusing on monopolizing domains of practice. The gap between the two groups and discourses was far less wide in the United States. Academic specialists expected to be called in by the attending generalist as a consultant in particularly difficult cases, and many addresses to professional associations reiterated this point. Elite obstetricians, like other academic specialists, were willing to concede normal cases to GPs; difficult births, however, needed to be assigned to "specially trained men connected with well-equipped hospitals." And these practitioners, it was sometimes suggested, should be allowed to practice only on the basis of licenses granted by state boards of health.[20] Other specialties were even more insistent on their right to treat difficult cases. A presidential address to the AMA Section of Laryngology and Otology went on at some length about the scientific contributions of specialties to the medical knowledge required by general physicians. Nonetheless, the speaker eventually slipped into this second mode by arguing that generalists needed above all to recognize when referral to a specialist was necessary. Here the justification was the greater skill and efficacy of the specialist. "He can not fail to recognize, therefore, the equally important fact that when years of tireless study and energy are concentrated on one special branch of medicine, the physician who devotes himself to this special study must needs be more capable of diagnosing and treating successfully the diseases comprised in that specialty."[21]

This understanding of specialties as forms of practice bringing greater efficacy could be expressed even more emphatically. In a speech of 1911, Hugh Cabot defined a specialty as a field devoted to an organ, organ group, or group of conditions. While he recognized the advancement of medical science as an important function of specialties, he also based his claim for their legitimacy on the development of "intricate and difficult methods of diagnosis and treatment." He argued, for instance, that specialists in urological surgery enjoyed greater success than general surgeons; in prostatic conditions, he claimed operative mortality for the former was 6 percent and for the latter, 15 percent.[22] This language of efficiency made increasing rhetorical use of such notions as "division of labor," "industrial efficiency," and "scientific management" as justifications for both specialization and new institutional arrangements.[23]

Ophthalmology presented especially grand claims to practical skills and physiological knowledge:

> In diagnosis the ophthalmologist must master special instruments and methods, the trial set, the ophthalmoscope, the perimeter, the transilluminator, the tonometer, the varied muscle tests. These diagnostic attainments cannot be surpassed for refinement and importance in any other branch of medicine. What procedures in surgery require such delicate exactness, more intelligent planning or more carefully elaborated technic than the extraction of cataract, iridectomy or the plastic operations in the lids?[24]

Little wonder that many of its practitioners were beginning to believe that ophthalmology could not be practiced without special and standardized training.

The years before World War I were transitional for the image of specialists. To a considerable degree, specialists continued to be identified with academic medicine, elitism, and knowledge production; practice outside the hospital meant consultation in difficult cases. A letter to *JAMA* in 1907 described the chief division within American medicine as one between "the Established Specialist and the College Professor," on the one hand, and the "General Practitioner or the Developing Physician," on the other.[25] Leaders of the AMA saw things rather differently, but nonetheless recognized that its specialty sections were poised delicately between two competing visions. In one, they provided specialist knowledge to GPs, and thus papers had to be of general interest. In the other, they had to appeal to those among AMA members who were among "the most highly trained medical scientists in the country," requiring "opportunity . . . to meet each other in discussion and to share with each other work of so highly special a nature that it is of necessity beyond the grasp of many members of the Association."[26] An indication that the traditional role of specialties in educating GPs was losing some of its pertinence was the decision in 1918 not to routinely publish in *JAMA* papers presented in the specialty sections; this decision was taken on the grounds that most of these papers were not in fact of interest to general practitioners.[27]

There were many reasons for the changing self-image of American specialists. The movement of patients from GPs to specialists, as well as the swelling tide of doctors into specialties, reflected the conclusive victory of the belief that specialized expertise was the highest form of scientific medical knowledge. There had always been specialists who were primarily practitioners. But their number grew with astonishing speed during this period, generating new forms of collective identity. Fields such as ophthalmology, neurosurgery, and radiology had in fact developed complex procedures that were difficult to master and that clearly set their practices apart from those of GPs. Public health measures and philanthropy allowed several other fields to become strongly oriented toward primary care.

Pediatrics constitutes a classic example of this last process. The development of the Infant Welfare Movement after World War I provided pediatricians with a practical basis for a new kind of identity based on specialist practice. Rather than on specific clinical or diagnostic procedures, pediatric practice and identity were based on advice offered to parents of healthy children, and on the "right and duty of the pediatrist to guide, direct and develop this educational work" by determining "just what is best and right to teach. . . . " One positive outcome of this work, it was suggested, would be to expand private pediatric practice among "the babies of the well-to-do."[28] Sidney Halpern has convincingly argued that child-health centers were in fact instrumental in creating new demand for private pediatric practice; the number of full- and part-time pediatricians rose from 879 in 1914 to 4,371 in 1938.[29] Much the same occurred in other fields such as psychiatry, given new life by growing concern with mental health, and orthopedics, stimulated by new interest in rehabilitating disabled soldiers and children.[30] Even so technical a field as cardiology, it has been suggested, grew initially out of public health concerns to provide care to the poor; the Association for the Prevention and Relief of Heart Disease, founded in 1916, which became the National Heart Association in 1925, was based on the model of the National Tuberculosis Association.[31]

The shift from an academic to a practice-oriented perspective was gradual. Rather than one vision replacing another, individuals and associations shifted from one to another according to context. Representatives of each specialty or would-be specialty continued to insist on the centrality of their organ to general medicine and to a wide variety of systemic illnesses. Questions about of the place of each specialty in the medical curriculum lost none of their pertinence. Medical schools in fact became collections of specialized departments, generating by the second half of the century serious problems for the development of a coherent medical curriculum.[32] However, other questions now assumed equal prominence. One of the most controversial had to do with determining precisely which procedures were parts of the recognized domain of any specialty. Specialists felt an almost reflexive need to expand the scope of their specialty practice. Roentgenologists insisted that their role was not merely to take pictures but also to function as consultant diagnosticians, utilizing not just roentgen rays but "all the latest forms of examination."[33] Dermatologists claimed surgery of the skin and anxiously asserted traditional claims over syphilis, burns, erysipelas, and other conditions that they feared were slipping out of their grasp.[34] Some pediatricians claimed child psychiatry, and gynecologists laid claim to all abdominal surgery.[35] Assertions of relevance to public health frequently accompanied such demands. Public interest in the rehabilitation of injured soldiers and child "cripples" during the interwar years provided orthopedists with the leverage necessary to demand responsibility for all serious fractures and industrial accidents.[36]

With endearing bluntness (and genuine sociological acumen) the chairman of the AMA's Orthopedic Section summed up the fundamental nature of competition among specialties:

So long as a specialty is contributing to the advancement of knowledge, it tends to hold its ground, and to advance its borders. When it stops, other specialties encroach on it. It must take up new ground to avoid absorption either piecemeal by other specialties, or bodily by general medicine and by general surgery. Such a change of ground we have witnessed recently in gynecology. Whether the gynecologists can maintain their new position remains to be seen. If they succeed to the field of abdominal surgery, they will succeed to it, not by claiming that they are entitled to it, but by demonstrating that they are best equipped to hold it. When in my childhood's happy days I would say to my esteemed parent that I was "entitled" to this or to that, he would answer: "My son, you are entitled to just what you can get."

Orthopedic surgery was born to a strenuous life, and has held its borders, never sharply defined, by constant struggle.[37]

The precise relationship between related fields such as gynecology and obstetrics, ophthalmology and ORL, psychiatry and neurology was also frequently a subject of dispute. Some of these will be discussed at greater length in chapters 10 and 11.

As increasing numbers of doctors presented themselves as specialist practitioners with unique skills, it became clear that many of them had little training to justify such claims.[38] As in Germany, and often in exactly the same terms, these "six-week specialists" and "pseudo specialists" were characterized as a menace to the public.

Furthermore, it was becoming evident that the number of specialists had become excessive. At certain elite schools from two-thirds to three-quarters of all graduates were becoming full-time specialists.[39] Demands for appropriate training inevitably led to an even more basic and relatively new sort of question: "Who, exactly, counts as a specialist?" Specialties that faced competition from other professions— ophthalmologists who competed against opticians, stomatologists who were seeking to integrate dentistry into medicine, pathologists and radiologists competing against nonmedical providers of the same technical services—were especially preoccupied by such issues.[40] But so were growing numbers of specialists in ORL, surgery, and other fields in which practitioners believed they possessed unique skills.[41]

Domains that led to government jobs, notably in public health, were at the forefront of graduate university training. By 1914, six universities, including Harvard and the University of Pennsylvania, had established programs leading to a doctorate of public health.[42] Also in 1914 the University of Minnesota established a two-year graduate course in diseases of the eye, ear, nose, and throat.[43] Other specialties were introduced, and by 1917, seventy-five Minnesota graduate students had passed through or were still in the program.[44] That same year, Minnesota granted its first degree of Doctor of Science in pediatrics; this was the first post-MD doctorate in a clinical subject.[45] The aim of the Minnesota program, which combined a clinical assistantship with research, was to train teachers and researchers who would then go on to train not GPs, but other specialists. "At the present time one may perhaps regard our effort as an officers' training school preparatory to the larger work that must attend the drilling of the entire army of specialism, a task gradually to be accomplished."[46]

Many strategies for implementing this task were proposed. Some, such as the Minnesota plan, focused on university postgraduate programs and aimed at producing a scientific elite; others proposed state licenses based on examinations; yet others thought that it might be possible for medical students to follow a specialty track within a reorganized undergraduate medical curriculum. But after much internal debate, the American profession eventually opted for certification controlled by specialty groups; these specialty credentials would lack formal legal authority but could be made effective through the coordinated action of elite medical institutions.

The rejection of mandatory state certification was in large part a product of political conditions in the United States. Because the states held powers in this domain, a national system was virtually out of the question. Even the less radical solution of establishing professional boards granting specialist certificates and then seeking to convince state licensing boards to make these certificates legal requirements for specialist practice was rejected, "[o]n account of the complete independence of state licensing boards with various standards . . . ."[47] At a time when government-sponsored health insurance seemed a terrifyingly real possibility, many in the profession, like their counterparts in Germany, were deeply hostile to the principle of state involvement in the training and recognition of specialists.

Toward Professionally
Controlled Certification

As would also be the case in France, pressures to identify competent specialists began with surgery, the area of medicine that had changed most radically during the previous half-century. Not only were surgeons now attempting many new and extremely dangerous procedures, but the number of full-time surgical specialists—traditionally small in the United States—was growing rapidly due to the widespread creation of new hospitals.[48] Furthermore, general surgery was gradually losing large areas of practice to narrower surgical specialties, including gynecology, ophthalmology, and neurosurgery.[49] These developments provoked concerns about the role that would be left for general surgeons if current trends continued. Solutions proposed in the name of protecting patients from unqualified surgeons included introduction of a referral system on the British model, restricting surgical appointments in hospitals to small numbers of highly qualified individuals (as was the case in much of Europe), and setting up a system of formal licensing. In the end, American surgeons took matters into their own hands and opted for a system of elite peer recognition that would serve as a model for other specialty groups.[50]

In 1913, the American College of Surgeons was established by a group of prominent surgeons inspired by the example of the British royal colleges. Those recognized as possessing appropriate surgical skills were appointed fellows of the College. Although its apparent elitism provoked considerable hostility, the College eventually proved successful because it was generous and inclusive in granting membership. Initially, 1,059 fellowships were awarded; by 1914, 2,700 fellows had been selected. Henceforth, examinations following the fulfillment of specific training prerequisites became the requirement for admission. The College also campaigned against fee-splitting in cases of referral, and for hospital reform and standardization. The latter movement was particularly critical because one of the major requirements for the certification of hospitals was that they hire College-certified surgeons.[51] Their success in this endeavor substantially advanced the cause of certification. The AMA remained for the most part friendly to the College, at least in part because of some overlapping of leadership between the two organizations; perhaps more crucially, the AMA was also being led by its educational policies in the direction of specialist standardization.[52]

The establishment by internists of the American College of Physicians in 1915 followed the model of the College of Surgeons but proved less influential. Internal medicine was at that point a smaller field than surgery and was dominated by academic physicians. The latter saw little need for a college providing recognition to competently trained practitioners since, like European academics, they were already distinguished by prestigious institutional affiliations. Although 518 fellows were appointed before 1920, examinations were not instituted. This college remained essentially a high-level specialty society that published the prestigious *Annals of Medicine*.[53]

Ophthalmologists were in a better position to advance the process of specialty certification. Not only did they constitute a high-status and relatively large specialty group, but they had for the past several decades been engaged in a struggle against opticians and GPs over who was competent to do examinations for refraction. Without recognized standards in ophthalmic practice, specialists were vulnerable to the charge that they had no greater claim to expertise than their rivals. In 1916, the American Ophthalmological Society, the American Academy of Ophthalmology and Otolaryngology, and the AMA Section of Ophthalmology collaborated in setting up a joint certification board. Most of the certificates were awarded on the basis of credentials and experience, and a few were awarded on the basis of examinations. By the end of 1925, these flexible standards had resulted in the certification of 501 physicians, over one-third of all American doctors who called themselves ophthalmic specialists.[54]

The AMA added a distinctive new element to the organizational efforts of specialist associations. The original justification for its own specialty sections was to present the results of specialist knowledge to general practitioners; but, as we saw, these sections were increasingly being run by specialists for specialists. The Association was already in a small way in the business of recognizing specialties and specialists. The pages of *JAMA* and the published *Proceedings* of the sections served as a major forum for the diffusion of specialist claims. The decision to establish a specialist section, or occasionally to eliminate one, was of momentous consequence for the status of a specialty.[55] The AMA even published a number of prestigious specialty journals, including *Archives of Internal Medicine, American Journal of Diseases of Children,* and *Archives of Neurology and Psychiatry.*[56] Equally significant for the legitimacy of specialty groups were the decisions of the *American Medical Directory* about which specialties it would recognize as legitimate categories for self-identification. By 1918, such decisions were being made by the AMA's board of trustees,[57] which in effect imposed conditions on who could call himself or herself a specialist in this significant publication. The *Directory* also distinguished between full-time and part-time specialists, which added potentially significant information to the informal judgments of specialist competence that doctors were constantly making. The AMA, within which specialists were becoming increasingly powerful, if not dominant,[58] was clearly moving in the direction of recognizing competent specialists in some more formal way.

As it turned out, the AMA proposed a rather different kind of certification procedure than did the specialty organizations. After 1913, the AMA's Council on Medical Education and Hospitals, largely dominated by medical academics, became seriously concerned with the standardization of graduate medical education. In 1916 it made a complete inspection of graduate medical schools, and repeated the exercise in 1919 and again in 1923. The Council's concept of specialty certification was the establishment of a national system, covering all specialties and controlled by university medical schools.[59] By 1923, many of the postgraduate schools had, on the Council's recommendation, discontinued certificate programs lasting less than six months.[60]

As was the case in other nations, America's entry into World War I added further urgency to concerns about specialist regulation. The surgeon-general cited "the modern development of specialism" to justify the establishment of a military Division of Internal Medicine that included more specialized sections. This reflected the traditional link between ideas of military efficacy and specialization, as well as the need to get highly trained specialists to apply for commissions by assuring them that they could continue to work in their accustomed fields.[61] To actually run specialized institutions of military medicine, the surgeon-general granted considerable power and recognition to leading specialists. This policy greatly disturbed the leaders of the AMA. Said one: "A small coterie of specialists, of gynecologists and surgeons, no matter how eminent or how successful they may have been as promoters and exploiters of special medical societies, can in no way in this great emergency and in this great democracy represent the medical profession."[62]

Nonetheless, the attitude taken by the military established clearly that specialist power in the United States resided in the leadership of specialty societies rather than in general medical associations. This situation, so different from conditions in Germany, would have a momentous impact on the form that specialist certification would eventually take. A more immediate effect was that specialist appointments to the military health service were determined by examinations; the results showed that large numbers of declared specialists were pretty much unfit to practice.[63] Those deemed "not qualified but . . . too good to be discarded summarily" were assigned to "salvage classes" where they were brought up to a minimally defined standard.[64] To deal with immediate needs, intensive training was provided for specialists in a variety of fields. This training underscored the need for clear standards of competence and simultaneously provided concrete and sometimes innovative models for specialist training.[65] In orthopedics, for instance, standardized training programs for military physicians were established at a number of university medical schools; by the end of the war, 700 medical officers had passed through them.[66] The military medical experience, it was later argued, changed the mentality of those who went through it; individuals "who experienced the profound comfort and satisfaction of thorough, accurate, scientific work, possible only in such groups of consulting specialists, are little likely to return with equanimity to their former custom of attempting individually to cover the whole field of medicine."[67] During the 1920s, the military continued to encourage specialization within its ranks. Courses of instruction leading to specialist posts in military hospitals were made available to Navy medical officers.[68] Developments in the military also influenced specialties in other ways. Jack Pressman has argued that the unification of military psychiatrists and neurologists, brought about by Thomas Salmon during the Great War, prefigured the coming together of these two fields in the postwar years under the aegis of Adolf Meyer's interpretive psychobiology.[69]

In civilian medicine, during the 1920s the regulation of specialties developed slowly, in part because so many institutions were pulling in different directions. In 1920, the AMA Council on Medical Education set up fifteen committees, each devoted to a particular specialty, to develop curricula for both undergraduate and graduate training. Eleven of these were devoted to clinical fields and four others were devoted to basic sciences such as anatomy and physiology. The committees initially published widely divergent training requirements, but in 1923 the Council published its *Principles Regarding Graduate Medical Education,* which set out optimal conditions for graduate programs concerning length of training, admission requirements, supervision, curricula, and qualified teachers.[70] On the basis of these guidelines, the Council inspected and approved graduate programs. From 1924, it also inspected and approved hospital residency programs, the other, and increasingly dominant, locus of specialty training.[71] The results of this work of inspection were published lists of approved graduate schools and residency programs. By 1925, the Council had approved thirty-five graduate schools and sixteen special hospitals.[72] Specialties with the largest number of programs were otolaryngology, surgery, ophthalmology, public health, and neurology/psychiatry.[73] Five years later, the Council listed 338 hospitals offering over 2,000 residencies.[74] And by 1940 the number had risen to 587 hospitals with 5,120 residencies and fellowships.[75] This represented an increase of eighty-four hospitals and over a thousand residencies from the year before.[76] And this growth showed no sign of abating. "A steadily increasing number of young physicians are seeking the direct approach to specialization without an intervening period of general practice. Their search for specialized training is causing more and more hospitals to enter on courses of graduate instruction."[77] The proportion of graduates who became specialists without a preliminary period of general medical practice rose from 30 percent in 1915 to 53 percent 10 years later; nearly one-third of the latter had some postgraduate specialist training.[78]

One factor behind these phenomena was that more and more specialty groups were introducing certification. Spurred on by developments in the closely related field of ophthalmology, which had always served them as a professional model, otolaryngologists moved toward certification. In 1924, five specialty societies combined to establish the National Board of Examiners in Otolaryngology. By 1928, 1,368 physicians had been certified, 354 of them by "invitation." During these same years, obstetricians and gynecologists were moving in the same direction. Unlike the American College of Surgeons, which tended toward inclusiveness and the imposition of minimal standards, these other specialty bodies were eager to restrict the numbers of practicing specialists.[79] The dangers for the profession of not acting quickly became apparent in 1929 when the New Jersey legislature debated a bill to create a state licensing system for specialists. Opposed by the medical profession, which feared political involvement in its affairs, the bill failed to pass; but it underlined the need for quick action.[80] The rapidly rising number of specialists served as yet another stimulus to the intensified organizational activities of the 1930s.

By 1940, 23 percent of active physicians in the United States were full-time specialists, and many others were in part-time specialist practice.[81] It was generally thought that this figure was far too high. Spurred on by the Great Depression and rising health costs, some efforts were made to consider specialties from the perspective of national medical priorities and needs. In the early 1930s, the Committee on the Costs of Medical Care (CCMC) represented the most serious and famous attempt to deal with specialization in the context of larger policy and manpower requirements. Both the majority and the minority reports that it produced, supported efforts to improve training and regulation of specialists within a broad context of national health care.[82] In the end, overwhelming medical hostility to all forms of government intervention, group practice, prepayment, and limits on individual initiative, in combination with the absence of relevant national administrative agencies, undermined this committee's efforts.[83] In any event, there is no evidence that members of this committee thought deeply about specialization.[84] The CCMC was primarily concerned with mechanisms for providing access to all types of health care; specialist training and certification seem to have been understood as an internal medical issue.[85] The regulation of specialties continued to be worked out through the actions of numerous professional groups, each pursuing its own special interests.

By the early 1930s, a variety of specialties were certifying competence. Following in the footsteps of ophthalmologists and otolaryngologists, other specialty groups contemplated, and a few actually set up, certification boards. Among these were obstetrician-gynecologists (1930), whose quest for certification, like that of their counterparts in Great Britain, was aided by the public health movement for maternal and infant welfare,[86] dermatologists (1932), and pediatricians (1933). These groups sought to control education standards while excluding from their midst GPs with specialist interests by insisting that full-time specialist practice be a requirement of certification. Eleven new boards were set up between 1934 and 1940.[87] All this activity created major conflicts of jurisdiction. Tonsillectomies, a major source of income for hospitals, became an activity over which otolaryngologists competed actively against GPs.[88]

The AMA and the Struggle for Regulatory Dominance

The AMA provided guidelines for all these developments. In addition, the organization began gradually to take a more direct role in the case of several small technical specialties where it was particularly difficult to impose medical authority. Its incursion into the realm of physical therapy stopped short of actual certification. In 1925, it established the Council on Physical Therapy to examine the huge number of machines that were coming onto the market. This council concluded that while manufacturers' claims were usually inflated, the majority of appliances had some therapeutic value and in most cases should be applied by competent specialists. It mounted as well a major effort to improve the teaching of the subject at both under-graduate and graduate levels of medical education.[89] Through its publications, in-cluding several editions of the *Handbook of Physical Therapy*, the Council sought to make known the advantages of physical therapy—simple methods such as heat, massage, and exercises that could be applied by any physician, as well as more com-plicated machines that required the expertise of medical specialists. "The use of these physical agents has become thoroughly established as an integral part of medical practice," claimed the Council's report of 1936. "The physician should no more condemn physical therapy in toto than [he] should condemn internal medi-cine, surgery, orthopedics or roentgenology in toto."[90] The Council eventually en-couraged the creation of numerous hospital departments of physical therapy under the direction of competent physicians. Such support was crucial for the develop-ment of the specialty because orthopedists were seeking to control the field by ar-guing that lay physiotherapists working under the supervision of orthopedists con-stituted the most efficient form of organization for this domain.[91]

The incursion of the AMA into this sphere was unique; to my knowledge, none of the other national medical associations in the countries under discussion did anything remotely similar. The AMA's actions were in part a consequence of the great popularity of such therapeutic methods during the 1920s and 1930s, and reflected the AMA's wider effort to distinguish useful treatments of all sorts from those that were not. Medical interest in physical therapy was also a response to two related developments: the decline of infectious diseases and the spread of alterna-tive forms of medical practice:

> There is no doubt that the failure on the part of the medical profession at large to employ all the means at its disposal to deal with chronic disease has been respon-sible for the growth of cults. The relief which many patients receive from the ad-ministration of the various kinds of physical and psychic therapy practiced by the exponents of these cults has resulted in the development of spurious practices which often are as injurious to the individual and inimical to the public health as they are lucrative.[92]

This initiative was also indicative of the AMA's willingness to become directly in-volved in the internal development of specialties. The Association went even far-ther along this path in the case of pathology. In 1923, the AMA's Council on Med-ical Education came to the aid of the two societies of medical pathologists that were seeking to stamp out pathological laboratories run by nonmedical personnel. Ini-tially the Council surveyed clinical laboratories and listed those which met with its approval because they were directed by MDs. In 1931 there was a change of strat-egy. Rather than listing recognized laboratories, the Council began to list annually qualified pathologists; these were licensed physicians evaluated on the basis of training and experience. Within a year, 538 pathologists had been recognized.[93] Only those with at least three years' experience in the specialty were deemed quali-fied for the directorship of a clinical laboratory.[94]

Similarly, the Council set out to defend the medical character of radiology against the claims of lay technicians. By agreeing in 1928 to list qualified laboratories, and later radiologists as well, the AMA hoped to discourage "the unreliable commercial laboratory operated by technicians and lay specialists," as well as unqualified physicians, from working in the field. The mechanism for this exclusion was supposed to be that physicians would utilize such lists in referring patients. The list of radiologists in 1933 contained the names of 1,200 physicians.[95] In that same year, the chairman of the Council on Medical Education and Hospitals, Ray Lyman Wilbur, announced:

> The Council is also prepared to extend to other special fields of medicine the service which it has rendered in the fields of radiology and pathology, to the end that members of the medical profession and others who may be concerned may be able readily to distinguish those who have received training in the various branches of medicine from those who are merely self-constituted "specialists."[96]

Indeed, efforts to provide certification for problematic specialty domains turned out to represent the thin wedge of a much more ambitious claim by the AMA: that it should prepare and publish all lists of qualified specialists. Not only was the AMA "in the best position to speak with the voice of the entire medical profession," but its biographical files and inspectors allowed it to verify credentials and its various publications could widely distribute such information. "The Council is already engaged in the preparation of lists of qualified specialists in two of the fields of medicine so that it is much more economical for it to extend its activities than for some new agency to be created."[97] Soon thereafter, the Council made arrangements for the *AMD* to include information about the specialist boards and, within the alphabetical listings of practitioners, to indicate those physicians with board certificates. (Unlike its German counterpart, the AMA did not forbid the uncertified from calling themselves specialists, even in its own directory.) As its claims to overall supervision of specialty boards intensified, the AMA gradually abandoned the task of directly approving radiologists as specialists.[98]

The AMA, however, was not alone in seeking to oversee specialist certification. Several different institutions set out to control and standardize the establishment of specialist boards; most of these joined together in 1934 to form the Advisory Board for Medical Specialties, in a bid to coordinate specialty development. However, the AMA Council on Medical Education harbored its own regulatory designs and refused to join this new body.[99] Its rationale was that, in view of the AMA's current activities in this area, the Advisory Board's function should be to aid in the practical operation of the boards and not to judge their results, a task that should properly be left to the Council on Medical Education and Hospitals:

> As an independent body, the purpose of which will be to maintain the operation of the certifying boards in the specialties at a high level both as to standards adopted and as to conduct, the Council on Medical Education and Hospitals could

hold no representation on this coordinating board. It may, of course, advise with the coordinating board at such times as its advice may be sought. It would hardly be in order for a body sitting in judgment to hold membership on a board whose work it was expected to judge.[100]

Soon after, the AMA made an even more powerful claim: "It is expected and planned that the Advisory Board for Medical Specialists will be reportable to and work under the general direction of the Council on Medical Education and Hospitals of the American Medical Association."[101] There were substantive issues as well as matters of jurisdiction at stake. The Council, claimed its head, Ray Lyman Wilbur, was concerned about the tendency for specialist societies to use the boards to "shut out" qualified individuals from specialties, and wished to guarantee free access.[102]

Despite these rocky beginnings, the two bodies gradually came to jointly elaborate a set of conditions necessary for the establishment of new specialist boards and specified the twelve (later fourteen) specialties that should be represented by such boards. As a result of these guidelines, the establishment of new boards intensified, and by 1940, fourteen specialty boards were in existence; by that date, they had issued 15,600 certificates, making nearly 40 percent of all full-time specialists board certified.[103] In that year, and despite the opposition of the AMA to such requirements, five boards insisted that applicants devote themselves exclusively to the practice of the specialty, and three others demanded at least 70 percent concentration in their field.[104] Starting in 1940, the Advisory Board published the *Directory of Medical Specialists*, which listed all those who were board certified. The AMA, meanwhile, found its niche:

> In connection with the advisory board on specialties, we have assumed certain powers in regard to them by not joining this advisory board but asking that each board submit to the Council its constitution and its program for the approval of the Council. Some of those who were reluctant to do so found that our power largely consisted in our ability not to list them in the directory [AMD], so that I think we can say now that all of the special boards are in a direct relationship to the Council.[105]

Although the creation of new boards freed the AMA from direct responsibility for certifying technical specialties operating in institutions—radiology, pathology, anesthesiology, and physical medicine—the organization continued to take a special interest in these new and vulnerable specialties, seeking, for instance, to standardize the relationship between these specialists and insurance plans according to principles of direct fee for service, and to stipulate work conditions in hospitals.[106]

World War II, like previous wars, further increased the status of specialties. The introduction of a series of graded categories based on professional qualifications, and accompanied by differential salaries and sometimes supervisory powers as well, created even more distinctions among doctors. Certified specialists were given higher rank than experienced general practitioners. Such recognition was especially important for boundary groups such as internists, who won the highest status as "consultants."[107] After the war, thousands of doctors received specialty training subsidized by the G.I. Bill of Rights. The number of hospital residencies rose from about 9,000 in 1946 to 15,000 in 1948.[108]

How is one to evaluate the activities of the AMA and other agencies behind the American system of specialist certification? On the one hand, the guidelines elaborated by the AMA and the Advisory Board, and apparently based on Danish professional regulations, were detailed and remarkably effective. A specialty board had to represent a well-recognized and distinct specialty; it should include more than 100 specialists, have the support of major specialty organizations and the related AMA section, and should determine necessary training, test ability, and certify competence. Three years of training following internship, along with membership in the AMA, were demanded of candidates. Even the appropriate specialty fields were designated, leading to extensive lobbying by those groups that had been ignored. In less than a decade, all the approved fields were represented by boards.[109] More important, the system limited the proliferation of unapproved boards, though it could not prevent it altogether. Perhaps most significant, a concrete definition of specialties and specialists now existed in the United States. A true specialist was someone who had been certified by a recognized board after training. In reality, doctors could practice as specialists even without board certification, but this was clearly a deviation from the accepted standard. The system of boards, moreover, left room for considerable variation in development of specialties. Internal specialties such as cardiology and gastroenterology tended to become subspecialties, while surgical fields were more likely to evolve into independent specialties.

The lack of interest shown by most medical schools in playing a more central role in graduate education resulted in the emergence of hospital residency programs as the chief form of training for specialists. By 1939 there were over 4,500 residency programs in existence, with nearly 1,800 of these lasting three years or more. Abandoned was the ambition to make these programs the equivalents of advanced university degrees. But academic programs continued to exist; in 1935 two universities had graduate schools of medicine and twenty-nine reported that they offered systematic courses of graduate instruction.[110] About 2 percent of the residency programs in surgery or the surgical specialties approved by the American College of Surgeons either required or made optional the pursuit of a graduate degree.[111] With the spread of training, the widespread nineteenth-century belief that specialization should grow out of general medical practice disappeared, to be replaced by the view that becoming a specialist was merely the continuation of undergraduate medical education. Discussing the claim that not enough residencies were open to general practitioners, an influential report of 1940 argued:

> There is a widespread impression that there are not enough residencies open to such men. Their experience in general practice is doubtless a valuable background for specialized training. However, there is now a growing belief on the

part of medical educators that the period in general practice has made adaptation to hospital routine and discipline difficult and has postponed unduly the entrance into a specialty, which even without this period occurs relatively late in life. Furthermore, the physician may have become less capable of absorbing the instruction offered by his teachers.[112]

Residencies, however, were unequally distributed; those in large fields such as ophthalmology and otolaryngology were recognized to be insufficient in number.[113] Residencies also varied widely in quality. In the absence of authoritative bodies cutting across individual specialties, little standardization of programs took place.[114] The AMA Council on Medical Education tried to become such an authoritative body, but failed because many of the specialist groups were mistrustful of it. But it was powerful enough to prevent other bodies from emerging to play this coordinating role.[115] The lack of national health insurance in the United States meant that what served as a powerful motive for standardization in other countries did not emerge in the United States. The culture of individual rights remained powerful throughout the profession.

Despite such problems, the American system of certification was in many ways a great success. It is difficult to overstate the significance of the changes that it brought about. In the space of several decades, the majority of specialists were transformed from generalists who gradually took on specialist work in the course of their careers to exclusive experts whose specialty training in hospital residency programs, followed by certification examinations, was the culmination of their medical education. In the context of this new form of training, part-time specialist work made very little sense, even when it was not expressly forbidden by a specialty board. Consequently, part-time specialists, who made up more than half of all specialists in 1925 and 1930, became increasingly rare; by 1945 they comprised a tiny proportion of the medical population.[116] Not all specialists, it may be objected, were certified, unlike the situation in Germany. But by 1960, most of those in large cities and quite a few in smaller ones were board certified, and the proportion increased in subsequent decades.[117] One institution after another made certification a vital career step. Encouraged by bodies such as the American Hospital Association, hospitals increasingly made board certification a requirement for appointing and promoting specialists.[118] Public programs of various sorts made use of board certification in choosing participating physicians, health insurers paid higher fees to board-certified physicians, and the military granted them considerable privileges.[119] By 1959, approved examining boards in the medical specialties had granted over 77, 000 specialist certificates.[120] Both the experiences and the meanings related to being a specialist were transformed to a remarkable degree in the space of a few decades.[121]

Nonetheless, this system also suffered from serious weaknesses. One of these, as Rosemary Stevens has pointed out, was that the Advisory Board had little influence on standards once a board was established. Not only was there enormous variability, but specialty boards have typically been made up of representatives of the medical faculties and residency programs they are supposed to be monitoring.[122] William Rothstein has argued that not only did this situation persist into the 1980s, but that there was in that decade a significant decline in the number of residency programs at a time when the number of residents was rising.[123] Furthermore, the tendencies toward professional fragmentation remained powerful. The Advisory Board was able to contain some of the pressure for yet more specialist boards by allowing primary boards to introduce subspecialty certificates. In 1940, it approved subspecialties within the American Board of Internal Medicine—in cardiovascular disease, pulmonary disease, allergy, and gastroenterology. Only 6,583 individuals took qualifications in these subspecialties before 1960, and these fields did not really begin to take off until the 1970s.[124] But although this subspecialty system allowed American medicine to recognize new developments in a way that the German system could not, it proved to be problematical and conflict-producing.[125] Furthermore, while the system successfully replaced most part-time specialists with full-time specialists, it failed to significantly limit numbers of specialists. The proportion of full-time specialists among all physicians rose from 11 percent to over 30 percent from 1923 to 1949, with another 12 percent in the latter year claiming to be part-time specialists. What is more, the figure was as high in smaller cities as it was in the largest ones.[126] To some degree this rise reflected the popularity of internal medicine—as was the case in Germany—as a primary care specialty. But as we shall see in the Epilogue, primary care also declined and the position of traditional GPs became increasingly untenable.

Most important, neither the Advisory Board, nor specialist boards, nor the AMA was in a position to deal with broader policy issues. The system, as Stevens has argued, was not able to address concerns with rationalization and manpower needs beginning to emerge everywhere. On one hand, there continued to be too many specialists relative to the most widely quoted estimates of health-care needs put forward by Lee and Jones in 1932. On the other hand, there seemed to be too few practitioners in a number of fields, including obstetrics-gynecology and neurology-psychiatry.[127] Regional distribution was another problem difficult to address through existing institutions. The system reflected professional perceptions and interests rather than what Stevens has called "the public interest."[128] This is certainly a loaded term, and there is no reason to assume that the "public interest" is better served by civil servants and economists than it is by doctors. But it does point to a real narrowness of perspective. If such a narrow medical orientation also characterized the German and French systems of specialist regulation, equally dominated by professional concerns, both of the latter were introduced in the context of a national health insurance system; such systems made it impossible to ignore wider policy concerns, and eventually granted political and administrative elites significant power in shaping institutions. While efforts to deal with such issues never ceased in the United States, the fragmented nature of institutional and medical authority in that country made effective action considerably more difficult.[129]

Conclusion

The American system of specialist regulation was, like the one set up in Germany, conceived and administered by the organized medical profession. This fact substantially facilitated its early implementation. In both countries, specialist regulation reflected the concerns of doctors to standardize specialist training, thereby reducing the number of specialists and decreasing competition while ensuring competence and protecting the health of the public. From the vantage point of professional leaders, this pretty much defined the "public interest," while further efforts to manipulate and control the practices and distribution of specialists most definitely did not. The two national systems, however, differed in fundamental ways. In Germany, specialists were certainly the more powerful force, but GPs nonetheless retained considerable leverage because of a widespread desire to preserve general practice and because of the monopolistic position of the DÄV, which represented medical practitioners rather than academic elites—who were in any event preoccupied with their status in educational institutions. In the United States, specialist organizations, led by larger, more amorphous, specialist elites wielded great power and forced the AMA to struggle for influence.

The American system of specialist certification and training was not unlike those of other nations, with the notable exception of Britain, in reflecting the narrow concerns of the medical profession. Individuals such as Ray Lyman Wilbur, who played a part in the AMA's certification efforts as well as a prominent role on the Committee for the Costs of Medical Care, certainly had a wider view of the medical needs of the American population. But it is not clear that either he or anyone else linked broad social issues to the question of specialist training, which was treated as a largely internal, technical matter. Furthermore, this medical domination of specialist training took place in a uniquely decentralized medical context in which power of all sorts was highly fragmented. Such fragmentation was intensified by American political debates over health policy during these years that, in the words of one historian, left American physicians "as the least constrained medical community in the world."[130] This convergence of circumstances would have major consequences for the development of American medicine during the second half of the twentieth century.

Chapter 8
The French Style of Regulating Specialists

We saw in chapter 1 that specialties were admitted to the Paris Medical Faculty during the 1860s. By the first decades of the twentieth century, all French medical schools had specialist chairs; in 1919, there were nine in Paris, eight in Bordeaux, and six in both Lille and Lyons. The nation's seven medical schools combined had eight chairs in clinical obstetrics, seven in ophthalmology, six in dermatology-venereology, and five in both psychiatry and pediatric orthopedics (an unusual chair by international standards).[1] Specialized medical practice spread as well. By the 1930s, almost half of all Parisian doctors and nearly as many in large provincial cities were calling themselves specialists in medical directories. Nonetheless, while specialist regulation was being set up in Germany and the United States in the 1920s, the subject in France was virtually ignored until the end of that decade. Full specialty certification was not introduced in that country until 1947. One should not overstate the significance of this French lag, which was, in the context of the full history of specialization, relatively brief. Nonetheless, it is suggestive of the unique logic of specialization in French medicine.

We must first dispose of three possible explanations for the French delay. First, French doctors as a group were not especially hostile to the regulation of specialties. Opposition from the medical profession did not, as one historian has claimed, prevent the introduction of specialty certification before 1947.[2] Second, the French delay cannot be explained, as I assumed initially, by the inability of the French medical profession to achieve consensus on this and other issues. On the contrary, we will see that the profession eventually achieved a very effective working consensus on this matter. Third, despite France's reputation for bureaucratic centralization, neither the political elite nor the state administration delayed specialist regulation; they in fact exerted relatively little influence over developments. As was the case in Germany and the United States, debate about specialist certification in France was dominated by professional associations with sporadic (though significant) input from state authorities, which most often showed little interest in this issue. When they did intervene, it was usually because specialties battling for turf attempted to use the legislative process to pursue their aims or, more rarely, because the specialty system had ramifications for more significant policy issues. Substantial state control over medicine affected the introduction of specialist regulation in more indirect, subtle, and interesting ways.

I will argue in this chapter that the structural characteristics of French medicine and the professional strategies that these fostered led French doctors to become interested in the question of certification somewhat later than their German and American colleagues; once they did so, they followed a very ambitious certification strategy—also in response to French institutional realities—that took nearly two decades to implement successfully.

Two linked factors were critical in pushing medical professions in Germany and the United States to quickly resolve the issue of specialist regulation: (1) the perceived urgency of the need for more general professional regulation and reform and (2) the existence of a national professional association capable of tackling these issues. The lack of licensing regulations in the United States for much of the nineteenth century, and the introduction in Germany of a free field in medical practice in 1869, led to unbridled competition among medical practitioners. In both countries, specialization became one of many issues that required resolution, and strong national associations arose to unify geographically fragmented medical professions. France, in contrast, had a long-standing system of state-sponsored regulation of doctors. State medical diplomas of one sort or another had been an official requirement for medical practice since the beginning of the nineteenth century. This requirement was, it is true, enforced badly; but demanding enforcement of existing laws—as French doctors did—was not the same as demanding wholesale reform. French medical associations thus focused on narrower trade union issues. The matter of specialist regulation was consequently treated in relative isolation and appeared less pressing. Furthermore, the regional decentralization of both the American and the German political systems, as well as profound hostility to government intervention in the health-care field, encouraged medical associations of various sorts to act unilaterally in setting up professionally controlled specialty training programs and diplomas. In centralized France, however, there was relatively little principled opposition to national educational credentials granted by the state, which constituted the normal mode of professional certification. Such credentials, however, would prove immensely difficult to set up.

Why Specialist Regulation Was Not a Priority in France

Specialization spread very rapidly after 1880 in the largest urban centers of France. Specialists were organized around a rich institutional network of specialty scientific societies, trade unions (*syndicats*), journals, and, for an elite, faculty and hospital positions.[3] All these groups and institutions were seeking to advance medical specialization in a variety of ways; but until the end of the 1920s, they showed little interest in formal specialty certification. Surgeons constituted the single exception; several years before World War I, their trade union examined the question of introducing a special surgical diploma, but did not push the matter very hard.[4] Several factors account for this relative indifference to an issue becoming increasingly contentious in other countries. All French doctors had, by virtue of their diplomas, the right to perform any and all medical procedures; consequently, specialization was perceived as a voluntary limitation of practice by individuals rather than as a right conferred by virtue of greater expertise. (It was this restriction of clientele rather than special competence that was cited in France to justify the higher fees that specialists commanded.) Changing this perception would have been particularly difficult before World War I because the medical world was torn apart by something like a civil war between elite and rank-and-file practitioners. The underlying conflict was about inequalities of privilege, status, and wealth, but the precipitating cause was an attempt to create a higher medical degree designed for future academic researchers. This was perceived as yet another barrier separating practitioners from the elite, yet another symbol of medical inequality. In this context, any measure to create formal specialty credentials would have had similar incendiary implications.[5]

Like specialists in other countries, turn-of-the-century specialists in France focused primarily on two issues: first, defining as part of medicine such domains as radiology and care of the teeth, in order to keep them out of the hands of nonmedical practitioners such as X-ray technicians and dentists; second, and even more critical, ensuring that their specialty was properly represented in elite hospitals and, especially, medical schools. These of course were the characteristic concerns of specialists in *all* countries, but for a variety of reasons, French doctors did not immediately respond to the rapid spread of specialists, as did their German and American counterparts, by pursuing a strategy of specialist training and certification.

One possible reason was the high status of French academic specialists. Hospitals were closed to rank-and-file physicians and were restricted to an elite recruited through competitive examinations (*concours*) that began in the first years of medical school when students competed for externships, and in subsequent years for even more scarce and prestigious internships.[6] Elite specialists did not require certification to distinguish themselves from the less well-qualified. They did, however, require the institutional posts that would make research and teaching possible, and such positions gradually came into being from the latter decades of the nineteenth century. The Paris hospital administration (*Assistance Publique*) officially recognized only about a half-dozen specialty groups, each of them recruiting through its own distinct competitive examinations.[7] But outside these specialty corps, there were in fact specialized hospitals in many fields; their staffs might be classified in official lists as general physicians or surgeons, but functioned in reality as specialists. Furthermore, the power of senior clinicians to choose their patients meant that many general medical and surgical wards became de facto specialty wards.[8] In the medical faculties, formal specialization was even more developed. Chairs in the major and quite a few minor specialties existed in Paris and were spreading to the larger provincial faculties as well.[9] The competitive examination leading to junior faculty posts, the *agrégation*, traditionally a test of general knowledge, was before World War I divided into twenty-one sections representing a wide array of specialties and disciplines.[10] The essential needs of elite specialists were thus being met.

Aside from their unusual success in integrating elite institutions, the French specialist elite was not much different from other European medical elites in showing little interest in specialist certification. The really significant difference had to do with rank-and-file specialists who drove the campaigns for certification in Germany and elsewhere because they faced competition from those they deemed totally "unqualified." French doctors were severely handicapped in this respect by the lack of a representative professional body comparable with the American Medical Association, Deutsche Ärztevereinsbund, or British Medical Association. The Association Générale des Médecins was largely a self-help group, and the Union des Syndicats Médicaux limited itself to trade union issues. The latter was in any event dominated by physicians in the provinces, where specialization was slower to take root. Nor did associations specifically representing nonelite specialists in political and economic matters emerge until relatively late. As a result of all these factors, training for elite specialists was being handled through competitive hospital clerkships (*internat*) and junior faculty and hospital posts, while the teaching of specialties to non-elite practitioners continued to be perceived chiefly as a means of producing competent general practitioners.[11] This view was also common in the wider scientific world. In 1909, the Academy of Sciences voted a resolution to the effect that the exercise of radiography should be considered a medical act reserved for doctors. However, it specifically rejected the creation of any special diploma for radiologists and suggested instead that radiography be given more time in the general medical curriculum.[12]

Educational reforms before World War I created a system of clinical rotations for those students (the vast majority) who were not hospital interns. Practical postgraduate clinical experience, when added to these rotations, provided a basis for non-elite practice. In addition, many hospitals and medical schools set up short courses, lasting from a few weeks to a few months, to teach the essentials of specialist knowledge to GPs as well as to future specialists.[13] Medical schools also set up a number of more formal programs leading to special "university" diplomas that lacked the rights associated with official state degrees. But these remained few in number and were usually awarded in fields where there were administrative job opportunities—public health, colonial medicine, forensic medicine, child health—rather than in clinical fields, represented among these diplomas only by electroradiology. General practitioners opposed the creation of such diplomas, which they feared might become an official requirement for public posts. Diploma holders did in fact regularly demand special consideration for such posts, but did not meet with much success.[14]

As in most other nations, the First World War increased the visibility and power of specialties in France. The Military Health Service, for instance, set up a special commission to supervise the treatment of nervous and mental diseases among soldiers and to oversee the neurology and psychiatry centers that were set up.[15] After the war, the government profited from wartime experiences and set up cancer therapy centers that, in the process, created a new specialty around this disease.[16] Nonetheless, it took another decade for the issue of specialty certification to emerge fully.

The Campaign to Regulate Specialties

Debate around specialty certification emerged in the late 1920s, for a number of reasons. First, the spread of specialization, which had been slow during the first two decades of the century, accelerated dramatically after World War I. In 1920 the proportion of specialists among doctors listed in the major medical directory of the period, the *Guide Rosenwald,* was only slightly higher than in 1905.[17] By 1935, however, over half the Parisian doctors listed (nearly 4,000 individuals) were labeling themselves as specialists. The proportion was similar among doctors in the largest provincial cities.[18] Specialist trade unions (*syndicats*) pursuing more narrowly economic and professional interests spread widely.[19] It was not just the number of specialists that was rising. Each day new and occasionally bizarre specialty categories made an appearance. The specialty list of the most important medical directory, the *Guide Rosenwald,* in 1935 contained no fewer than thirty-six specialties. When directed at the general public rather than medical professionals, specialty lists could be even more fragmented and outlandish. In 1921, for instance, a general directory of Parisian occupations included a medical list presenting physicians divided according to specialties; the list was split into no fewer than 120 categories.[20] The directory caused some consternation in certain medical circles, where it was cited as an example of the most absurd excesses of specialization.[21]

Defending against such inflation of specialty claims seemed even more imperative to many because of what was perceived as an oversupply of doctors. This was of course a traditional complaint of doctors everywhere throughout the nineteenth century. But it is certainly true that the number of doctors in France increased by nearly 70 percent between 1896 and 1931.[22] This perception of overcrowding called forth defensive reflexes. The profession as a whole vigorously sought to exclude foreigners from its midst;[23] and specialists began to agitate in order to reduce competition from those they regarded as unqualified. Most specialty *syndicats* had for some time been selective in their recruitment, admitting as members only those individuals who could in some way demonstrate special competence (variously defined). From this type of selection, it was a relatively short step to campaigning for some kind of formal certification.

Furthermore, the postwar period was a time of rapidly expanding social welfare programs, some of which involved payment to doctors for medical services.[24] State programs of medical assistance (particularly benefits to veterans of the First World War and worker compensation), insurance companies, and above all the new system of health insurance in the process of being set up, were all distinguishing between acts performed by specialists and those performed by general practitioners; for the same procedure, specialists were often paid considerably higher fees.[25] This provoked a good deal of intraprofessional tension[26] and highlighted the need for some unified professional structure to deal with these changing conditions. It also raised the obvious question of how to determine who in fact was a specialist.[27] One of the chief functions of the specialty *syndicats* was to attempt to negotiate conventions establishing fees and conditions for specialty status with various agencies and insurance plans. It is no accident that similar discussions about specialist status had occurred in Germany two decades before as a consequence of the expansion of that nation's health insurance system, and in Belgium during the 1930s as that country set out to introduce social insurance measures.[28]

As a result of such issues, the traditionally fragmented medical syndicalist movement in France attempted to consolidate itself both nationally and internationally. Nationally, negotiations were initiated in 1924 to allow the trade unions of specialists to join the larger medical trade union movement, although conditions of specialist membership in the Union of Medical Trade Unions proved very troublesome.[29] When the medical trade union movement split in 1926 in a disagreement over the best way to respond to the probable creation of a health insurance system, the specialist *syndicats* left the Union and formed their own autonomous organization in 1927.[30] This Groupement des Syndicats des Spécialistes rejoined a medical confederation that was reconstituted at the end of 1928 and functioned within it despite the fact that the place of specialists within the confederation was never satisfactorily resolved.[31] Consequently, the growing concern of specialty *syndicats* with certification spread to the general medical trade union movement, which, now representing about 80 percent of all French doctors, began to wield some of the influence of comparable national associations in other countries while retaining a much narrower trade union focus.

Like the question of fees, these trade union maneuvers and negotiations raised the question of who, exactly, was a specialist and how he or she differed from the general practitioner.[32] At one its first meetings the Groupement des Syndicats des Spécialistes defined specialists as doctors who practiced a specialty exclusively and who possessed some qualification. A qualification was defined in one of two ways: it could be *practical*, such as the fact of practicing a specialty for at least five years or, for the elite, *technical*, defined as professional experience sanctioned by a title, such as that of an *interne des hôpitaux*, who spent at least three years in a specialty clinic, or the even more senior *chef de clinique*, who spent at least two.[33] This definition, opposed by many doctors, inevitably became an issue in trade union negotiations and gradually took on a life of its own.[34]

One manifestation of growing concern with specialization was the setting up of an international association, the Association Professionnelle Internationale des

Médecins (APIM) in Paris in 1926, under the direction of a leading French medical syndicalist, Dr. Fernand Decourt. Extending the aims of medical syndicalism to the international arena, the APIM sought to defend doctors' interests more effectively and published its own journal.[35] Since specialty certification was a critical issue in several countries where it had been recently introduced or was contemplated, it became important as well for the APIM and its largely French leadership.[36] One of its first projects was the publication of a lengthy international survey of the status of specialization and specialists in Europe, written by Decourt on the basis of responses to a questionnaire by representatives of affiliated national associations.[37] Decourt divided European countries into three groups: those with laws regulating specialization (Czechoslovakia, Hungary, and Yugoslavia), those with professionally organized and widely obeyed conventions of specialist practice (six countries, including Germany and Sweden), and those with no regulation whatsoever (seven, including France and Great Britain). The APIM followed this survey with a discussion that produced some practical conclusions: the practice of specialization should be regulated according to plans developed by medical organizations; the number of specialties should be kept as low as possible; specialization required special studies and training in hospital clinics, but there should nonetheless be ways for autodidacts to become specialists; all practitioners could perform specialized acts, but only those fulfilling specific conditions could publicly call themselves specialists.[38] These conclusions were very similar to the principles that would be embraced by the French medical trade union movement. Equally important, the report provided an international framework that would henceforth be utilized and cited in French discussions of specialization.[39]

In the following years, traditional concerns such as fighting off nonmedical competition to specialists continued to channel considerable energies; in the mid-1930s, dermatologists became agitated about competition from beauty salons and other nonmedical practitioners.[40] However, what directly precipitated debate about specialist regulation and certification was the long-standing and acrimonious dispute between dentists and doctors practicing medicine of the mouth and teeth.

For most of the nineteenth century, dentistry in France was unregulated. It was practiced by some doctors but also by unlicensed practitioners. Reforms in 1892 created a modern dental profession. All MDs continued to be free to practice dentistry, but anyone else needed to obtain a newly created diploma in dental surgery granted by the state medical faculties.[41] From the beginning, there was violent conflict between dentists and doctors calling themselves first odontologist and then stomatologist. Each group demanded a monopoly for its members. Stomatologists insisted that their field was a medical specialty and that dentists were second-rate practitioners who should be eliminated. Dentists insisted that a dental diploma be required of all practitioners, including MDs, because special technical skills were required to care for the mouth and teeth. There were moderates in both camps who dreamed of unifying the two professions as a single specialty of medicine. In this view, future dental specialists could be trained as doctors on condition that transition measures would safeguard the dignity and professional status of dentists currently in practice.[42]

After nearly three decades of fierce conflict, matters came to a head in the mid-1920s. In the face of persistent rumors that dentists had succeeded in winning political support for a mandatory dental diploma,[43] stomatologists in 1928–29 succeeded in getting legislation introduced in the National Assembly that required an MD degree for the practice of dentistry. This involved the provision of dental training for doctors and raised the issue of specialist training more generally. It thus unleashed a wave of discussions in medical journals and trade union circles.[44] Although the question of dentistry remained central to discussions of specialization during the next decade, primarily because dentists and stomatologists came very close to actually engineering a merger of the two professions, the issue of specialist certification quickly took on life of its own.

First surgeons joined the fray in 1928 by submitting a demand in the Academy of Medicine for a special surgical diploma that would be mandatory for the practice of surgery. They argued that technical advances had made surgery so complex and dangerous that lengthy training was now necessary to ensure competent and safe practice. The Academy voted down the principle of an obligatory surgical diploma because this would violate the unity of the existing MD degree. But it did express support for some nonobligatory form of certification that would distinguish those individuals who were fully qualified in surgery.[45]

Surgeons continued to agitate for some form of certification, and their trade union threatened sporadically to go it alone by granting its own specialty certificate. But the issue was quickly appropriated by the General Confederation of Medical Trade Unions, which transformed it into a professionwide issue. This had major strategic implications. Since the Confederation represented most sectors of French medicine, it had to elaborate a proposal capable of generating broad consensus. This proved to be a laborious undertaking. The Confederation began deliberations on the issue in 1931. On several occasions it came up with proposals, only to abandon them in favor of an entirely different concept of certification. Not until 1938 was a workable plan finally achieved; and by then Europe was on the brink of war.

The Long Road to Professional Certification

The process of crafting a suitable model of specialist regulation was dominated by the General Confederation of Medical Trade Unions. The government and politicians more generally played a supporting role in the process, rubber-stamping the Confederation's proposals (and later those of the Ordre des Médecins) or occasionally adding political muscle to the demands of one professional group or another. Although the insurance system served as a key impetus for professional efforts to regulate specialists, its administrators seem not to have intervened in the ensuing deliberations, making their own quiet and usually unilateral decisions about the provision of and remuneration for specialist services. A few medical academics participated in the regulation debates but most did not, and medical schools as a bloc did not support any specific set of proposals.

As in most nations, general practitioners in France tended to oppose specialty certification because they feared that formalizing existing divisions would freeze them out of many lucrative domains of practice and turn them into second-class doctors. The Confederation recognized the legitimacy of such fears and never considered any obligatory form of certification. But its leadership consistently supported some form of nonobligatory certification that would ensure appropriate standards of practice. In its view, medicine was a single profession, and all doctors were permitted to perform all procedures for which they felt qualified; specialty certification, however, would set apart those individuals who met nationally defined criteria of appropriate training and exclusive practice of the specialty. Only certified individuals, it was quickly established, would be permitted to publicly identify themselves as specialists. Furthermore, in order to prevent professional fragmentation and keep as much medical work as possible within general practice, it was widely accepted that the number of recognized specialties should remain small (with numbers ranging anywhere from four to ten, depending on the plan). Fields most often recognized as legitimate specialties were based on hard-to-master instrumentation (electroradiology, ophthalmology) or skills (surgery). With time, specialties based on other criteria also achieved recognition. Apart from seeking to elaborate a plan for specialist certification, the Confederation exercised some limited control over the proliferation of specialties by admitting or not admitting specialist *syndicats* into its midst. Thus the association representing gynecology was refused admission because it did not require its members to limit themselves exclusively to the practice of their specialty.[46] Overall, the goal of certification was as much to *limit* the spread of specialization and specialties as it was to raise specialist standards.

Led by the powerful Medical Federation of the Paris region, opponents of certification remained unmoved by such concessions. Their continued hostility reflected the belief that, at best, a two-tier system of medical practice would be set up. They insisted, moreover, that despite the theoretical right of all doctors to perform all medical procedures, the insurance system would, by controlling payment of honoraria, effectively limit general practice and destroy the integrity of the MD diploma. Even more serious was the danger that law courts, traditionally severe with doctors in matters of malpractice, would inevitably act harshly against the noncertified brought before the justice system for performing specialty procedures. Finally, not all opposition was totally self-interested. A strong case was made that specialization would fragment medicine as self-interest turned every doctor into a specialist, leaving no one to assure the primary care of the whole patient.[47] This concern became increasingly prominent during the 1930s as an influential holistic movement developed within French medicine. The disappearance of the *médecin de famille* came to symbolize all that was wrong with a reductionist and fragmented medical system. Opposition to specialty certification never dissipated, but it was powerless to prevent the Confederation from taking a forceful stand in favor of nonobligatory certification.[48] The major difficulty, rather, lay in the choice of an organizational modality from among the many alternatives available.

In its initial deliberations of 1932, the Confederation's Commission of Labor Law voted in favor of a trade union approach to certification.[49] Only a small number of specialties would be officially recognized. Practitioners would obtain certificates of competence from the Confederation of Medical Trade Unions, based on the judgments made by the national specialist and local general medical trade unions. Either a hospital clerkship or a longer period of private practice as a specialist would normally be sufficient to obtain this credential.

A year later, the administrators of the medical education system began planning a reform of medical training that included efforts to reorganize programs of specialty instruction.[50] In response, the Confederation's Commission on Medical Education elaborated a second and very different proposal that centered on the state medical faculties.[51] Its plan called for *state* certificates in a small number of specialties. Eventually these would be obtained through formal programs of postgraduate study set up in medical faculties. As a transitional measure, however, the faculties could grant these certificates to doctors who had practiced as specialists for at least three years. Such state diplomas granted by faculties would make it possible to introduce formal examinations, central to French elite culture. Faculties, it was also argued, were in a better position than trade unions to impose uniformity of credentials on a national scale and keep the number of recognized specialties small.

Considerable opposition to this proposal emerged within the Confederation, whose Central Council resoundingly rejected the concept of state specialty certificates.[52] But in the face of repeated threats by the trade unions representing surgeons and otorhinolaryngologists to create their own specialty certificates,[53] the Confederation quickly came up with a modified plan for national certification.[54] According to this third proposal, specialization could occur within the framework of the existing MD degree; the diploma of the graduating physician would in this plan specify whether it covered general medicine or one of the recognized specialties. Clinical clerkships in specialties would begin during the course of medical studies, normally in the sixth and final year. For most specialties one year of training would be sufficient. For a few others, notably surgery, several more years would be required and graduation would thus be delayed. This would not be a major inconvenience, it was suggested, since such delays were already the rule for elite interns, who put off graduation until internships were completed. The great advantage of this plan was that it guaranteed equality between GPs and specialists since everyone would hold the same MD degree. It was presented as a means of avoiding the emergence of a higher caste of practitioners with postdoctoral certificates while still keeping certification in the hands of state faculties that could ensure objectivity and high standards.

That controlling the spread of specialties was a major aim of the educational administration was made clear by a reform of the *agrégation*, which regulated entry to the lower ranks of the professoriate, that was promulgated in 1934.[55] This measure eliminated nine of twenty-four specialized competitions (*concours*) that had led to "a hasty and excessive specialization to the detriment of general culture." Among the subjects eliminated were hygiene, bacteriology, legal medicine, neurology and psychiatry, dermatology and venereology, hydrology and climatology, and urology. This left fifteen *concours*, mostly in basic science disciplines; among clinical specialties only surgery, ophthalmology, otorhinolaryngology, and obstetrics continued to be foci of elite recruitment. Although this did not imply a repudiation of specialization, the reform clearly aimed at creating more unified and broadly educated medical elites.

The Confederation's proposal for certification more or less disappeared from view during the next few years, as difficult negotiations between stomatologists and dentists and the deliberations of an interministerial commission to elaborate a legislative bill took center stage. In the former case, the thorniest disagreement was over whether dentists could be allowed to call themselves "doctor" or even to trade in their diploma for an MD, as they desired; stomatologists (and most doctors) were violently opposed. Finally a compromise was reached in 1936: during the transition dentists might call themselves *docteur-dentiste*. This term could *follow* an individual's name, but the word *docteur* could never *precede* the name.[56] In exchange for this concession, dentistry would gradually become a medical field, thereby creating significant new career opportunities for doctors at a time of professional overcrowding.[57] Haggling among all parties continued for nearly two more years until, in March 1938, a law creating a system of specialist doctorates while at the same time eliminating the profession of dentistry was finally introduced in the French Senate.[58] Unfortunately, just at that moment the agreement that had been worked out between dentists and stomatologists fell apart over the issue of whether dentists currently in practice would have the right to transform dentistry degrees into the MD.[59] This destroyed the rationale for the proposed law and sent everyone back to the drawing boards.

The Confederation took advantage of the need to produce new legislation that avoided the issue of dentistry to further refine its proposal.[60] After much discussion it introduced two particularly significant wrinkles. First, specialty qualification was detached from the MD degree and embedded in independent specialist certificates that could be obtained either before or after the MD degree.[61] Certificates were exclusively geared to specialists and, unlike the earlier plan focusing on the MD diploma, contained no recognition of general practice. Second, in its desire to keep the number of specialties small[62] and yet satisfy all the specialties clamoring for professional recognition, the Confederation introduced the notion of a second tier of specialties whose use could be authorized by the medical trade unions and which had different status from specialties certified by state faculties. In spite of substantial opposition within the medical community,[63] the new proposal was sent off to the government with the hopeful comment: "If the national and international political situation remains stable, one can predict reform for the year 1939."[64] In this perspective, yet another unsuccessful effort was made to negotiate a unification of medicine and dentistry.[65]

The War and Postwar Years

The situation of course did not remain stable, and war delayed reform for nearly a decade. But one consequence of the French defeat at the hands of Nazi Germany was to simplify the process of establishing specialty regulation: the wartime Vichy regime finally established the long-awaited Ordre des Médecins to govern the profession. This national institution had, among other powers, the authority to introduce specialty certification by administrative means, thus bypassing the treacherous and lengthy political process (though it did not eliminate the exercise of political pressure). It also began its existence with ambitious, indeed visionary, plans to restructure and revitalize French medicine. Among the reforms that it immediately began to consider were the promulgation of a code of medical deontology, the reform of medical education, reform of hospitals, and specialist certification. In June 1941 the National Council of the Ordre published a draft plan for a system of certification based on the Confederation's plan of 1938.[66] Instead of the original seven recognized specialties, this plan called for nine. (Obstetrics-gynecology and dermatology-venereology were the two added categories.) A second tier of "free specialties" that could be combined with general practice was fully defined and was integrated into the state system rather than being left to *syndicats*.[67] But regular meetings of the National Council from March through December 1941 did not get very far in deciding how to implement the reform. Many Council members saw specialty certification as part of a much grander renewal of French medicine that did not translate easily into simple administrative measures. The problem was made even more intractable by the wide variety of ideological visions represented on the Council.[68]

The more down-to-earth National Councils that succeeded this one and that were dominated by the medical trade unions continued to work behind the scenes on this reform.[69] But they were not able to advance the process of implementation under the unsettled wartime conditions. In 1942 a plan to train surgeons in a number of special schools was introduced, but nothing came of the initiative. Two years later a modified plan for surgical training was again introduced, but with no more success.[70] During the same period, the National Council began urging the regional branches of the Ordre to identify and qualify specialists in five of the most important specialties.[71] But again, under wartime conditions most regional councils failed to respond to central directives.[72] The Ordre, much to the consternation of some doctors, did, however, attempt to ensure that all specialists received the highest possible fees, introducing in the process even larger discrepancies between health insurance fees paid to specialists and those paid to GPs.[73]

During the final chaotic months of the Second World War in France, a special section of the National Council was organized under the direction of the surgeon and medical trade unionist Serge Oberlin, to attempt once again to implement specialist certification. The framework of this reform of 1944 was slightly altered from that of 1941: there were now ten full-fledged specialties that had to be practiced exclusively (the new one added was phthisiology). Six were explicitly justified by special techniques, and the four others by their importance for public policy. There were nineteen second-tier specialties.[74] In the various circulars that the National Council sent out, regional councils were again urged to begin the process of qualifying practitioners in the five major specialties. Adding a new twist to the process, Oberlin instructed the councils simply to register as specialists anyone claiming such status who had established a medical practice in the region before 1939, but to investigate the credentials of anyone who had begun practice in the region after that date.[75]

By the end of the war, the Ordre had little to show for its efforts to regulate specialties. But the general principles governing specialist certification were by now well established and widely accepted. After the liberation of France, a reconstituted Ordre quickly resumed efforts to introduce specialty certification, pushed to some extent by the imperious need of a greatly expanded health insurance system to identify specialists.[76] In close cooperation with the Confederation of National Medical Trade Unions, the Ordre came up with a proposal that was discussed during much of 1947. This plan introduced a system of specialty certification that was a refined version of the one originally proposed in 1938, published in 1941, and modified in 1944. Without formally limiting the right of doctors to practice medicine as they wished, the proposal called for two levels of specialists, defined by postgraduate training and certification: (1) full specialists and (2) holders of specialty "competencies" that could be combined with general practice.[77] (The latter could also be practiced exclusively, in which case practitioners, although not considered real specialists by the Ordre, were treated as full specialists for the purpose of health insurance fees.[78]) Both forms of specialty status were granted by the Ordre; eventually specialty qualification was to be based on specialty diplomas or certificates awarded by medical faculties, but in the short run they were accorded by local commissions set up for the purpose. These commissions made judgments on the basis of criteria that varied from one specialty to another but that normally included either hospital experience or private practice in a specialty for specified periods of time.

The Ordre shrugged off vigorous opposition to specialty certification[79]; the proposal went forward and was gradually implemented after 1947. Nonetheless, the process was far from simple. Definitions needed to be made precise. It was decided that specialists were required to practice a specialty exclusively and had to be capable of performing all acts associated with the specialty. A *médecin à compétence* was a GP who had special knowledge of a branch of medicine that he or she preferred to practice and who was permitted to advertise that fact. A consultant was defined as having special expertise, and could be either a specialist or a generalist.[80] It was resolved not to attempt to legally restrict specialty practice to the certified—even in such cases as major surgery, where it was clearly desirable to do so for reasons of public safety; it was decided instead to rely on fear of legal consequences for unsuccessful treatment to deter the unqualified.[81] It was also necessary to organize transitional measures to satisfy the health insurance system until faculty programs for the training of specialists could be fully organized.[82]

The most controversial issues had to do with deciding which were full specialties, which were competencies, and which were neither. After some debate, urology was deemed a competency rather than a specialty. Both homeopathy and rheumatology were denied either status.[83] Although special technology and skill remained the major criteria for full specialist status (with surgeons serving as the prototype of specialists),[84] social significance was also recognized as a significant criterion that justified specialty status for obstetricians, psychiatrists, and dermato-venereologists. In response to a request from the Ministry of Youth, the Ordre agreed to a competency médico-sportive for the 200 or so doctors who had public functions in this area.[85] Other socially relevant domains, such as pediatrics, whose practitioners wanted to be considered specialists were at first recognized only as competencies. An important consideration in such decisions was whether a government department specifically requested specialty status for practitioners in domains where it ran programs; this was the case for obstetrics, psychiatry, and dermato-venereology but not for pediatrics.[86] By the end of the initial process, there were seven exclusive specialties (surgery, ORL, ophthalmology, biology, electroradiology, gynecology-obstetrics, and stomatology),[87] four that could be practiced as either specialties or competencies (pneumo-phthisiology, dermato-venereology, neurology, and psychiatry), and twenty-one competencies that could be combined with general practice or could be practiced exclusively.[88]

Commissions representing each specialty spent much of 1948 elaborating detailed educational proposals that could be developed by medical schools.[89] Fee schedules were worked out with the health insurance administration. During this time, local commissions were certifying specialists in active practice. These varied considerably in their degree of restrictiveness. Certification in surgery pretty much required that a candidate be a former surgical intern in a city with a faculty of medicine (a very restrictive condition, indeed). In contrast, an electroradiologist could follow a variety of career trajectories to certification, including having practiced as a specialist for five years.[90] By October 1948, 2,375 specialists had been certified out of 2,709 who had applied. Two months later nearly 5,000 specialists had been certified.[91] In 1950, faculty programs began operating, and possession of a specialty certificate granted by a faculty became the primary mode of specialty qualification in all but a few cases. Most significantly, surgeons refused to create academic programs, on the grounds that training as an intern in a faculty city was the most pertinent criterion for certifying surgeons.[92] By early 1954, there were twenty-three specialty or competency certificates conferred by faculties after two or three years of training.[93] Over 13,000 doctors in France, about one-third of the medical population, were known to have qualified in one way or another as either specialists or *compétents*.[94] Three years later there were 14,700 specialists or *compétents* in a medical population of a little over 42,000 (35 percent).[95]

Specialist categories continued to evolve. After its initial rejection, pediatrics finally won recognition as a full specialty in the later 1950s, amid much controversy and thanks largely to political intervention justified by fears of a declining French population.[96] At that time, rheumatolology was also admitted as a competency, while other categories initially recognized as competencies, such as thermal medicine, were eliminated. Neurology and psychiatry were combined into a single specialty, neuropsychiatry. Gynecology, which when combined with obstetrics was considered a specialty and when practiced separately was considered a competency, was subject to particular pressures from its heterogeneous community of practitioners; these pressures eventually succeeded in dividing the field into three categories: obstetrics and gynecology combined, medical gynecology, and surgical gynecology.[97]

In the years that followed, there was much criticism of the new system. This is not surprising in view of the fact that a single set of detailed national regulations had to apply to a wide variety of professional groups and administrative bodies within a complex set of legal jurisdictions. Although the Ordre des Médecins set overall policy, it was dependent for implementation on powerful institutions, such as the insurance system and medical schools, over which it had little control. Respect for acquired rights had to be reconciled with the desire to restrict the number of specialties and specialists. Some doctors voiced approval of the Belgian medical profession, which had also begun discussing specialty certification in 1929 but which had resoundingly and repeatedly rejected the proposal.[98] Most criticisms, however, had little to do with the principle of certification, but instead concerned details of implementation. For instance, it was argued that transitional measures for naming specialists were too lenient and did not always guarantee real expertise. In other cases, the Confederation of Medical Trade Unions argued that conditions were too severe and did not respect the acquired rights of individuals who had practiced as specialists.[99] One legal expert accused the Ordre of practicing a systematic "Malthusianism" designed to restrict the admission of young doctors to specialist status.[100]

More seriously, it eventually became clear that there were *two* authorities in matters of certification whose policies occasionally conflicted: the various levels of the Ordre des Médecins, which certified doctors. and the Sécurité Sociale, which administered the health insurance system and had its own mechanisms for determining which doctors fit into its various administrative categories. For instance, the Sécurité Sociale did not in some cases recognize doctors with a "competency" that they practiced exclusively as equivalent to specialists in matters of fees; the Ordre, however, did. Nor did the Securité Sociale recognize, as the Ordre did, medical biology as a specialty. Urology, in contrast, was recognized only as a competency within the Ordre's classification but as a full specialty by the Sécurité Sociale. The same was true of gynecology and obstetrics when they were not combined.[101]

Local hospital administrations that named specialists to hospital positions added a further level of possible conflict. In one well-publicized case, a local hospital administration tried to take away the right to do caesarean sections from an obstetrician who had obtained qualifications as a *compétent* rather than as an exclusive specialist. In 1958, the health bureaucracy made it clear that hospital administrations did not need to take account of specialty certificates when recruiting hospital specialists by traditional competitive examinations (*concours*).[102] And once the faculty programs got under way in the 1950s, vigorous complaints were heard about variations in standards among different specialties and faculties.[103] The complex legal basis for such an elaborate regulatory system administered at the national level proved to be a serious problem as well; on several occasions, either the Council of State or law courts found the existing procedures for specialist qualification to be illegal according to French administrative law. This forced major administrative modifications to be introduced on three different occasions.[104]

Above all, the higher fees granted specialists—for standard consultations they were double those of GPs, and commonly referred to as "C2"—were a constant source of tension; they seemed to sanction the inferiority of general practice and to encourage ever greater numbers of doctors to become specialists.[105] Those justifying disparities in fees tended to alternate between the older argument that it was necessary to compensate doctors who were drastically limiting the number of patients they could see, and a newer one in which higher fees were the reward for special education, greater skills, and more complicated procedures. Specialists also argued (and GPs denied) that the expenses of specialty practice were greater and that consultations were longer. As many writers pointed out, however, fee differentials had long preceded, and owed little to, the new system of medical certification.[106]

GPs were not the only ones who were unhappy. Stratification based on specialty status (often thought to be unearned) had, it was argued, destroyed traditional forms of distinction that had permitted some individuals to charge higher fees: public notoriety, training as an elite *interne des hôpitaux de Paris*, or service in hospital posts in general medicine.[107] Former interns were especially vocal in trying to protect their status. Faced with a choice between lobbying for the recognition of elite general medicine as a specialty in the form of internal medicine (as was the case in Germany and the United States) or extending the special rank of "consultant" generalist that already existed for faculty professors and hospital physicians to all former interns and those who had achieved "notoriety," the association of interns selected the latter option. This position was supported by the Confederation of Medical Trade Unions in 1954, but without much effect.[108] In contrast, former interns did win the right to have their internships considered equivalent to faculty certificates in a number of specialty fields.[109] Some specialists felt that the refusal to legally restrict certain difficult acts to trained specialists undermined the whole principle of certification.[110] Just about everyone believed that specialization was excessively widespread. By 1960, a high-profile medical mandarin, Henri Pequignot, could refer to specialization as the "internal gangrene of the medical profession."[111]

Specialty certification was thus a typical French compromise reform that left many deeply unsatisfied. Despite the barrage of criticisms they regularly faced, the leaders of French medicine nonetheless seemed rather proud of the system they had constructed. At a congress devoted to medical ethics that was held in 1955, one of the preliminary reports described the recently created system of specialty certification.[112] The subject may seem to a reader in the first years of the new millennium to have been somewhat out of place in a meeting about medical ethics. But the French system of specialization was perceived by its authors not merely as an administrative compromise among different professional groups and interests but as a measure reconciling many different rights and obligations. It thus represented professional ethics at the most practical level.

Conclusion

The lack of specialty regulation in interwar France does not require elaborate cultural theories about the French character. Nor can it be explained by the hostility of the French medical profession or by its fragmentation and inability to achieve consensus. On the contrary, the profession eventually achieved a rather effective working consensus in spite of substantial opposition. The relative tardiness of the French is best explained by the ambitious quest of the organized medical profession for a national system of state certification rather than the easier-to-achieve systems of professional certification implemented decades earlier in Germany and the United States. Achieving this goal required years of discussion within the national association of medical trade unions and difficult choices laboriously made among several competing regulatory models. Necessary legislative intervention was complicated and delayed by rivalries between doctors and dentists, each group having its political supporters. It took the creation of a new administrative body, the Ordre des Médecins, with the authority to impose specialist certification outside of the political arena, to successfully complete the process after World War II. The same ambitions that delayed the introduction of certification were responsible for the administrative problems and professional complaints that such a complex and unwieldy apparatus provoked throughout the 1950s. But this quest for a uniform national system seemed an appropriate strategy to apply to the centralized national system of medical institutions that had evolved during the previous century.

Chapter 9
Regulating Specialists in the British Manner

In Germany, France, and the United States, organized medical professions orchestrated the regulation of specialties while navigating among a host of external forces and pressures. Doctors justified specialty regulation on the grounds that it was (1) needed to protect the public from untrained specialists and (2) imperative to restrict competition within the profession. These requirements seemed so overwhelming that little thought was given to the larger context of population health needs. In Great Britain, however, the pattern of development was different. Despite the efforts of certain specialist groups, the profession as a whole showed relatively little interest in formal specialist certification because neither competition nor dangers to the public seemed particularly salient. Specialist numbers were contained because the specialist was usually defined as someone with a hospital post. Hospital staff and administrators thus determined how best to meet their need for specialists. There were of course specialists without hospital posts, but they functioned in a different professional sphere and went largely unrecognized.

By the 1930s, the British Medical Association began to identify specialists in order to fulfill the needs of public and private health insurance programs, as well as various public health initiatives. This was the model that continued to be followed during the following decade, with one big difference. Rather than merely identifying specialists for the health services, it was now thought necessary to *produce* them. The organization of specialties in Great Britain was in large measure a *by-product* of plans to provide comprehensive health services to the population, culminating in the postwar National Health Service. The purpose of regulating specialties was to ensure that personnel requirements for these services would be adequately met. From the beginning, notions of administrative rationality and planning were joined to traditional ideas of medical hierarchy to produce a broad consensus about the need for a clear division of labor between specialist consultants and general practitioners. The foundation upon which the eventual organization of specialists would rest was thus not formal certification but rather the time-honored practices of the British medical elite adapted to new administrative realities: appointment of specialists to hospital posts through informal modes of decision-making by members of the hospital elite, acting in association with the health bureaucracy.

Behind these developments lay another institutional peculiarity of British medicine. While academic elites in France and Germany collectively had little to do with the professional politics of specialization, and whereas such elites in the United States were very active but functioned primarily through relatively fragmented specialist societies or private national associations, the consultant hospital elite in Britain wielded enormous political influence through the powerful and prestigious royal colleges that they controlled.

The Belated Acceptance of Specialization

In the twentieth century the British medical profession accommodated itself to specialization; but it did so belatedly, less thoroughly, and quite differently than medical professions in other nations. British practitioners in such fields as cardiology and neurology achieved international recognition in their fields, in spite of the fact that many did not think of themselves as specialists.

Overall, specialism before 1920 was less visible and less developed in Britain than elsewhere. In 1915, Abraham Flexner could describe British teaching hospitals in the following terms:

> . . . as a rule, the hospital and its outpatient departments contain material enough for the purposes of instruction, but this material has not been carefully differentiated. Medicine, surgery and obstetrics are recognized as separate divisions; but there is little intensive specialization, and research suffers in consequence. The English hospital also lacks the laboratory equipment and staff needed for the critical study of disease.[1]

At the time Flexner wrote these words, World War I was already subjecting British medicine to military forms of administrative rationality and substantially furthering the specialization process. Early in the war, four separate types of hospitals for officers suffering shell shock were established. The goal was to "classify them [officers] as soon as possible so that each might be brought at once into an environment best suited to recovery."[2] Large numbers of cardiac problems in the British army, conditions popularly known as "soldier's heart," led to the creation of special hospitals whose staffs after the war formed the core of the "new cardiology."[3] Special orthopedic hospitals were established to deal with amputees. The *Journal of the American Medical Association's* (*JAMA*) regular contributor from London wrote in 1916: "One of the new features of army medical organization is the extent to which the War Office has used specialists of all kinds. Our leading orthopedic surgeon, Mr. Robert Jones, has been appointed inspector of military orthopedics."[4] Special hospitals were also created to treat head and facial injuries, tuberculosis, and epilepsy.[5]

After the armistice, specialists remained influential as military models of organization were integrated into civilian life. The Ministry of Pensions utilized specialists extensively to determine who was eligible for disability pensions for such conditions as soldier's heart and shell shock.[6] The War Office continued to appoint specialists to fill vacancies in general hospitals authorized as military establishments.[7] The government also moved large numbers of soldiers from general to military orthopedic hospitals, much to the distress of general surgeons. The treasurer of the Radcliffe Infirmary wrote:

> The speed at which "orthopaedic" surgery has taken over the care of practically the whole body is remarkable; with the result that general surgeons of ripe experience and approved ability are no longer considered fit to give a prognosis or to treat active or discharged soldiers; and a branch of surgery which began with treatment of bones has now extended its sphere of operations into almost every portion of the body, even tracing paralysis to its source. . . . [8]

The Royal College of Surgeons (RCS) intervened with the director general of the Royal Army Medical Service, stressing the need to associate general surgeons with the care of wounded soldiers so that advances in knowledge and treatment would become available in civilian medicine. The letter also protested against use of the term "orthopaedic" hospitals to identify military institutions. The military leadership responded by changing the name of these institutions to "special military *surgical* centres" but remained committed to the principle of specialist military institutions.[9] The attractiveness of orthopedics to government officials and its capacity to challenge general surgery would prove to be short-lived.[10] But the military and administrative logic behind its fleeting popularity would continue to advance specialization.

Postwar prospects for expanding state involvement in health care added more enduring impetus to the rhetoric of administrative rationalization that was calling for a sharper and more efficient division of labor between GPs and specialists and among different types of specialist institutions.[11] Growing public and private sponsorship of medical research promoted similar processes of differentiation. In 1925 the Middlesex Hospital Medical School received a private gift worth $100,000 to support an institute devoted to research in the diseases of the ear, nose, and throat.[12] But if the need for teaching specialties was increasingly recognized, accepting specialties as legitimate forms of medical practice occurred slowly in Britain. As late as 1949, Sir Henry Cohen could tell the Medical Section of the Royal Society of Medicine, at a meeting on the subject, that if research in a narrow field was justified by the demands of science, the same was not true of medical practice.[13] Notwithstanding the pervasiveness of such sentiments, specialization gradually did gain acceptance as a legitimate form of medical practice.

Postgraduate training was established in late 1890s. This included supplementary training for GPs but also short training programs for specialists. Because of the importance of the imperial enterprise, tropical medicine became, with the establishment of special schools in London and Liverpool, something like a specialty with short training programs and special diplomas.[14] Other training programs also proliferated; in 1935 Hammersmith Post-Graduate School was set up to centralize and expand such training.[15] Despite the growing acceptance of specialist practice, however, Britain remained unique among our four nations; no attempt at an overall system to train and certify specialists was contemplated before World War II, despite the efforts of several specialties to establish their own regulatory mechanisms. After the war, a rather unusual approach to specialist regulation was eventually worked out.

There are many reasons for the distinctive evolution of specialization in Britain. The establishment in 1911 of a national health insurance system, which served elsewhere as an impetus to identify and define specialists, did not initially perform this function in Britain because hospital and specialty services were specifically excluded from coverage. The social structure of the medical profession was an even more determinant factor.

University/hospital elites *everywhere* showed little interest in certification because clerkships, honorific titles, and posts in hospitals and medical schools were the key markers of elite specialist status. Everywhere, early training programs were short and geared to more modest practitioners rather than the elite, and were thus not taken very seriously. (In Britain, almost none of the many specialty diplomas established after the turn of the century were even allowed by the General Medical Council to appear in the *Medical Register;* the only exceptions were those of public health or state medicine, as a direct consequence of the law of 1886.[16]) In most countries, it was not the elite but less well-established specialists, threatened by competition from the totally untrained, who most vigorously advocated certification as a form of occupational self-defense. Such practitioners certainly existed in Britain, but the widespread convention that the only specialists who counted were hospital consultants prevented the emergence of the kind of grassroots specialist movements that occurred in other countries. Furthermore, the fragmentation of specialists everywhere was exacerbated in Britain by the separation in different royal colleges of surgical specialists from medical specialists in such fields as neurology, cardiology, and otorhinolaryngology.[17] With such divided interests and loyalties, many specialty groupings had difficulty elaborating common professional strategies.

This narrow definition of specialists as hospital consultants also served to obscure and perhaps actually to moderate one of the chief imperatives for certification in other countries: the unbridled spread of specialists. After 1890, more and more practitioners unquestionably chose to practice as specialists; the need to staff hospitals in provincial cities and towns was a major impetus for the emergence of GP-specialists, including many who practiced surgery part-time.[18] Nonetheless, the initial attitude of much of the profession was that these were GPs with a "special interest" and therefore not particularly threatening. This attitude began to change only in the 1920s, when certain specialties began campaigning actively to remove certain practices from normal GP work (see below). By then, the National Health Insurance was also beginning to place restraints on the specialist practice of GPs through capitation fees that did not reward specialist acts; specialist practice by GPs, moreover, was increasingly becoming unnecessary financially as panel practice successfully raised their incomes.[19] This left specialties largely in the hands of consultants, who were appointed to hospitals according to the time-honored and informal criteria of the medical elite: general qualifications in medicine or surgery, followed by junior hospital training posts, followed by more senior posts that demanded as a prerequisite the higher *general* fellowships of the royal colleges and that were awarded through a process of informal judgment by peers. Consequently, pressure for certification remained restricted to isolated specialty groups.

Finally, the forces that since the nineteenth century had attempted to move British medicine toward greater unity remained powerful and militated against any *formal* recognition of divisions among medical practitioners. The British acceptance of specialties continued to be based on certain fundamental conditions: that they remain firmly rooted in a united profession (hence the significance of the unification of specialty societies within the Royal Society of Medicine) and that they not be too visible (hence the opposition to visible identification in medical directories). This outlook permitted growing support for a "rationalized" division of labor in which GPs referred patients to consultant specialists. But certifying these specialists seemed to go much too far toward granting each category a separate and autonomous identity.

The editorialist of the *British Medical Journal* (*BMJ*) who responded in 1908 to the movement developing in Germany to regulate specialties lucidly expressed this combination of attitudes:

> British experience does not suggest the need for these regulations; but in Germany it is the custom for specialists to indicate their line of practice on their door-plates and so advertise themselves directly to the public, a plan which is not regarded here with favour. With us a specialist looks to his professional brethren for the recognition of his qualifications, and his practice depends upon their being convinced that he possesses the necessary training and experience. It is rare for anyone to start practice as a specialist without holding a hospital appointment, and this in itself affords some guarantee of his having the requisite knowledge and skill.[20]

To sum up, the key distinction in Britain was a *functional* definition of specialists as general physicians or surgeons who performed particular tasks based on the requirements of their hospital appointment but who remained essentially indistinguishable from their peers. Where such a clear-cut functional definition did not exist (the case in most other nations), specialists had to seek out identifying features: they had to insist on full-time practice as a specialist, membership in an elite national specialist society, or, ultimately, some form of certification or diploma.

Institutional Realities

Making possible this constellation of attitudes were some unique institutional realities. Chief among them was the dominance of the royal colleges in the granting of postgraduate diplomas. Other institutions also granted such diplomas, but these were usually of lesser stature. A joint, persistent effort by the two London colleges could certainly have produced a system of specialty certification that would have been widely accepted, but the colleges for a long time showed little interest in this task. From their perch at the very summit of the profession, college fellows felt no particular competition from half-educated practitioners calling themselves specialists. They remained deeply attached to the vision of a unified medical profession and to a view of elite practitioners as generalists who, in many cases, just happened to be performing specialist functions. They gradually began to offer specialist diplomas for rank-and-file doctors but insisted on higher general credentials for those who wished to join them in the consultant ranks.

The British Medical Association (BMA), for its part, saw itself as representing the general practitioner and had little reason to become involved in what seemed essentially a consultant issue. If the question did come up, the Association was hostile to certification, not only because it was committed to a unified profession but also because such certification threatened to limit the sphere of activity and lower the status of GPs. Discussing projects for certification in Germany, an editorial in the *BMJ* commented:

> The circular speaks of the late increase of specialists as a grave matter, but it is questionable whether the actual number of practitioners who bear the appellation without being properly qualified to do so is really large enough to justify the proposed changes. Moreover, the difficulties connected with the official lists of available institutes, etc., are likely to prove serious. Where and how would the line be drawn? Institutes and specialists not mentioned in the lists would be, so to speak, denounced as unfit.[21]

As a matter of principle, BMA leaders in the 1920s defended the right of GPs to assume specialist functions and activities, although this attitude would change in the following decade.[22]

There is one final and, in my view, especially noteworthy reason for this unique British attitude to specialties. In other countries, pressure for certification followed full acceptance of academic specialization by professional elites. Once specialties were fully accepted as subjects in the medical curriculum, which occurred in most countries by the first decade of the twentieth century, more and more doctors began calling themselves specialists; the training and certification of these specialists thus moved to the forefront of pressing issues. In Britain, however, the initial process of academic acceptance took considerably longer and continued to be a dominant concern. Most specialties had little place on curricula and examinations, and those having any place at all were not well integrated within educational programs.[23] Even representatives of ophthalmology, arguably the most prestigious of the specialties in Britain, were still contending in 1919 that courses and examinations in the subject should be a requirement for medical students. Using comparative data, they concluded: "Great Britain stands almost alone in granting diplomas to practice medicine without evidence of an adequate knowledge of diseases of the eye."[24] In this larger context, seeking certification seemed either beside the point or positively counterproductive.

At the annual meeting of the BMA in 1912, the Section of Laryngology and Rhinology met in joint session with the Section of Otology to discuss education for their specialties. An overview of the situation in continental European by a Danish physician[25] was followed by an examination of British conditions, presented by P. Watson-Williams, lecturer in this specialty at the University of Bristol.[26] After emphasizing the relatively poor standing of these specialties in Britain as compared with the Continent, the speaker made three practical suggestions:

1. That the undergraduate medical curriculum give due recognition to these specialties
2. That special departments in teaching hospitals should be better equipped and organized
3. That future specialist formation should be based on systematic postgraduate training that would result in a distinctive degree or qualification. Such training would be much more extensive than existing programs and would be equivalent to the stringent prerequisites that were required of consulting surgeons and physicians. A major justification for this third innovation was the current convention that higher training in general surgery was the criteriona for hospital posts in ORL; this meant that the entire medical side of the specialty was being neglected.

In the discussion that followed,[27] the first two proposals received general assent. But the reaction to the third was mixed; some speakers agreed, but the majority did not. Aside from general hostility to the multiplication of diplomas, a common theme was that the specialty first had to raise its status within the profession by gaining an adequate position in the medical curriculum. Sir St. Clair Thomson of London is reported to have said, "Until they had raised their own standard and dignity, and until they insisted on the absolute necessity of otolaryngology for all pass examinations, he thought it unreasonable to put forth a demand for a separate and particular examination for a specialist. They must first improve themselves and their work, and the material out of which specialists were made, before they tried to mark them off by examination."[28]

Herbert Tilley of London agreed, and argued for the conventional approach to specialist formation: "the specialist was born not made, and for any special line in medicine or surgery to secure the respect of the general profession, those who elected to work in it must necessarily have had a good training in general medicine and surgery, and then by their own good work so advanced the knowledge in their specialty that they would command the honour and goodwill of the general profession."[29] Another London specialist also associated himself with this view and pinpointed the informal selection mechanisms that, in Britain, constituted the essential elements of professional recognition: "the genuine expert specialist was made not by diploma but by a process of natural selection, and he thought that the committee which nominated for hospital appointments formed the chief instrument for the advancement of that natural process."[30]

Twenty-four years later, a radiologist suggested that respectability for specialists could be achieved only by traditional means: "The higher [general] degrees [of the colleges] are the key to our final status, particularly in hospitals and schools. They transform the radiologist into the physician in charge of the radiological department."[31] Despite such views, radiologists in fact opted for special diplomas relatively early. Other marginal specialties resisted this trend. In the 1930s, specialists in physical medicine initially expressed reluctance to introduce a specialist diploma, on the grounds that they would lose their status as physicians and become mere technicians. This had economic implications since it would "tend to narrow the field of their work into the limited specialty of physical medicine."[32] But it was above all a matter of professional stature: "Every effort which has recently been made to elevate the status of this subject has been directed to incorporating it as a branch of general medicine, as against an isolated technical specialty. . . . who except a technician would wish to take such a degree? . . . it would deprive the consultants of their chance of equal status with other physicians, and it would ruin their chances of [hospital] beds. . . . "[33]

The result of all these forces was that during the first decades of the twentieth century, educational institutions created specialist training programs rather haphazardly. They were initially short and aimed primarily at general practitioners. By the 1920s, even the royal colleges were establishing conjoint diplomas of this sort in the major specialist subjects.[34] As time went on, the colleges targeted a wider clientele that might also include potential consultants. The RCS took the lead, its Committee of Management explaining in 1920 that since other examining bodies were already providing such diplomas, "it may be considered advisable that the Royal Colleges which together grant by far the largest number of qualifications, should offer to their Diplomates the opportunity of obtaining advanced Diplomas in Special Subjects." Since facilities for specialized practice were increasing, "[i]t is believed that the possession of a Diploma or Certificate of Proficiency as evidence of special Post-Graduate study, would be welcomed by many who desire to possess evidence of efficiency in their own subjects and by those who hope to obtain Hospital Appointments in Special Departments." Perhaps most germane was the attitude of public authorities, particularly those responsible for health insurance. The College's report pointed out that a conference organized by the National Health Insurance Commission for the provision of "expert service" had decided that a general practitioner might be considered an expert if he had special postgraduate training, or held a hospital appointment that offered opportunities to acquire experience, or was recognized by the local profession as an expert. Certificates granted by the royal colleges "might well be considered by the Ministry of Health as fulfilling the conditions requisite to hold the position of Member of the Expert Medical Service." If the need to remain relevant to government plans was not a sufficient incentive to action, the report also noted that since November 1919, specialists in the Army Medical Corps received higher pay than GPs.[35]

Some of the diplomas thus created became indispensable for certain institutional posts: medical officers of health, the Colonial Medical Service, hospital radiologists, asylum physicians, to name the most important. However, in mainstream clinical medicine their usefulness was less clear. If it was sometimes acknowledged that graduates of these programs often functioned as poorly trained specialists, this was not seen as a major problem because unofficial recruitment standards usually kept these graduates out of major urban hospitals. It was also the case that such practitioners were usually confined to certain specialties compatible with insurance practice. The single effort in 1919 to establish a truly high-level specialty certificate, the fellowship of the RCS with special mention in ophthalmology, managed to attract only one candidate during the next few decades because its requirements were so stringent; the examination could be obtained only *after* the passing of all regular exams for the FRCS.[36]

In London, efforts were made to coordinate and standardize the programs that had been created. From 1898 to 1913, the London Postgraduate Association—representing most of the undergraduate medical schools and several specialist hospitals—tried to fulfill this role. In 1918, the Fellowship of Medicine and Postgraduate Medical Association attempted to assume the same role, but without success.[37] The Athlone Report of 1921 expressed the extent to which education had succumbed to the prevailing rhetoric of rationalization and efficiency. Its primary recommendation was the establishment of a postgraduate medical school attached to large hospitals: "The school should be the center of a great teaching organization, in which the special Hospitals of London, the Poor Law Infirmaries and the Medical schools with their clinical units and research departments would all find their place. As an integral part of the organization there should be a bureau or central office established under a wisely appointed committee of management to coordinate the whole system . . . ."[38]

In 1925, the Ministry of Health appointed yet another commission, the Greenwood Committee, which sought to implement the recommendations of the Athlone

Committee. Its deliberations led to the establishment of the British Postgraduate Hospital and Medical School at Hammersmith Hospital in 1935.[39]

Rationalizing British Medicine

Most energy continued to be expended on efforts to improve the status of specialties within general hospitals and programs of medical training. This sometimes provoked turf battles over specific practices. Conflict between surgeons and orthopedists that had begun during the war continued. In 1925, the sections of Surgery and Orthopedics of the BMA engaged in a lively debate about whether special wards dealing with fractures should be established in hospitals under the direction of orthopedic specialists.[40] But the key effort remained focused on gaining an enhanced role in the curriculum and examinations for general medical training, symbolizing acceptance of the field by the medical elite. This issue came up regularly between the wars in conjunction with numerous plans to reform medical education. As in other countries, educational reform focused chiefly on the need to find room in the curriculum for the recent explosion of new medical knowledge and particularly the laboratory sciences. It also had to do with expanding the role of medical research that had brought so much prestige to Germany and, now in the twentieth century, was doing the same for the United States. The specialties were brought into the discussion as components of general medical training that needed to be improved, particularly in domains, such as obstetrics and pediatrics, with important public health implications. New regulations introduced by the General Medical Council in 1922 and again in the mid-1930s significantly improved the status of specialties in medical training.[41]

The problems of British health care, however, extended well beyond medical training. According to one historical survey, "Health care provision after World War I was a patchwork of ramshackle and uncoordinated services."[42] The problem was recognized, and generated a widespread desire to unify and rationalize the various services that had developed during the previous century through a process of accretion, and that continued to multiply at a rapid rate.[43] Hospitals constituted an especially troubled sector where the rhetoric of administrative rationalization was used to promote reform. The reorganization of the chaotic hospital system seemed particularly urgent because of financial difficulties in the voluntary hospital sector and because there seemed to be a shortage of beds and services in spite of (or because of) the many different kinds of institutions and authorities in existence.[44] Efforts at change began in the late nineteenth century but met with little success.[45] After World War I, one parliamentary commission after another examined the organization of hospitals.[46] And pressure increased as a result of the Local Government Act of 1929; poor-law hospitals were taken over by county governments, raising the prospect of competition between municipal and voluntary hospitals.[47] Furthermore, this reform created powerful administrative bodies responsible for coordinating large numbers of hospital institutions; the London County Council, for instance, took over responsibility for seventy-six hospitals with 42,000 beds.[48]

This gave rise to immense pressures for institutional restructuring. All these issues and problems extended far beyond specialists, who were nonetheless deeply implicated. For one thing, rationalization was frequently identified with more organized and better-organized specialty services. The London County Council divided its hospitals into six categories, including those devoted to children, maternity patients, and mental patients.[49] In the voluntary sector, the existence of numerous specialty hospitals and specialty wards in general hospitals, as well as the fact that specialists such as pathologists, anesthetists, and radiologists were among the first staff of the London hospitals to be employed full time,[50] put the issue of specialists near the center of personnel concerns. The same was true in the provincial cottage hospitals. Turf battles among specialties for wards and services were often cast in the language of hospital reorganization and efficiency, as Roger Cooter has shown in the case of orthopedics.[51]

These pressures were intensified by two other factors. The first had to do with growing pressure to expand the services of the National Health Insurance (NHI) through a variety of local and national plans. The second was connected with the efforts of certain specialist groups to cope with growing professional competition by seeking to regulate training and certification for specialist practice.

In regard to the first factor, almost as soon as World War I ended, pressure began to build for a comprehensive health insurance program including hospitals and specialist services. One official committee after another dealt with the issue without bringing about the desired changes.[52] Nonetheless, these committees' reports had important repercussions. A strong administrative orientation focusing on the unification of health-care institutions within a rational hierarchical framework became firmly established; this was exemplified by the Dawson Report of 1920, which defined separate primary and secondary health-care roles and promoted the distinctions between GPs and consultants that were in the process of being established.[53] Many new programs were introduced—from workman's compensation to rehabilitation services—that extended beyond the boundaries of the NHI. These programs frequently included the provision of relatively inexpensive consultant and specialist services to those eligible for benefits. In the mid-1920s, the BMA drew up a list of ophthalmologists throughout the country (500 in 1926, increased to 800 several years later) to whom insurance societies could send patients for a cost of only 1 guinea. The goal was to ensure that such patients were not sent to opticians without medical qualifications.[54]

In a response to efforts by the Hospital Savings Association to arrange special consultation fees for its members, the BMA rejected the idea of a restricted panel of specialists and in 1932 drew up a comprehensive Consultants and Specialists List for London that provided the names of 380 competent individuals willing to treat such patients at a reduced rate.[55] It was also hoped that the scheme would attract patients away from hospital outpatient clinics, where free care was provided.[56] A year later the BMA made an effort to extend the scheme to the provinces, but this proved unsuccessful; many provincial consultants believed that the plan would lower their incomes.[57] But the London plan continued and, for a while, placed the BMA at the center of efforts to identify specialists.

The BMA's list of London specialists was republished in 1938 with over 600 individuals included.[58] It was meant, as the cover prominently announced, "_For Circulation to Members of the Medical Profession Only_" (italics and underlining are in the original) and was designed to facilitate referrals. Practitioners were divided into nine categories: medicine, surgery, obstetrics-gynecology, ophthalmology, dermatology, otorhinolaryngology, pathology, radiology, and physical medicine. What is more, considerable numbers of individuals in the first three categories—particularly in medicine—identified themselves as having a further specialist interest.[59] The list was established by a "consultants board' made up of representatives of the BMA and the royal colleges, with input from the Royal Society of Medicine. They examined carefully all applications for inclusion on the list; as in the earlier edition, the applicants had to satisfy "one or more" of the following three criteria:

1. That an individual had held a hospital or other appointment affording the opportunity to acquire some special skill and had exercised this skill in recent practice
2. That this individual had pursued special academic or postgraduate study in the area which he or she was practicing
3. That other practitioners in the area recognized the individual as having special proficiency in the area.[60]

Since specialists were being asked to treat certain patients for much less than normal fees, these criteria were relatively liberal; the board, moreover, had considerable leeway in making choices.[61] It might reject an application, request documents and testimonials, ask the opinion of an eminent specialist, or force an individual who wished to be in two categories to choose one or the other.[62] But the board nonetheless granted something like official recognition of specialty status. It also decided what counted as a specialty—rejecting, for example, "neurasthenia" and deciding that individuals might include under the "physical medicine" rubric the terms "therapeutic movement" and "electrotherapy.' The board considered, but decided against, distinguishing full-time from part-time consultant specialists (as the American Medical Association was doing).[63]

Other programs fulfilled a similar role in identifying competent specialists. The BMA's list of ophthalmic surgeons evolved into a National Eye Service to make refraction services by physicians more affordable, thus undercutting opticians.[64] Discussions about the creation of a National Maternity Service, begun in 1935, raised all sorts of questions about the future of GPs in obstetrics.[65]

Parallel to these developments, in regard to the second factor, some of the larger specialties—particularly those associated rather uneasily with surgery—began after World War I to introduce specialist diplomas. Such efforts seem to have aimed mainly at raising the status of specialized practitioners and delegitimizing those considered less well trained.[66] But they could also be justified by the growing need to identify specialists for service within the expanding national insurance system and the hospitals. These efforts were further advanced by growing, if not always enthusiastic, acceptance of specialization by the medical profession, in spite of the fact that Britain in the early twentieth century probably led the world in the number of public orations that warned against the dangers of excessive medical specialism. By the 1930s, it was common to speak of "consultants" and "specialists" as overlapping and closely related professional groups with common aims and interests.[67] An editorial in the *BMJ* in 1937 argued that most general consultants were specialists in some branch, to some degree, and that most specialists were consultants.[68] This was not an idle claim, as the Consultants List of the BMA showed clearly.[69] This blurring of distinctions went hand in hand with the growing status of specialties. In 1935, a proposal to reorganize the consultant services of the municipal hospitals of Manchester involved tripling spending in order "to ensure that every patient suffering from acute illness shall receive specialist attention as a matter of course."[70] Attitudes in London may not have been quite so enthusiastic, but they were not notably different. Specialized medical care was increasingly considered optimum medical care.

Different specialist groups reacted very differently to the prospect of organized training. Dermatologists and urologists showed little interest in creating special diplomas. Practitioners of physical medicine initially hesitated, then tried but failed. Some of the larger and better-established specialties were able to establish new diplomas through established channels.[71] A degree in orthopedics, for instance, was set up at Liverpool University in 1924 with significantly more elaborate requirements than other existing specialty diplomas. The royal colleges established eight conjoint specialty diplomas by the mid-1930s.[72] Near the end of World War II there were, excluding the membership and fellowship diplomas of the royal colleges, nearly forty postgraduate diplomas of this sort.[73]

Nonetheless, some specialties found it impossible to function within existing frameworks. Obstetrics was the most significant. Since the nineteenth century, its practitioners had been divided among three groups: those who wanted to combine traditional midwifery with gynecological surgery; those more traditional obstetricians who saw their field as a branch of physic and had no desire to pursue gynecological surgery; and those who saw gynecology as merely a branch of general surgery. As Ornella Moscucci has shown,[74] in the mid-1920s, a proposal to place gynecological surgery under the tutelage of the Royal College of Surgeons provoked a countermovement to combine obstetrics and gynecology under the jurisdiction of a new independent college. This latter effort was advanced by two factors. First, obstetrics was the oldest of the specialties, and thus had some leverage not enjoyed by newer fields more closely tied by tradition to either the Royal College of Physicians (RCP) or the RCS. Second, it also benefited from extensive political and public concern with high rates of maternal mortality. There was thus considerable political support for arguments that the existing royal colleges had not done enough to improve obstetrical training and that a special college might do considerably better. In 1929 the British College of Obstetricians (the title "Royal" was added in 1938) was established. Following the model of older colleges, it established a diploma aimed at GPs, who were supposed to deal with most normal births, and a membership examination for consultants, who were to deal with difficult births and gynecological surgery. Neither diploma had any legal status for practice.[75] In some ways this development was very traditional, following in the tracks of the royal colleges. The primary focus of the field remained the training of GPs and midwives in obstetrics. GPs, however, soon became convinced that obstetricians were seeking to elbow them out of midwifery practice by moving birthing into hospitals; indeed, a significant current within the specialty advocated precisely that policy.[76]

The case for the independence of radiology was strong, since the field was clearly distinguished by its technological focus. By the 1920s its status was rising, and full hospital rank was increasingly granted radiologists. Cambridge established a diploma in 1920, and several other universities (and, eventually, the royal colleges) followed suit. London University in 1930 created a chair in radiology. Still, radiologists lacked either the historical legitimacy or the public health visibility of obstetricians. They also faced unique professional problems because radiological practice was fundamentally unlike practice in the clinical specialties. An attempt to establish an independent "college" was vetoed by the royal colleges. Later, however, the amalgamation of several associations led to the founding in 1939 of the autonomous "Faculty" of Radiologists.[77] Just after World War II a Faculty of Ophthalmology was also constituted.

The BMA and the Beginnings of Specialty Regulation

By the early 1930s the issues surrounding specialization had become ubiquitous enough to convince leaders of the BMA that the Association could influence the various changes under way only by making more room for specialists and consultants. Consequently, in 1934 the Association established a Consultants and Specialist Group with direct representation on the governing council.[78] One of its first acts was to define the terms "specialists" and "consultants" in order to determine who could be a member of the group. For purposes of eligibility in this section, consultants and specialists were defined by full-time practice in one of four categories: medicine, surgery, obstetrics-gynecology, or the specialties; prospective members had to sign a statement that they fulfilled these conditions.[79] This was very different from the BMA's Consultants List, which was open to part-time GPs; the Group in fact tried unsuccessfully to impose similar restrictive criteria on the Consultants List being drawn up.[80] The Group's definition of "consultants and specialists" is interesting is several respects. It treated specialists as comparable with consultants in general medicine and surgery, indicating the changes in attitude that had transpired since the end of the war. This definition also made no mention of hospital posts, one of the traditional definitions of the term in Britain; it is likely that this represented a deliberate effort to exclude the many GPs who now served as consultants and specialists in small provincial hospitals. This did not deter many GPs from seeking to become members of the Group and then complaining bitterly when they were refused.[81]

Through this and other BMA committees that were being established, specialists became directly involved in policy discussions. They dealt with the salary demands of employed specialists, the representation of specialists on boards of examiners for medical diplomas, the right of full-time hospital staff to make home visits, and the place of consulting and specialist services within the evolving insurance and hospital systems.[82] The Consultants and Specialists Group also helped to define criteria for those to be included in the revised Consultants and Specialist List.[83] During World War II, specialists in the BMA became directly involved in such governmental programs as the Emergency Medical Service. They served as well on the various planning commissions that were established to review the status of health services.[84]

The Consultants and Specialists Group was only one of several representative clusters of this sort in the BMA. Special groups had earlier been created for pathology, spa medicine, and physical medicine. In the years that followed, groups representing radiology and psychological medicine were set up. Homeopaths unsuccessfully petitioned for such a group on the grounds that they constituted a specialty.[85] All of these specialist categories were fairly marginal in the British context, and members probably hoped to gain greater recognition and influence through such independent groups. Rules for membership were somewhat more lenient than for the Specialist and Consultants Group because "predominant" as well as "exclusive" practice of the specialty was accepted as a criterion for membership.[86] Other specialties were represented by committees formed around specific issues; the Ophthalmic Committee, for instance, was mainly concerned to administer the BMA's program of eye examinations but was seen by many as the representative of the specialty within the BMA.[87] This did not prevent some ophthalmic surgeons from seeking to establish a separate ophthalmic "group."[88] The Ophthalmic Committee was called upon to consider the request and decided, in the "interests of unity," to support its establishment. But the BMA Council decided instead to review the overall organization of specialist groups within the Association.[89] The result was the new Special Practice Committee that came into existence in 1938 with the purpose of representing all the emerging special groups and reporting directly to the BMA Council.[90] A General Practice Group was simultaneously established. But individual specialist groups continued to exist, and the Ophthalmic Group was soon approved, becoming by far the largest such group in the BMA, with 352 members.[91] It was quickly joined by groups representing orthopedic surgeons and, later (1945), dermatologists. In each, members were required to "predominantly" practice the specialty.[92] By 1939 over 1,100 individuals in England and Wales, as well as 150 in Scotland, were members of the Consultants and Specialists Group. After World War II, part-time specialists sought unsuccessfully to gain recognition as a group within the BMA.[93]

The fact that specialists were organizing in the context of a general administrative reform of health insurance and hospital services had profound implications. The status of specialties was raised because specialization had, within an administrative logic of resource distribution, significant practical advantages. Furthermore, specialization in Britain, far more than in the other three countries under examination, came increasingly to be seen through an administrative lens focusing on manpower needs. This reinforced traditional tendencies to view specialism in functional terms, with the difference that function now signified the provision of services within regionally coordinated hospital systems, a development furthered by the development during the war of the Emergency Medical Service.[94] A postwar report by the Ministry of Health commented on these wartime changes:

> As a result of this co-ordination of hospitals it was possible to arrange for special treatment centres in many of the medical and surgical specialties . . . .The advantage to the nation in the saving of life and the restoration of physical and mental efficiency that resulted from these special centres points to their continuance on such a scale that they will be available throughout the country to any patient who requires them.[95]

One hundred and twenty of these centers were set up during the war years; the two largest categories, with twenty centers each, dealt with orthopedic surgery and skin diseases. Equally important, the principle of public payment for specialist work in hospitals was firmly established.[96]

An important expression of all these new forces was the report of the Special Commission on Medical Education (known as the Goodenough Report), published in 1944 after extensive consultation with the medical elite.[97] Unlike previous reports on education, which had focused primarily on undergraduate medical training, this report also dealt extensively with the postgraduate training of specialists. Even the long discussion of the undergraduate medical curriculum was informed by a new perspective. Specialization, in the Goodenough Report, was presented as an all-pervading reality, a defining feature of medical life. The Report provided the traditional warnings against the dangers of narrow specialism but added that in future, virtually all the teachers of medicine would be specialists. How, then, could the medical curriculum retain coherence and unity? This was a crucial problem for which the authors suggested several types of remedies.[98] But the most original aspect of the Report was its emphasis on postgraduate training: "A nation embarking on a comprehensive health service cannot afford to do without a comprehensive system of post-graduate medical education," and had to remedy "the insufficiency of competent specialists in certain branches of medicine and surgery."[99] It made the following proposals based on "a large consensus of opinion":

1. Qualifications and standards should be determined by "some suitable central machinery."[100] The form this would take was not specified, but the Report expressed the hope that the royal colleges would collectively administer this mechanism.
2. The primary requirement should be four or five years of postgraduate training following registration as a physician, and a resident hospital appointment in general medicine and surgery.
3. The universities, in consultation with the profession, should set up a national system of specialized postgraduate institutes built around specialist hospitals. The Report insisted on the need for major investments in such hospitals.

The manpower needs of an expanded health-care system was the predominant concern of the Goodenough Report. Specialists were seen as consultants requiring lengthy training and quite possibly the high-level qualifications in general medicine and surgery conferred by the royal colleges.[101] Here notions of administrative efficiency seem to have been shaped by the traditional attitudes and values of the hospital elite.

From 1944, the training of specialists became an integral element in plans to establish a national health service. In the absence of existing standards, different medical bodies came up with their own criteria for defining a specialist. These ranged from the simple insistence on hospital appointments, to the relatively loose criteria that currently applied for insurance practice, to inclusion on the Consultants and Specialists List.[102] The royal colleges, at the Ministry of Health's urging, undertook (unsuccessfully) a national survey of consultants and specialists.[103] The general conclusion reached was, in the words of Lord Moran, president of the RCP and head of the Consultant Services Committee, that to the question of how one defined a consultant or specialist,

there is at present no satisfactory answer. A considerable number of those who now practice as consultants and specialists are not recognizable as such on paper. Their colleagues, in the course of time, have come to accept them in this role on account of their sagacity in consultation or their proficiency in some technique. This difficulty in saying who is a specialist and who is not means that any estimate of the total number of specialists in this country is only an approximate figure.[104]

Specialists and the National Health Service

Much has been written about the creation of the National Health Service (NHS).[105] It is well known that consultants and specialists, represented by the royal colleges rather than the BMA, were treated very generously by the government and, on the whole, supported its plans; GPs were treated less well and expressed greater opposition.[106] Leading consultants such as Lord Moran served as trusted advisers to the administration, while leaders of the BMA did not. Not only were preexisting divisions within the profession significantly widened, but the consultant elite managed to eliminate a major source of competing power: local authorities who had, with lay officers in voluntary hospitals, traditionally played a dominant role in hospital administration. Early plans had placed most health services in the hands of county and municipal authorities, and the wartime coalition government had planned to consign hospitals to the jurisdiction of thirty-five to forty local administrative bodies. However, leading consultants and their administrative supporters insisted that local jurisdictions were too narrow to provide uniform, high-quality care. As a result, hospitals were nationalized. The postwar Labour government placed hospitals and related institutions under the jurisdiction of fourteen large regional boards centered on universities and extending far beyond the jurisdictions of local authorities. Aside from considerations of efficacy, Lord Moran admitted, "it was only by giving the Regions power that doctors could be protected from lay interference in the conduct of their professional duties."[107] Furthermore, teaching hospitals were granted their own administrations, independent of even these regional structures. At the end of the day, consultants won considerable freedom from any "lay" interference.

This is not the place for a detailed discussion of the newly established NHS. I will limit myself in what follows to its features that were particularly significant for the development of specialties.

First, the blending together of consultants and specialists that had begun during the 1920s culminated in virtual fusion. As Lord Moran's quote above indicates, the words "consultant" and "specialist" came to be used interchangeably, especially among politicians and administrators.[108] The Health Services Act consistently used the word "specialist" rather than "consultant."[109] Both terms were defined by possession of hospital posts and patient referral, and the status of both as salaried hospital employees distinguished them sharply from GPs and panel practice. The nationalization of hospitals under regional boards and a national income structure that was far higher than that for GPs further welded them into a coherent and privileged interest group, despite persisting inequalities among them.[110] As the rift between consultant-specialists and GPs widened during the postwar years, relations between the royal colleges representing the elite and the BMA with its mandate to speak for the entire profession became strained. Who would speak for the profession in dealing with government became a controversial issue, requiring in the end a joint committee representing all the involved institutions and groups.[111] Tensions arose as well among different kinds of specialist-consultants. One axis of division was between the traditional elite of teaching consultants and specialists centered in the royal colleges, and nonteaching specialists who tended to gravitate toward the BMA.[112] Another was between general and specialist consultants. The BMA's Consultants and Specialists Group came out against any attempt to differentiate between general consultants and specialists in matters of fees,[113] but as we shall see, serious inequalities remained.

Second, workforce concerns preoccupied the administrators of the system. The immediate goal was to increase the number of consultant staff and improve their distribution through the creation of salaried posts on the basis of local needs.[114] Nonetheless, the central government left a great deal of scope to regional bodies in organizing services. The Ministry of Health provided detailed guidelines but hastened to insist that its various missives were merely "suggestions" and not "instructions."[115] It went on to spell out clearly the Ministry's moderately decentralized vision of health services:

> There is no wish to standardize consultant services throughout the country and each region will be able to plan these services in the way best suited to the local organizations and need; indeed experiment and variation between regions are essential to future developments. There are, however, general principles which will be applicable in all regions and it is probable that broadly similar plans will emerge in each.[116]

Third, personnel needs were to a significant degree understood from the traditional perspective of the medical elite. Consequently, there was deep reluctance to subdivide general medicine excessively; the Ministry of Health viewed certain specialties as special interests within general medicine or surgery. Thus neurology, cardiology, and hematology could be part of the work of general physicians, while genito-urinary surgery and gastroenterology remained part of general surgery.[117] During the next few decades, few individuals would enter these fields as exclusive specialists.[118] Nonetheless, unfettered by the traditional concern of medical associations to limit the development of new specialties, civil servants displayed characteristic administrative faith in solving problems through more elaborate specialization. Instructions to regional authorities designated no fewer than twenty-six "consultant services," and they insisted that many of these services needed to be staffed by exclusive specialists either immediately or at some point in the future. Thus pediatrics, dermatology, and diseases of the chest were recognized to be exclusive of general medicine, while gynecology, orthopedics, neurosurgery, and thoracic surgery were considered distinct from general surgery.[119] It was emphasized that special consultants were needed for hitherto marginal fields such as physical medicine and anesthesia. Diagnostic radiology was distinguished from radiotherapy, and both were treated as exclusive specialties.[120] Traumatic and orthopedic surgery was charged with the treatment of all diseases and injuries of the "bones, joints and associated structures," finally winning its long battle against general surgery.[121] Overall, the system of specialist regulation in Britain was unique to the extent that the goal was not to limit the spread of specialties but, on the contrary, to train many more specialists to satisfy the needs of the health services. Charles Webster makes the conservative estimate that between 1949 and 1958, the consultant labor force increased by at least 30 percent.[122]

Fourth, in one respect, however, the traditional preference of the medical elite was respected: informal mechanisms of selection to hospital positions were maintained. Regional hospital boards and boards of teaching hospitals were responsible for determining standards of specialist appointment and practice.[123] The General Medical Council had proposed in 1944 that a statutory register of specialists be established and that appointments be made from individuals on this list[124]; some specialty groups, such as the radiologists, had approved this suggestion.[125] But a register was never implemented for several reasons. The royal colleges tried to prepare such lists for the Ministry of Health, but gave up because any specific criteria would have excluded too many individuals. In any case, it was argued, "there are neither standards nor criteria that can be applied at the present time . . . "[126]; consequently, decisions could be based only on local medical opinion. Furthermore, a register would have required rigid definitions of specialist status and the consequent inflexible classification of practitioners into different categories. This provoked widespread opposition from the royal colleges and the BMA.[127] The *BMJ* spoke of general consensus among these institutions that "there should not now be established a statutory roll and that appointments boards acting in the hospital regions should make their appointments on the merits of the applications without seeking to apply some nationally imposed standard."[128] A report by the Medico-Psychological Association emphasized that "the chief criteria for eligibility to specialist status must always remain a man's contribution to his subject and the standing he enjoys among his colleagues. . . . "[129]

To some degree, this flexibility was justified by immediate manpower considerations.[130] Politicians and administrators desired the greatest possible flexibility in satisfying personnel needs, and thus avoided rigid definitions of terms such as "consultant" and "specialist" that would have restricted their room to maneuver. A report of 1948 by the Ministry of Health clearly expressed this view while shaping subsequent policy:

> No general criterion of specialist status can be laid down—a proper assessment can be arrived at only after a consideration by professional advisors of the qualifications and experience of each practitioner. . . . It is clear, however, that the determination of status cannot depend solely on the possession of post-graduate qualifications, but must take account of experience which may itself suffice to warrant acceptance as a specialist; and that practice exclusively as a consultant or specialist cannot be applied as a criterion, since a number of practitioners engaging in other medical work may be qualified as specialists by experience or otherwise, and their service will be essential for the adequate staffing of hospitals.[131]

Some powerful figures, notably Lord Moran, saw this flexibility as a temporary expedient, so that "those who seek to enter this field [specialties] in the future will be required to satisfy the proper authority that they are suitably equipped. . . . It is very necessary if the standard of consultant practice is to be maintained that this training should be jealously supervised and that the criteria which permit a doctor to specialise shall be laid down by the consultants and specialists themselves."[132] In fact, postgraduate institutes (the British Postgraduate Medical Federation, BPMF) were set up, starting in 1948, to fulfill these tasks.[133] Nonetheless, the preference for flexible human evaluations in opposition to "some nationally imposed standard"[134] ran very deep among members of the British medical elite. Such fluidity carried a price, however. Specialist groups complained constantly that regional boards did not consult them about appointments made in their field.[135] Others grumbled about the unfairness of procedures.[136] Nor did authorities necessarily restrict their choices to individuals listed on the BMA's Consultants Roll or even the part-time Consultants Roll listing individuals willing to treat patients at a reduced fee.

Fifth, consultant status was set at a high level and was determined by the holding of hospital posts. The royal colleges suggested that appointment to such posts should require at least five years of postgraduate training at an approved hospital as well as the traditional general higher diploma of one of the royal colleges.[137] Within the BMA there was great concern to safeguard the interests of GP-specialists.[138] But despite much discussion, hand-wringing, and resolution passing, the main result was an attempt to accommodate some GP-specialists, as well as local government medical officers, by establishing a lower hospital grade, "senior hospital medical officers," who were to practice as full-time specialists. And the establishment of this category was dictated as much by workforce needs as by anything else. Specialists without hospital posts from the prewar years were defined out of existence in the new NHS.[139] Thus specialist status would not depend on self-identification, as in the past, or on professionally controlled systems of certification that functioned in most other countries. In the words of the secretary of the BMA's Central Consultants and Specialists Commission: "There is no definition of a specialist. The effect of this is that the decision by a board to appoint a practitioner to a specialist post on a hospital staff confers specialist status. To this extent the number of specialists is controlled by the established number of specialist posts as well as by the fitness of an applicant to fill such a post."[140] As Rosemary Stevens has pointed out, the traditional mode of appointment to voluntary hospitals had become universally applied and regionally controlled.[141]

Efforts continued, however, to create higher specialist diplomas replacing the general diplomas granted by the colleges (FRCP and FRCS). In the RCS, at least four specialist groups lobbied vigorously for higher degrees. Two of these, in ophthalmology and otorhinolaryngology (the largest of the specialty groupings), managed to obtained variants of the FRCS with a mention of their specialty. Anesthesiology and dental surgery were constituted as separate faculties within the College; these faculties awarded their own fellowships, which constituted the higher degrees for these fields. There was much less pressure for such arrangements in the RCP, where practitioners in fields such as neurology and pediatrics showed little interest in differentiating themselves through separate qualifications; they seemed to have shared in the generalist culture of the College and continued to perceive themselves as generalists "with a special interest."[142] It was not until the 1960s that pressure from psychiatrists, pediatricians, and pathologists began to mount.[143] In any event, it is not clear whether the higher specialist diplomas that did come into existence constituted a significant advantage to individuals applying to hospital boards for consultancy positions.[144]

Efforts were also made to provide adequate postgraduate specialist education. The British Postgraduate Medical Federation was established in London in 1945. This combined several preexisting institutions, notably the British Postgraduate Medical School, which had been in existence since 1935.[145] Several years later, the "institutes" that had been called for by the Goodenough Commission were established within the Federation. By the 1950s, there were two general and thirteen specialty schools, all associated with hospitals. But they did not become major foci of specialist training.[146] In fact, during the 1950s there was no coordinated system of postgraduate training, a situation that would prevail for much of the twentieth century.[147]

Unlike medical systems elsewhere, the British system did not have an overabundance of specialists. In 1963, only 31 percent of the doctors in England and Wales were specialists.[148] But, as was the case in other countries, specialization in Britain had its characteristic problems. The extraordinary distance, both social and administrative, between general and specialist practice was unprecedented in other countries, and over the years provoked a wide variety of well-documented problems. Furthermore, there were clearly discrepancies between the manpower needs of the health insurance system (as defined by administrators) and the imperatives of professionally controlled institutions of training. In particular, setting the training bar at such a high level made it difficult to satisfy personnel needs. The distinction between teaching and nonteaching hospitals also provoked considerable discussion and disagreement.

One of the most controversial aspects of the British system had to do with remuneration. There existed a system of salary levels that was uniform for all specialties (though distribution of levels could vary sharply among different specialties); generous Distinction Awards, which significantly raised incomes, were also presented to those designated as having special proficiency. A special committee of leading consultants, led for many years by Lord Moran distributed these awards in the characteristically informal, peer-group style of the British elite. The workings of this committee were regularly criticized.[149] Indeed, the analysis of the distribution of awards by specialty is indicative of how little the real distribution of power and resources had actually changed. Of approximately 2,400 awards handed out in 1964, general medicine and general surgery, providing 21 percent of all consultants, received 38 percent of the awards. Over 50 percent of all individuals in these two categories received such awards. Of even greater significance is the distribution of the highest Distinction Award (the extremely generous "A+"). Of ninety-one awards, more than half went to three groups—general physicians, surgeons, or obstetricians—out of twenty-three listed specialties.[150] *Plus ça change.* Charles Webster remarked: "In effect liberal distribution of 'glittering prizes' to the consultant elite purchased their compliance with the NHS and this brought in the entire support structure. Unfortunately the severe imbalances of remuneration soon became institutionalised and although recognized as a major injustice they have never finally been erased." [151]

Conclusion

The regulation of specialties in twentieth-century Britain differed substantially from the processes that occurred in the other nations we have examined. It grew out of the needs of a new administrative system rather than from the aspirations of the medical profession. Today, the United Kingdom is unique among Western nations in the relatively small size of its specialist population. This results from the narrow definition of specialists as hospital consultants who do not engage in primary care. The U.K. model is of course relatively cheap, as every health economist knows. The separation of functions also has the virtue of being immediately intelligible to administrators. GPs act as gatekeepers, which reduces the number of patients who receive expensive specialist services. Unlike the situation in many other countries, British specialists do not compete directly against GPs in the domain of primary care. Finally, the system permits the consultant aristocracy to remain small, privileged, and exclusive, though perhaps overworked.

Administrative advantages, however, cannot explain everything. Comparative analysis has highlighted the uniqueness of the British model and the difficulty of imposing rigid functional distinctions on unruly medical professions or their patients. One must try to imagine how things might have turned out had large numbers of non-elite British doctors claimed and successfully built their identity around specialist status, as was the case in France, Germany, and the United States.

There are many reasons why this did not occur in Britain. The hostility to specialization among British doctors throughout the nineteenth century may well have played a role in keeping the number of specialists relatively low. Refusal to recognize as specialists those without hospital posts also inhibited many from making the claim. More important, however, was the long process that unified a deeply fragmented medical profession around the principle of patient referral. This was a compromise that turned out to be beneficial for all parties concerned; and it was not congruent with the dual development of specialties both as consultant activities and as direct forms of primary care that was occurring in other nations. But it certainly was congruent with the ideology of "efficiency" and "rational organization" that underpinned the development of the NHS. Finally, I would suggest, in a more speculative mode, that the hierarchical stratification of British medicine was not the primary factor behind the success of the consultant elite in appropriating specialties; such stratification was hardly unprecedented in the European context. Much more central, I would contend, was the degree of professional power that this elite could exercise through the prestigious royal colleges that had no equivalent in the other nations under discussion. Equally critical, I suspect, were uniquely close relations between medical elites and the British governing classes. Just as in the nineteenth century they were united by a culture of general education and gentlemanly virtues that inhibited specialization, so they were joined together in the twentieth by a widely shared culture of public service that somehow combined, while blurring the boundaries between, notions of administrative and social rationality, expert knowledge and traditional elite privilege. The British system of specialties reflected this broader elite culture of public service.

Part III

MEDICAL SPECIALTIES IN
COMPARATIVE PERSPECTIVE

Chapter 10

From Divisions of Medicine to Specialties

For much of this book, nations have served as our fundamental units of analysis. We have discussed specific specialties insofar as they played a particularly significant role or illustrated particular themes of national medical development. I should like in this chapter and the next to change focus by examining a number of specialties in an explicitly comparative framework. My starting point will be the medical directories that I have cited so frequently in this book. The quantitative data for the mid-1930s calculated from these sources provide a very rough estimate of the general distribution of specialists and specialties in the countries under examination. I begin by looking at a new group of specialists just beginning to appear on the scene: women. I then go on to examine a number of specialties or groups of specialties as they developed in our four countries. Each one faced particular kinds of difficulties and each evolved rather differently from one country to the next. I begin with domains that from the beginning were considered basic divisions of medicine before being transformed into specialties. I continue in chapter 11 with some fields that emerged somewhat later. I do not present an exhaustive history of these fields, but place each specialty in a broad international and comparative context that illuminates themes that are largely invisible in purely national studies.

Looking at Some Data

Appendix 1 (pp. 257–258) is calculated from national medical directories and from some statistics of the period; it summarizes information about specialist populations in three of our four countries in the mid-1930s. British data vary so wildly from one source to another as to be almost unusable. I have presented them separately in appendix 2 (p. 259). Given the different criteria used to identify specialists in each national directory, it would be foolhardy to attempt a rigorous statistical comparison.

German sources count certified specialists, while French data are based on both self-identification of specialists and editorial selection, with little in the way of limiting criteria. American figures include both board-certified specialists and the self-identified, with both categories and conditions for using them predefined by the AMA. Despite all these caveats, these data suggest a number of general observations.

First, by the 1930s specialization had become international. Specialties that existed in one country usually existed in all. There are a few striking exceptions, often small, marginal categories that continued to exist in countries such as France, as yet without a regulatory system, but that had been rendered invisible in those nations where they were excluded from newly established systems of certification. These included fields such as thermalism or spa medicine, nutrition, and organ specialties that in other countries had become subfields of internal medicine. In the United States, the *American Medical Directory* recognized some specialties with very small numbers of practitioners and with a place in clinical medicine that was then problematic; these included anesthesiology, public health, and pathology. One suspects that the reasons for this were in part political and had to do with affirming the medical character of these domains in the face of competition from non-MD practitioners including nurse-anesthetists and pathological technicians. Specialist categories that existed in some countries but not others were characteristically practiced by small numbers of individuals; nonetheless, there were several important exceptions. Internal medicine—a major category in Germany and the United States—did not exist in France or Britain; in contrast, stomatology was not recognized in the United States. Electrical medicine was not visible in directories anywhere except France, where it claimed a significant number of practitioners.

Second, specialties that attracted large numbers of practitioners in one country usually attracted large numbers in other countries as well. This is hardly surprising. Not only was there an international culture of specialties that was in large part driven by academic medicine, but patterns of disease or use of medical resources were not, as far as we know, dramatically different from one country to the next. Diseases of women and of the ear, nose, and throat were common everywhere, and thus the specialties around them characteristically attracted large numbers of doctors. Surgery was a staple of virtually every hospital, and so its practitioners were numerous in all four nations. Nonetheless, there are several cases where major discrepancies of scale exist from one country to the next. The number of dermato-venereologists in Germany; the number of gynecologists, obstetricians, and electroradiologists in France; and the overrepresentation of ophthalmologists in Britain are among the more glaring examples. Such discrepancies are not mere artifacts; they may or may not reflect real functional differences, but they certainly express national variations in institutional arrangement and modes of classification. We will discuss some of these cases in greater detail below.

Third, discrete specialties were often practiced in combinations, some of which became authoritative everywhere. The combination of care of the ear, nose, and throat is one example. Other combinations were common in most countries but not in all: venereology and dermatology were associated nearly everywhere (despite the claims made by urology to treat venereal disease) except in Britain. Large numbers of doctors combined gynecology with obstetrics. But this was becoming the formalized norm only in Germany. In Britain, such dual practice was restricted to the elite, while separate practice of each specialty remained common in both France and the United States. Likewise, psychiatry and neurology were moving closer together, but this was the formal norm only in Germany, where the two subjects were combined for purposes of training and certification.

As I suggested earlier, there were two distinct logics of specialty development. Elite medical careers depended on acceptance in the institutions defining elite status: medical schools, hospitals, dispensaries, and scientific societies. Different professional groups possessed unequal resources for pursuing advancement in this sphere. Among the factors that counted were the theoretical knowledge that a specialist group had produced, as well as the more practical techniques that had emerged from its work and that its members alone could teach the rest of the profession and perform in complicated cases; public interest in social problems or types of patients associated with specific specialties; the social and educational characteristics of the individuals attracted to different specialties.

Different specialties thus had unequal access to elite institutions. Surgery, we shall see, was especially rich in such opportunities, as were several other specialties. Within this elite sphere it often did not matter whether a particular kind of problem was widespread or not. There might be a niche for small numbers of high-level specialists devoting themselves to relatively rare problems. Those fields that became subspecialties of internal medicine in some countries but were autonomous categories in others—gastroenterology, nephrology, cardiology—are particularly good examples of this sort of development. In France, for instance, these were predominantly specialties for relatively small numbers of hospital practitioners.[1]

Elite posts attracted affluent private patients to the lucky specialists who held them. But a very different logic was characteristic of doctors in private medical practices. Here the crucial variable seems to have been the incidence of particular health problems or the number of potential patients that doctors could treat; conditions perceived to be widespread tended to attract many physicians. Gynecology serves as an especially visible example of this kind of specialty since it targeted half the population. Pediatrics as well offered a huge clientele on condition that other specialties were not competing for the right to care for children. Government might radically recast such opportunities by establishing state programs of prevention or cure directed at specific problems such as child health or venereal disease. Illness thus constituted something of an evolving market, and practitioners can be conceptualized as seeking to find a niche in that market. I emphasize, however, that this framework is an abstraction that attempts to account for large-scale, collective patterns of career choice. Individual physicians chose specialties for the most varied and personal of reasons.

If all specialists faced similar sets of choices, there was one group of specialists that had to deal with unusual conditions and challenges: women. Data here are very scattered and are not included in the appendices. Women did not begin entering medicine in significant numbers until the last decades of the nineteenth century (the first decade of the twentieth in Germany). By the 1930s the proportion of women in the medical profession was about 4–5 percent in the United States, 6–7 percent in France, and 7–8 percent in Germany (where, however, many women were not in active practice). In Britain about 10 percent of those listed on the Medical Register in the mid-1930s were women.[2] In the decades that followed, the number of women in medicine grew at a modest rate. By the early mid-1960s, the proportion of women in national medical professions had risen to roughly 15 percent in France, West Germany, and the United Kingdom[3]; in the United States, the figure was substantially lower, and had in fact changed little since the 1930s.[4] Only in East Germany, which followed the pattern of other Communist states, was the proportion of women substantially higher: 27 percent in 1964.

Whether women entered specialties or practiced as generalists depended to some extent on the degree of specialist regulation. In France, for instance, a majority of women doctors called themselves specialists because there were no constraints on specialist self-identification.[5] Among German women doctors, in contrast, only about 25 to 30 percent of women physicians practiced as specialists during the 1930s, once the Bremen Guidelines defined strict criteria for specialist practice.[6] In the United States, the exclusion of women from most residency programs made it particularly hard for women to become specialists.[7] The proportion of specialists among women doctors in the United States, according to one survey, was 5 percent in 1939, about the same as twenty years earlier.[8] (One would of course expect much higher figures in large cities.) In Britain, since specialist status in most fields was tied to hospital consultant positions, relatively few women were identified as specialists.

Women specialists tended to be concentrated in a small number of fields that had to do with the care of children and women. In 1905, 76 percent of Parisian women specialists labeled themselves as gynecologists and 49 percent as pediatricians, with many claiming both categories. By 1935, this concentration had become less overwhelming but remained substantial, with over one-third of all women specialists in gynecology and another third in pediatrics. The only other large concentration of women was in orthopedics-physiotherapy (at around 15 percent of specialist women, with most in physiotherapy rather than orthopedics). During this period, women also had a moderate presence in dermatology (8 percent of all women specialists) and ophthalmology (9 percent).

The situation looked broadly similar in Germany, except that close to half of all the women specialists were in pediatrics.[9] The care of children was simultaneously a traditional female activity, an increasingly important public health concern providing salaried jobs, and a relatively low-status specialty that competed with general practice. According to official statistics of the period, gynecology/obstetrics was much less popular (at around 13–14 percent), most likely because the constitution of the specialty as a combination of gynecology and obstetrics with a strong surgical orientation was either unattractive to women or because German obstetricians joined other surgical specialists in keeping women (and Jews) out of their domain. Internal medicine (another field that competed against general practice) attracted about 9 percent of those in the national sample. The two other substantial fields in the national sample were dermatology/venereology and ophthalmology, at around 9 percent each of women specialists.[10] It is worth noting that almost all of these specialties also attracted disproportionate numbers of equally marginal practitioners: Jews.[11]

Our knowledge of the choice of specialties made by American women doctors is very patchy. But it is clear that obstetrics/gynecology, which initially loomed large, declined markedly as a specialty for women in the decade before World War II. A survey done in 1940[12] found that this field ranked only sixth among specialties for women, which probably reflects the surgical orientation that had become predominant. The most popular specialty among American women, as among German women, was pediatrics. It was followed by psychiatry/neurology and pathology.[13] Pathology was in large measure a salaried service specialty with insecure professional status. The popularity of psychiatry/neurology is distinctive in the international context and is explained by a fairly unusual set of circumstances. After 1880, some 200 women doctors worked in state asylums and reformatories. Their effect was thought to be so beneficial to women patients that, despite opposition from asylum directors, eleven states (mainly in the Northeast) required that asylums employ women.[14]

We know relatively little about British medical women. Given the identification of specialists with hospital posts, one would expect numbers to be small except in certain fields where hospitals were frequently run by women (pediatrics and gynecology)[15] and in public health, which provided low-status jobs and fixed incomes. Various sources confirm this pattern. Among the small number of women medical graduates in Glasgow from 1898 to 1910, the two largest groups were in public health, particularly maternal and infant care (27 percent), and general practice (23 percent). Only eight (13 percent) were listed as working in voluntary specialist hospitals (mainly women's and children's). As was true for men, positions in anesthesia were fairly accessible to women, reflecting the general lack of professional recognition for this field.[16] Among women graduates in Manchester before 1938, about half were in general practice and a quarter in public health.[17] These figures are not notably different from those for men. A survey published in 1936 looked at careers of women medical graduates of St. Mary's Hospital between 1916 and 1924[18]; out of 230, 38 percent were in general practice and 14 percent were listed as "specialists (consultant, academic or research)." Since another category, "full-time hospital posts," also included specialists, specialists probably made up over 20 percent of the women in the sample, with another 5 percent listed as having full-time public health posts. Within the narrow category of "specialists," there was only one gynecologist; the largest group of women practiced anesthesia (five out of thirty-two), and four each practiced ophthalmology, psychotherapy, and pathology. There were two surgeons as well.

Overall, the numbers and distribution of women specialists look similar in all four countries. Numbers, while small, grew during the 1930s (except in the United States), with a varying but significant proportion of women entering specialties. In nearly all countries, it was relatively low-status specialties such as pediatrics that were the most popular career choices among women. But one also finds some interesting differences due to contingent local differences, among them the large number of women psychiatrists in the United States and women public health specialists in Britain.

To summarize, by the 1930s, considerable international standardization of specialties had taken place, and this standardizaiton would become more pronounced as the century progressed. However, significant national variations remained, and some of these would continue to be significant for many years to come. We can get a better sense of them by examining a number of individual specialties in greater detail.

The Original Branches of Medicine Become Specialties

In most nations, official healing in the eighteenth century was divided into two branches, medicine and surgery, the former focusing on medications or diet taken internally, and the other, on the external parts of the body or those few internal parts directly accessible to the surgeon's knife. (In Britain things were more complicated because apothecaries had become recognized medical practitioners.) Long existing as separate professions, the two fields were everywhere drawing together by the early nineteenth century and surgery was taught in many medical schools, though separate surgical schools continued to exist. The institutional separation of these fields never really took hold in North America because populations, both general and medical, were too sparse. This distinction would be abolished in France in the early nineteenth century and in Prussia in 1852. But even where it persisted legally and institutionally, the two sectors were increasingly perceived as two branches of a single medical profession and science, a factor, we have argued, that served as one important precondition for the emergence of specialties. By the same token, however, the rise of specialties also had profound effects on these original divisions of medicine: surgery everywhere, and internal medicine in some countries, were gradually recast into specialties.

German and American surgeons and internists were gradually redefined as specialists. The same process occurred in France in a partial and idiosyncratic way. In Britain, however, the shift from general branches of medicine to specialties was altogether more problematic. For reasons we have already discussed, British surgeons and physicians resisted thinking of themselves as specialists, the dominant self-image in Britain remaining that of generalist consultants with "special interests." Initially, specialties here were seen as subdivisions of either general medicine or general surgery, under the jurisdiction of the Royal College of Medicine or the Royal College of Surgeons, respectively. This framework proved too constraining for certain specialties, which then sought recognition as autonomous categories.

Surgery

As surgery became increasingly technical, complex, and radical, it also became increasingly distinct from general practice. From the 1860s, surgeons established their own journals and associations.[19] But even with all its distinguishing features, it remained possible for some time to perceive surgery as one of the two central divisions of medicine that included more restricted surgical specialties that might occasionally achieve an autonomous identity. In France the uncertainty was especially evident; an early medical directory of the 1880s referred to specialties as "spécialités médico-chirurgicales" and omitted surgery from the list of specialties. In the early twentieth century, two major Parisian medical directories included surgery on their list of specialties while a third, the *Guide Rosenwald*, did not.[20] By the 1930s what remained of this ambiguity was gone and surgery was clearly considered a specialty in France, as it was in Germany and the United States. Only British surgeons continued to resist the tendency to see themselves as specialists, but this resistance was to some extent masked by appeals to the more ambiguous concept of "consultant."

Despite such variation and uncertainty about how to define surgery, the proportion of surgeons among specialists remained remarkably constant. Surgery was always among the largest of the specialties. During the first four decades of the twentieth century, surgeons fluctuated at around 15 percent of all specialists in the large cities of France and Germany. The proportion tended to be higher nationally because statistics included smaller cities with fewer specialists, so that surgeons loomed larger; in Britain and the United States nationally, the percentage of surgeons hovered around 20 percent (see appendices 1 and 2) but was lower in Prussia. The continual emergence of new specialties providing doctors with many new career alternatives might have led to a decline in the proportion of surgeons among specialists, but this did not occur because possibilities for surgical work continued to expand as a result of new technical developments and the dramatic multiplication of hospitals throughout this period.

Although not all specialties were represented in smaller hospitals, surgery, as a core hospital activity, usually was. Similarly, it was everywhere among the largest disciplines represented in medical schools. Consequently, surgery was ordinarily a highly elitist specialty, containing a large proportion of individuals with hospital and academic posts.[21] In Paris, the proportion of surgeons listed in the *Guide Rosenwald* who had hospital or faculty posts declined from 52 to 36 percent between 1920 and 1935, largely because anyone could call himself or herself a surgeon.[22] In Prussia, where certification limited the right to identify oneself as a specialist, the proportion of surgeons with hospital appointments rose from 40 percent in 1903 to 51 percent in 1937.[23] Military need for surgeons, and the training programs organized for this purpose, also kept numbers high during the first four decades of the twentieth century. In the first years of Nazi rule in Germany, surgery was one of the few fields in which the number of practitioners continued to expand in spite of a general decline in the number of specialists (due to the exclusion of Jewish physicians).[24] It was also one of the specialties with the fewest Jewish and women practitioners. This most likely reflected conscious professional strategies of exclusion.

Although the number of surgeons was certainly influenced by the availability of hospital posts in different locales, significant numbers of surgeons did not have hospital or faculty appointments. The figure was about 40 percent in Prussia in 1938 and about 64 percent in Paris in 1935.[25] Private hospitals and clinics may have provided an alternative location in which surgery could take place, but the radical decline in private clinics in Germany after World War I suggests that this is at best a partial explanation. Clearly, much surgery was still practiced in the home or doctors' offices well into the twentieth century.[26]

Surgery seems to have been particularly well remunerated. This had always been the case for a small minority of elite surgeons on whose manual dexterity life and death frequently depended.[27] Higher incomes became more generalized as a result of the surgical innovations of the late nineteenth and early twentieth centuries. War also reinforced the status of surgery, the specialty most intimately identified with the dramatic saving of life. In a survey of the estates left at their deaths by French doctors who had been members of the Paris Academy of Medicine in 1900, it was found that surgeons transmitted considerably more wealth to their heirs than did other academicians.[28] Bradford Hill's famous study of medical incomes in Britain concluded that surgeons had a substantially larger proportion of high earners than other specialists; only gynecologists came close to matching surgeons in this respect.[29] Data from the United States showed much the same pattern; the only specialists who came close to surgeons in achieving high levels of income were orthopedic surgeons (a small group) and radiologists (who would have had high capital costs for equipment to deduct from gross incomes).[30] More fragmented German data from the war years show a similar pattern.[31] Such aggregate data, of course, need to be carefully scrutinized because of significant income inequalities among surgeons. A German surgeon complained in 1935 that it was primarily directors of hospital departments who earned above-average incomes and that life for the rest was very hard; this, in his view, explained why they tended to combine surgery with related fields such as gynecology, orthopedics, and urology.[32] Such economic competition may explain the spread of literary stereotypes that portrayed surgeons as money-grubbers in such novels of the early twentieth century as *Arrowsmith* by Sinclair Lewis and *The Citadel* by A. J. Cronin.

General surgery, like internal medicine, faced the constant eruption within its ranks of subgroups seeking to break free and become autonomous specialties. This process necessarily resulted in the shrinking of the original domain and frequently provoked resistance from the parent group. Outcomes of these confrontations varied, depending on how vigorously separatist tendencies were combated. Results might also depend on the institutional power of national medical associations and emerging regulatory bodies such as the Advisory Board for Medical Specialties in the United States—which usually tried to constrain specialty fragmentation.[33] As a general rule, surgeons opposed new surgical specialties in the nineteenth century but became selectively tolerant in the twentieth as techniques became more advanced and distinctive. In Britain, the Royal College of Surgeons (RCS) was especially flexible and made a point of finding ways for autonomous specialties—and in the case of dentistry, separate professions—to remain part of the institution and of British surgery more generally. But where territorial claims of newly autonomous domains had the potential to cut substantially into traditional surgical work, resistance could be very fierce indeed.

Surgery lost a string of domains as ophthalmology, gynecological surgery, and ORL split off into separate fields. In the twentieth century, the rise of orthopedics provoked major disputes because of the scope of the claims made by its practitioners, weak and largely unrepresented in medical schools though they were. In Germany, some orthopedists claimed nothing less than exclusive care for all organs of mobility and stability, and for everything to do with "cripples."[34] Despite much controversy, they were notably unsuccessful in their aims before World War II. An "agreement" between professional associations in 1937 pretty much allocated all operations to surgery, and mechanical manipulations and appliances to orthopedics. In Britain, orthopedists first claimed jurisdiction for all injuries to locomotor organs and then, somewhat more modestly, to hospital treatment of fractures. In neither case were they very successful until the creation of the National Health Service (NHS) satisfied many of their claims.[35]

Internal Medicine

According to one leading historian, "internal medicine has been in constant search of its own definition."[36] In the words of another, "[t]he formation of internal medicine might then be conceived as a series of historical contingencies."[37] It is evident that we are not dealing with an easily defined specialty. Internal medicine was from its beginnings a problematical category because, unlike surgery, it lacked the striking distinguishing features that could set it clearly apart from general practice. Consequently, conflict between generalists and internists over control of primary care became very intense in certain countries. Furthermore, internists had to deal with specialist categories that emerged simultaneously or, in some cases, even earlier, and that threatened to deprive them of significant parts of their vast domain. Some of these, such as neurology and pediatrics, achieved autonomy everywhere; pneumology and gastrointestinal medicine were "captured" by this imperialistic new field in the United States, but in Germany were among the specialist categories recognized for certification by the Bremen Guidelines in 1924. Finally, unlike surgery, which produced striking innovations during the last decades of the nineteenth century, internal medicine produced relatively little in the way of dramatic new therapies. Its claims to scientific status were thus fragile.

In Germany and the United States, the development of a specialty called internal medicine neatly solved the dilemma of the elite generalist who aspired to be something more than a GP. Internal medicine was defined as the general practice of elite physicians able to utilize sophisticated scientific techniques, particularly those of the laboratory, ordinarily unavailable to general practitioners. These scientific techniques distinguished them from general practitioners and guaranteed the quality of their work. And internal medicine held together within a single common specialist category many of the developing organ-based fields, which now had less incentive to secede in order to attain specialist status. The unity of a large segment of the profession was preserved, as was the integrity of the individual, "whole" patient. The language of wholeness as an alternative to the treatment of "organs" by other specialties was deeply ingrained in German internal medicine.[38]

Internal medicine emerged relatively late in the development of specialties. The first association in the field, the Verein für Innere Medizin, was founded in 1881 and provoked vehement protests from other medical societies.[39] In subsequent years, the term spread through German academic circles; in 1894 the *Centralblatt für klinische Medicin* became the *Centralblatt für innere Medicin*.[40] But this remained a problematic category in its country of origin; it was initially small and controversial because it threatened the livelihood of GPs in ways that surgical specialties did not.[41] In 1903, internists made up only about 5 percent of Prussian specialists, far less than the largest specialty groups. But internal medicine expanded significantly in the three following decades, becoming one of the largest of the specialties (16 percent of all specialists in the 1930s) in that state.[42] While the growth of hospitals accounts for part of this development, as does the very large number of internists in German medical schools (who were in a position to train more internists),[43] it seems that an important contributing factor was the appropriation of this title by non-elite private practitioners. The proportion of German internists in private practice rose from 43 percent in 1903 to nearly 70 percent in the 1930s.[44] This suggests that as specialization spread and became increasingly prestigious, practitioners who would have once been satisfied to remain GPs took on the specialty title most compatible with traditional general practice. We saw in chapter 6 that one the most serious problems surrounding the implementation of the Bremen Guidelines had to do with the conflict between GPs and internists.

The Association of American Physicians was founded in 1885, a few years after the appearance of the German association. It represented "the new generation of European-trained scholar-clinicians."[45] Based on the German model,[46] internal medicine was not immediately recognized as a specialist category in the medical directories of the late nineteenth and early twentieth centuries. The *American Medical Directory* (*AMD*) did not introduce the internal medicine designation until 1914, five years after specialist listings were first included. Nonetheless, by 1935, it was one of the larger specialties in the United States, though mainly in the major cities.

(Internists constituted 9 percent of specialists nationally but close to 15 percent in New York City and Boston [appendix 1].) One suspects that, as in Germany, the rapid spread of internal medicine in the United States was due to its capacity to provide visible and increasingly prestigious specialist status to *both* the academic elite and those private practitioners who in earlier years might have been content to remain GPs. Nonetheless, elite academicians provided leadership for the emerging specialty in the United States. Benefiting from prestigious institutional affiliations, this leadership saw little need to distinguish internists from other practitioners. Consequently, a certification board in this specialty was introduced rather late, in 1936.

In Britain and France, internal medicine did not become an accepted specialist category. In Britain, this reflected the broader tendency to keep specialism at a distance, even though general medical consultants in Britain likely played the same functional role as did internists in Germany and the United States. British consultants in general medicine had such high status as hospital-based consultants that they had no need to think of themselves as specialists until the two terms became virtually synonymous after World War II. Even when they did specialize in narrower domains, as most in fact did, many continued to think of themselves as generalists "with a special interest." As a result of the sharp administrative division between consultant work and primary care institutionalized by the NHS after the war, the position of general consultants became rather redundant. This category has gradually disappeared from official statistics. By 2001, a "General Medicine Group" comprising twenty-eight narrow specialties had replaced it. It consisted of 5,677 individuals (23 percent of all consultants). Within that group there were only 129 consultants in the field of "general (internal) medicine.' (A year later, this category had completely disappeared from official statistics.) In contrast, there were nearly 1,400 general surgeons listed among the nine specialist fields making up an equivalent "Surgical Group."[47]

In France, internal medicine did not emerge as a specialty because it simply did not make much sense in that nation's institutional context. When elite physicians in France chose to specialize (which was in most cases), they selected from a variety of organ-based specialties focusing on the gastrointestinal tract, the liver, the kidneys, or the heart. (If lumped together, these made up pretty much the same proportion of specialists as did internists in Germany and the United States.) These fit the reductionist and high-status pattern of specialty development far better than did the comprehensive but murky notion of "internal medicine." It is certainly significant that hospital and academic practitioners dominated these organic internal specialties, for it was precisely in these institutions that research and reductionism went together. And it helped that it was relatively easy for hospital practitioners to shape their wards along specialized lines by controlling the admission of patients. As for nonelite physicians, their need for primary care specialties was met by such fields as gynecology, pediatrics, and ORL, all of which attracted large numbers of practitioners.

In France, therefore, surgery eventually came to be considered as a specialty while internal medicine did not. That, at least, was the case until the 1960s, when an effort was made to follow American models by creating a specialty of internal medicine. This effort was not very successful. There were about 2,000 internists in the country in 1989, out of a total specialist population of 69,000.[48] In 2000, there were 2,500 internists, making up only 1.3 percent of the specialist population in France.[49]

In those countries where the category existed, internal medicine had an acute problem keeping control of its constituent subdomains. Constant effort was required to prevent internal medicine in the United States and Germany from breaking apart. The unity of the field was a regular theme of the annual meetings of the German Society for Internal Medicine.[50] Many German internists never quite got used to the developing association between neurology (which they viewed as part of internal medicine) and psychiatry, or to the growing autonomy of pediatrics.[51] The loss of pediatrics was particularly hard for German internists to bear, although by the twentieth century, the shared status of the two specialties as targets of the wrath of GPs was bringing them closer together. The desire for professional unity manifested by the major medical association, the DÄV, led to a reform in the late 1920s that required training in pediatrics and gastroenterology to include significant time spent on internal medicine.[52] Little more could be done for fields that had already developed autonomous identities by 1924. However, the DÄV was firm in opposing the breaking away of newer fields such as cardiology and nephrology.

Internal medicine remains a contested specialty in today's Germany. Its "unity" must be defended regularly, as must its status as a mixed specialty, some of whose practitioners provide consultative services while others—probably the majority— engage in primary care.[53] Professional rhetoric manages a complex balance between emphasis on scientific techniques that separate it from general practice and stress on care for the whole individual that distinguishes it from organ specialties; this middle ground is difficult to hold due to the fact that an increasingly specialized technological orientation seems increasingly characteristic of the eight fields recognized as subspecialties. (Gastroenterology and pneumology, originally autonomous fields, have been integrated as subspecialties.[54]) Nonetheless, internal medicine is a huge specialty; its practitioners constitute no less than 22 percent of the specialist population in Germany, about twice the proportion of surgeons.[55] We shall see in the Epilogue that internal medicine is now at the center of political conflicts over the reform of primary medical care in Germany.

In the United States, internal medicine also pursued a policy of comprehensiveness, with the support of national professional associations. Well-established fields such as pediatrics were left on their own, but smaller fields already in existence, such as gastroenterology and cardiology, were captured by internal medicine and turned into subspecialties.[56] This set the pattern for the development of newer fields such as nephrology. This strategy has maintained the formal unity of the field; it has also improved career prospects by allowing practitioners to divide their time between general internal medicine and narrower subspecialties that could not provide full-time work for so many practitioners. Nonetheless, this system has had its problems. These subspecialties have achieved far more status than general internal medicine and have led to considerable bureaucratization of the field.[57] Since at least the 1970s, fierce conflict over reimbursement, institutional resources, and power among the different groups making up internal medicine has been the rule. Powerful subspecialties such as cardiology have long sought recognition as autonomous specialties.[58]

As in Germany, internal medicine in the United States is a huge specialty that holds together primary care physicians and consultants. Since subspecialists frequently spend part of their time practicing general internal medicine, the role of the general internist has become problematical despite the recent political climate that supports increased resources for primary care.[59] While some have yielded to despair,[60] others suggest possible solutions; one is to valorize careers in general internal medicine by establishing separate training programs for this field alone.[61] A variant of this proposal elaborated in Canada would turn general internal medicine into a subspecialty equal to other, more technical subspecialties.[62] Yet others suggest, more modestly, that their field should become more closely focused on geriatric care, the newest growth field.[63] As we shall see in the Epilogue, internal medicine is deeply implicated in the larger problem of primary care provision in the United States.

Obstetrics and the Complex of Women's Specialties

By the early nineteenth century, obstetrics was considered by many as a third major branch of medicine. This status was explicitly recognized when medicine was united with surgery in Prussia in 1852; henceforth, medical graduates received a single diploma identifying them as "Arzt, Wundarzt und Geburtshelfer."[64] Nonetheless, the status of obstetrics, which had emerged relatively recently and dealt with only a small part of medical practice, was clearly different from that of the much larger fields of surgery and internal medicine. Once specialization became an accepted medical reality, obstetrics was quickly recast as a specialty. While it did not have quite the large, tangled web of connections with other specialties and subspecialties that characterized the two older fields, it was closely associated with several categories of practice relating to the care of women.

High infant and maternal mortality rates everywhere during the eighteenth century generated public concern to improve birthing techniques. Consequently, lying-in hospitals were established and obstetrical teaching of various sorts was introduced; initially the men providing the teaching were seeking to train midwives, and themselves intervened only in difficult cases. But by the end of the century, they were training male doctors as well and were increasingly involved in routine deliveries. By the early decades of the nineteenth century, there existed in every country faculty chairs, hospital clinics, and maternity hospitals that provided a rich institutional basis from which specialist identity could emerge. Specialty societies in obstetrics began to form everywhere during the middle decades of the century. The field was recognized in 1845 as a distinct section of the major German scientific association, the Versammlung der Deutschen Naturforscher und Ärzte (VdNÄ), and became an autonomous examination subject in 1852.[65] In Paris, chairs in obstetrics had existed since the establishment of the post-revolutionary Faculty of Medicine; during the 1850s the hospital administration began to distinguish hospital obstetricians from surgeons and physicians in official lists of personnel. In London, the Obstetrical Society, established in 1858, was one of the first British specialty societies.

The field of birthing was crowded with practitioners. Virtually everywhere, midwives remained key birthing attendants for significant parts of the population. American obstetricians sought to eliminate midwives, but for their European counterparts the issue was more commonly how to organize the division of labor between the two groups so that midwives were properly trained and under medical supervision. Furthermore, birthing was frequently viewed as part of general practice. The Obstetrical Society of London at its origins aimed to bring new clinical information to GPs, "upon whom the responsibilities of midwifery fall even more heavily than those of medicine or surgery."[66] Although obstetricians gradually expanded their activity to normal home births, the role of GPs remained significant. Charlotte Borst has shown that in early twentieth-century Milwaukee, certain GPs in ethnic neighborhoods might attend far more births than many of the individuals who called themselves obstetricians.[67] Well into the twentieth century, significant numbers of obstetricians continued to see themselves as academic specialists providing obstetrical training for GPs. But in every country, some groups of obstetricians argued that infant and maternal mortality could be lowered only if birthing was taken over by specialists. The movement to transfer birthing to hospitals provided considerable impetus to such efforts.[68] In the mid-twentieth century, Britain's National Health Service distinguished between "domiciliary service" provided by midwives and GPs and "institutional midwifery," the responsibility of consultant obstetricians.[69]

To some degree the number of practitioners in obstetrics depended on this field's relationship to the emerging specialty of gynecology. Internationally, gynecology was not originally associated exclusively or even most closely with obstetrics. In the eighteenth and early nineteenth centuries, specialists in women's diseases might be surgeons, physicians, or *accoucheurs*. Nonetheless, obstetrical practitioners and societies frequently included diseases of women and children as part of their domain, and the subjects were commonly combined in medical education.[70] From the 1860s on, as medical specialists of all sorts proliferated, gynecology became a distinct field and one of the largest of the new specialty groups that formed. In most large cities, doctors identifying themselves as specialists chose "diseases of women" in disproportionate numbers; practitioners in this category usually constituted from 10 to 15 percent of the local specialist population and were frequently the largest specialist group.[71] It is not difficult to understand why. Women made up half of the total population and were widely considered during the nineteenth century to suffer from intractable medical problems originating in their reproductive systems. Gynecology was also a protean activity that provided an enormous field of activity to medical practitioners. It could be, and frequently was, combined with general practice, surgery, obstetrics, pediatrics, neurology, electrical medicine, and later radiation, as well as with urology or venereology.

Because it could be combined with so many specialties, there was no necessary identification of gynecology with obstetrics, even though many practitioners combined the two activities. The dominant tendency almost everywhere in the second half of the nineteenth century was to claim for gynecology status as an autonomous specialty based on innovative surgical procedures.[72] Obstetrics, in contrast, had to contend with declining birthrates, competition from both midwives and general practitioners, and relatively few technical innovations. Everywhere from 1850 on, independent gynecological clinics, chairs, and societies appeared in major cities. Nonetheless, winning recognition from national bodies was not easy. The British Gynaecological Society (founded in 1885) sought from its inception to win recognition for an autonomous section in this field at annual meetings of the British Medical Association (BMA). In addition to its 300 members, it could point to international developments, notably the planned formation of a separate section of gynecology at the forthcoming International Medical Congress, to be held in Washington in 1887.[73] Despite such arguments, the BMA did not create such a section. Gynecology would have to function for a few more years within the Section of Obstetrics. And by the late nineteenth century, the pendulum was swinging back as internationally, pressure to unify the two fields intensified for a number of reasons.

First, to the extent that women's diseases were defined primarily by the female reproductive system, it seemed to make little sense to distinguish between specialists dealing with this reproductive system before and after childbirth and those concerned only with childbirth. It was not just that many gynecological problems were sequelae of childbirth, while gynecological problems frequently complicated birthing[74]; separation, it was argued, would have a negative impact on the scientific character of both fields. In his presidential address to the American Gynecological Society, J. Whitridge Williams claimed that Americans had made little contribution to obstetrics for a number of reasons, but chiefly because of the existing division between gynecology and obstetrics:

> But I know that in this country neither gynecology nor obstetrics will take its proper place until a body of men has been developed who will be interested in and devote themselves to the study of the problems connected with the entire sexual life of women. I hope I may live to see the day when the term "obstetrician" will have disappeared and when all teachers, at least, will unite in fostering a broader gynecology, instead of being divided, as at present, into knife-loving gynecologists and equally narrow-minded obstetricians, who are frequently little more than trained man-midwives. [75]

Second, this issue had significant political implications as well. For many, the whole point of gynecological care in young women was to ensure healthy reproduction. At a time when national elites were troubled by falling birthrates and high infant mortality, such arguments were increasingly convincing. Ornella Moscucci has argued that political concerns of this sort were central to the unification of gynecology with obstetrics in Great Britain during the interwar period.[76]

Third, as national medical associations began to grapple with ways of regulating specialties, they became concerned not just with limiting the number of specialists but also with keeping the number of specialties manageably small. This proved to be enormously difficult as both knowledge and the number of doctors grew. One way of keeping the number of specialty categories under control was to unite specialties with visible and defensible links into a single category. Wherever national medical associations addressed the issue seriously, they preferred to treat gynecology and obstetrics as a single unit. For similar reasons, associations usually encouraged the combination of diseases of the ear with those of the throat and nose and, in some countries, of psychiatry with neurology.

Fourth, more was at stake than just keeping down the number of specialties. Gynecologists tended to have low status within the medical profession.[77] During the last decades of the nineteenth century, this was mainly due to the field's association with unnecessary and mutilating surgery of the reproductive system. Though such surgery tended to decline gradually, the specialty also became associated with questionable electrical machinery, claims for which smacked of charlatanism. Its low status was reinforced in the early twentieth century by the sheer size of the gynecologist population and its relative lack of representation in academic and hospital institutions. In this context, combining gynecology with obstetrics, a very well established, rather staid field that had excellent and long-standing representation in academic and hospital medicine, could be seen as a way of "domesticating" a rather wild and woolly specialist group.

Fifth, the other side of these professional strategies to regulate specialties was to discourage—indeed, forbid—the combination of specialties considered discrete and unrelated. Gynecologists were particularly known for these sorts of combinations.[78] As professional policies began to have an effect and gynecologists were forced to abandon many of their traditional combinations, they increasingly took on the one supplemental field they were allowed and even encouraged to assume, obstetrics. Furthermore, formal recognition of this combination by professional associations had the added benefit of protecting gynecology from the ever-present danger that the powerful and imperialistic general surgeons would progressively absorb it.[79] Obstetricians, for their part, were given access to a potentially lucrative set of gynecological activities that did not involve the long hours and physical difficulty of attending childbirth and that promised to open up their rather traditional field to new and exciting surgical developments. Unity, finally, solved the technical problem of how to train doctors in obstetrical surgery, given the relatively small number of these operations that were performed; gynecological surgery provided the occasion for training young doctors to operate on the reproductive system.[80]

The German medical profession was the first of the four under study to move decisively to unify obstetrics with gynecology. The major scientific association, the VdNÄ, set up a separate Section of Gynecology in 1858, but only six years later reunited it with obstetrics.[81] By the early twentieth century, university chairs throughout the country combined the two fields, with a single professor usually directing separate teaching clinics in each subject.[82] The *Reichs-Medizinal-Kalender (RMK)*, the major German medical directory, which closely mirrored the views of the leading professional associations, provided only a single pictogram depicting a combined gynecological/obstetrical specialty. The Bremen Guidelines of 1924 made obstetrics-gynecology a single field of training and certification. It was initially possible to combine this specialty with surgery, but the combination was disallowed in 1933.[83]

In Britain, convergence of a slightly different sort took place. The merging in 1907 of the Obstetrical Society with the British Gynaecological Society as a single section of the Royal Society of Medicine heralded this change and prefigured the establishment two decades later of the College of Obstetricians, unifying the two fields.[84] As in other countries, public authorities supported this unification as a way of battling against high infant and maternal mortality rates. However, the College maintained an essential distinction between the two fields, granting lower-level diplomas only in obstetrics and restricting gynecological surgery (along with difficult births) to those who had passed its membership examinations.[85] This came to mean that GPs continued to perform routine obstetrics while hospital consultants combined the two fields. Planners of the postwar National Health Service affirmed the unity of these fields among consultants, declaring that these "two allied subjects constitute one specialty, although rarely a consultant may concentrate on one or the other side. As the service develops, gynaecology will cease to be undertaken by general surgeons."[86] In the subsequent half-century, this indeed seems to have occurred. Obstetrics and gynecology have merged, under the influence of the Royal College, into a single specialty that is not large, with about 1,300 consultants in 2001.[87] The continued role of midwives and GPs in routine childbirth certainly contributes to these small numbers.

In the United States, separation of the two fields was the rule early in the twentieth century. Medical schools rarely combined them; J. Whitridge Williams found that only eight out of forty-two medical schools that he surveyed in 1912 had a single department uniting the two specialties.[88] Practitioners could choose whether to announce that they combined the two fields or specialized in only one of them. The *AMD* thus provided three different abbreviations that listed practitioners could choose.[89] Nonetheless, the American Medical Association (AMA) always insisted on a unified section at its annual meetings, and pressure to bring together the fields increased during the 1920s. The establishment of a single certification board in

1930 lent considerable weight to the movement to combine the two specialties; this board insisted that specialists be certified in both subjects and promoted the unification of fields in medical schools and hospitals.[90] By 1935, at the national level those practicing the fields separately outnumbered those combining them (6 percent combined; 5 percent obstetrics; 3 percent gynecology). However, the situation was quite different in large cities of the Northeast, such as Boston and New York, where combination was far more common than separation (appendix 1). In 1943, 60 percent of American medical schools had combined departments, and a decade later the proportion had risen to 73 percent.[91] Nonetheless, the issue remained contentious. Pressure to grant separate certification for each field continued to be applied. At the Johns Hopkins Medical School the departments remained separated until 1959.[92]

In France, separation of the two fields was especially striking. Those practicing gynecology significantly outnumbered gynecologist-obstetricians, especially in Paris (appendix 1), and they frequently combined their field with a variety of other specialties. The high number of gynecologists in Paris was connected with the extraordinary medical competitiveness of the French capital and the resulting tendency for practitioners to combine claims to the lucrative market for female maladies with a variety of other specialty appellations. This practice was less common in provincial French cities, where medical density was not so high.[93] Such combinations were simply not an option in the more regulated confines of American and German directories.

All the pressures toward unification that I have described in Germany, Britain, and the United States operated in France. Declining population made infant and maternal mortality a central political issue. French gynecologists were widely perceived as out of control and badly trained. In 1931, for instance, when a national federation of specialist trade unions was established, the trade union representing gynecologists was the only one denied admission because it did not demand that its members practice their specialty exclusively.[94] And in 1930, when the Confederation of Medical Trade Unions began the long discussions that would eventually lead to specialty regulation in France, obstetrics and gynecology were consistently treated as a single specialty for the purposes of eventual certification. However, things turned out rather differently for several reasons.

The most serious was the historical separation of obstetrics from surgical gynecology in Paris hospitals. During the 1870s, the hospital administration decided to create an autonomous corps of obstetricians. Hospital surgeons agreed only on condition that gynecological surgery was rigorously excluded from obstetrical wards, which characteristically lacked operating theaters.[95] Consequently, as this separation spread to other French cities, elite gynecology developed a professional identity quite distinct from that of elite obstetrics. At first this identity was largely surgical, but in the early years of the twentieth century, gynecologists gained access to organic extracts, sulfonamides, and hormones that allowed gynecology to take on a more pronounced medical orientation.

A second historical contingency that permitted gynecology to survive as a separate specialty had to do with the way in which specialties became regulated in France. When specialist regulation was implemented after World War II, political pressures came heavily to bear and forced major modifications in the original proposal developed by professional associations. It was difficult for a state-sponsored institution such as the Ordre des Médecins to ignore pressure from interested ministries and legislators. One result of this process is that the original plan for a single specialty in ObGyn became modified so that four distinct groups were eventually established. The combination of obstetrics and gynecology was recognized as a full specialty that had to be practiced exclusively. Three other categories were defined as *compétences* that could be practiced either as exclusive specialties or in combination with general practice. These were surgical gynecology, obstetrics, and medical gynecology. Despite administrative distinctions, all four came to be seen as specialties, although ObGyn was clearly the highest-status option and would gradually assume a dominant position on the French medical scene. Nonetheless, France remains, to my knowledge, the only country that continues to have a specialist group in "medical gynecology." We will briefly discuss its fate in the Epilogue.

Obstetrics-gynecology was not the only specialty constellation within which relationships among categories evolved over time and assumed a variety of shapes. In the following chapter we shall examine several other cases of this sort.

Chapter 11
Division, Unification, and Competition

S pecialties associated with women were not alone in coming together and separating during complex processes of professional gestation. In some fields, unfolding patterns were common to all four countries discussed in this book. In others, significant national variations emerged. Specialties focusing on the organs of the head fit into the first of these categories, while venereology provides an example of the second. We then go on to examine the case of a specialty group, stomatologists, who competed against another occupation, dentists, while seeking to remain within mainstream medicine.

The Organs of the Head

The specialties that dealt with diseases of the eyes, ears, nose, and throat were large and institutionally significant almost everywhere at the beginning of the twentieth century. Ophthalmology was one of the very first fields to develop as a specialty and enjoyed significant academic stature. It began to emerge as a discipline during the eighteenth century, as a result of the development of new methods for treating such conditions as cataracts (extraction as opposed to couching), infections, and even blindness (artificial pupils); these were complicated and, by the standards of the time, reasonably effective. A vigorous medical literature in this area was being produced by the second half of the century, and the subject began to be taught in institutions of medical education. In 1765, for instance, a chair in ocular surgery was established at the Collège de Chirurgie at Saint-Côme.[1] By the end of the eighteenth century, surgeon-oculists were using complex new techniques that were not easily available to itinerant practitioners.[2]

At the same time, there existed in many countries considerable public anxiety about blindness, a common result of eye disease that could destroy the economic viability of families. According to Helen Corlett, eye diseases and oculists appear regularly in English poor law records, and schools and asylums for the blind developed in many countries.[3] In Britain, however, ophthalmology grew primarily through the establishment of private eye hospitals, a type of institution that became common in the United States somewhat later. In both countries, such hospitals were characteristically financed privately; being able to claim procedures that could prevent "blindness" was a uniquely effective way of appealing to philanthropists.[4] In the German-speaking world, the early development of ophthalmology depended not on hospital philanthropy but rather on its early acceptance in medical education. Vienna had a chair of ophthalmology in 1818, and by 1873 all Prussian universities had professorial chairs.[5] For reasons that remain obscure, ophthalmology did not emerge as an important field in France. In 1800 a proposal to establish a special hospice for eye diseases was rejected by a special commission of the Paris Faculty of Medicine asked to review it. While the commission was not hostile to the principle of a special hospital, it concluded that existing general hospitals already satisfied the needs of both patients and medical training; it also suggested that eye diseases were often the consequences of internal diseases and were thus best treated by generalists.[6] In subsequent years, the famous Paris surgeon Alfred Velpeau devoted much energy to preventing the separation of ophthalmology from general surgery. Much Parisian clinical research in this subject took place at an asylum for the blind, the Quinze-Vingt, rather than in hospitals. Foreign observers found Paris ophthalmology to be rather mediocre at midcentury, and in years that followed the specialty did not achieve the prominence in France that it enjoyed in Britain or the German-speaking world.

By midcentury, a variety of innovations, notably the ophthalmoscope (invented in 1851) and knowledge of refraction, greatly extended the scope of the field, even as anesthesia and antisepsis expanded opportunities for surgery on the eye. Despite its limited development in France, the intellectual stature of ophthalmology was widely recognized, and it was the first specialty field to be granted a professorial chair at the Paris Faculty of Medicine (in 1876). However, the number of practitioners in Paris continued to be relatively small by international standards. In early twentieth-century Prussia, by contrast, ophthalmology was the largest specialty, practiced by 15 percent of all specialists; complaints about overcrowding in the field were quite common as a result.[7] One reason for the specialty's popularity was its ubiquity within the university system; virtually every medical school had an ophthalmology clinic with one or two assistants who went on to specialist practice.[8] In the 1930s, the Ophthalmological Group of the British Medical Association (BMA) was by far the largest specialty group in that organization, and ophthalmologists constituted, after general surgery and general medicine, the largest single group of consultants on the BMA's Consultants and Specialists list. When the National Health Service (NHS) was set up after World War II, specialists in this field were significantly overrepresented among hospital consultants (appendix 2).[9] In Prussia, the proportion of ophthalmologists among all specialists dropped from 15 percent in

1903 to only 8 percent in 1937. The proportion of eye specialists in Britain declined to the levels characteristic of the three other nations considerably later, after the creation of the NHS, which favored the expansion of other fields.

Ophthalmology was rich enough in knowledge and difficult techniques to make efforts at combining it with other specialties relatively rare. The major exception was the amalgamation of this specialty with diseases of the throat and ears that emerged in the early twentieth century in both Germany and the United States (but not in France). These latter two fields had developed separately during the 1860s. Laryngology followed the model developed by ophthalmology; instruments—the laryngoscope and rhinoscope—provided new views and new understanding of these organs and their diseases.[10] Originally, laryngology—usually including treatment of the nose—was distinct from otology. In Germany, laryngology grew out of internal medicine, while otology was considered a surgical field. Following a widespread strategy of claiming proximate organs, some practitioners of these fields drifted up to care for the eyes, particularly in the United States (appendix 1)[11]; others drifted down into the respiratory system.[12] But the predominant pattern was the combination otology and laryngolgogy. In 1884, for instance, the International Medical Congress offered for the first time a section devoted to both fields.[13] The question of whether these should be unified or separated specialties was hotly debated in Germany. For some, separation was a sign of scientific seriousness; for others, it led to unnecessary fragmentation and served as too narrow a basis for both medical teaching and practice.[14] In the first years of the twentieth century, the *Reich-Medizinal-Kalender (RMK)* had separate pictograms for the ear and for the nose and larynx (though they frequently appeared in combination). Before World War I, smaller faculties combined teaching of the two fields, while large ones kept them distinct.[15] The Bremen Guidelines of 1924 confirmed the unity of these three organs within a single specialty.

Much the same process occurred in Britain. When the BMA created a Section of Otology in 1885, it was proposed that the field of laryngology be added to it, but this proposal was defeated.[16] In subsequent years, each field had its own section at BMA meetings, with laryngology associated with rhinology.[17] Similarly, the Royal Society of Medicine had from its inception two separate sections: one in laryngology and rhinology, and another in otology. Leaders of each field such as Sir Felix Semon in laryngology, continued to insist on the advantages of separation.[18] Nonetheless, membership in both sections was common and collaboration was not infrequent. The two sections, for instance, campaigned successfully in the early 1920s to make otolaryngology a required subject in the medical curriculum. Soon after, the Conjoint Board of the Royal Colleges began granting a diploma in laryngology and otology. Despite their continued separation in the Royal Society of Medicine, the two fields in subsequent decades grew closer together, with most hospital posts covering both domains.[19] The BMA Specialist List in 1938 treated it as a single specialist category, as did many of the planning reports for the National Health Service.[20]

In France and the United States, the combination was widely accepted by the start of the twentieth century. France's *Guide Rosenwald* treated it as a single category in 1905, as did the *American Medical Directory* from the time it published its first specialist list in 1909. Combining these fields made the resulting specialty more attractive by appealing to much larger patient populations. Almost everywhere this new combined field was one of the largest of the specialties. Its practitioners made up 14 percent of all specialists in Prussia in 1903 (making it the third largest specialty) and 11 percent in 1937 (fourth largest).[21] It was not quite so large in France; its practitioners constituted 11 percent of the specialist population in 1905 and 9 percent in 1935.[22] Otorhinolaryngologists (including those who also practiced ophthalmology) made up 13 percent of American specialists in 1935 (appendix 1).

Venereology and Dermatology

The combination of dermatology with venereology was common, though by no means universal. There was initially no particular institutional link between the two fields. Each had its own special hospitals that generated quite distinct professional identities. The practical basis for association between the two fields was the need to distinguish venereal lesions from other sorts of skin lesions. The discovery that microorganisms were frequently responsible for both categories of disease strengthened the rationale for combining them. Finally, as sexually transmitted diseases became increasingly perceived as a national danger requiring massive governmental intervention, it became useful for dermatologists to associate themselves with this field despite the moral opprobrium sometimes attached to it. The development of the Wassermann test and Salvarsan allowed venereal disease to be more widely perceived as a medical rather than a moral issue, and further increased the attractiveness of the field for dermatologists. Nonetheless, unification did not occur everywhere, and patterns of development varied widely.

In France the predominant tradition during the nineteenth century was separation of the two fields, which were based in different Parisian hospitals (St. Louis for skin diseases and Midi for venereal diseases). Professors at the Paris Faculty of Medicine in the mid-1870s, we saw in chapter 2, supported the creation of a chair of dermatology but did not think that venereology either constituted a part of dermatology or was worthy of its own chair. The national government literally forced a recalcitrant Faculty to accept a chair combining the two fields because of what it perceived as the public health importance of venereology. Then, to boot, the government appointed the venereologist Alfred Fournier to fill the chair. Henceforth the two subjects were irrevocably linked, at least educationally. Fournier, we saw, made unsuccessful efforts to establish a corps of elite venereologists in the Paris hospitals on public health grounds, an indication that some distinctions remained. This is confirmed by the fact that as late as the 1930s, a sizable proportion of doctors identified themselves in medical directories as either dermatologists or venere-ologists, and not as both (appendix 1). Nonetheless, the system of certification introduced after World War II definitively combined the two fields.

The number of French practitioners of these two specialties, whether separated or combined, does not seem to have been large. One reason may have been the limited scale of public health interventions—and consequently of public posts—in the domain of venereal disease. Although French authorities after World War I undertook educational campaigns to fight venereal diseases, as was the case in many other countries, there is little documentation to suggest extensive government commitment to medical treatment. This may well reflect governmental reliance on the traditional method of controlling syphilis though the regulation of prostitutes.[23]

In Germany as well, the two fields were initially separated. Skin diseases were associated with internal medicine, while venereology grew out of surgery. In 1825 an independent venereal clinic was set up at the Charité Hospital in Berlin, and a few years later another was established at the municipal hospital in Munich. The pattern changed first in Vienna, where in 1849 a combined ward was set up at the Allgemeine Krankenhaus under the direction of von Hebra. Gradually, this model spread throughout the German-speaking world. In 1869 the *Archiv für Dermatologie und Syphilis* was established, and in 1885 the Versammlung der Deutschen Naturforscher und Ärzte (VdNÄ) established a single section combining the two fields.[24] As in France, the discovery that microorganisms were frequently responsible for both kinds of maladies provided a scientific basis for this connection, while the social consequences of venereal disease added political relevance to dermatology. In 1900 for instance, the Prussian Ministry of Religion, responsible for public health, issued a decree that physicians working in the service that regulated prostitutes should have training in venereology. In 1901, a half-year practicum in dermato-venereology was made a requirement for medical students and venereology became part of the final examination in surgery.[25] Two years later, a reform of health insurance legislation ensured that VD patients were entitled to the same benefits as other members of health insurance plans. This represented a notable transition from the notion that VD was a moral issue to the view that it was a medical and public health concern. It also provided the specialty with a major boost since any member of a health insurance plan was, if infected, obliged to consult an approved specialist.[26] The desire of the profession to restrict the number of recognized specialties played a role as well in the merging of specialties. The *RMK* treated the two as a single specialty for purposes of self-identification from the beginning of the twentieth century. In 1924, the Bremen Guidelines would do so as well by including the combined field among the authorized specialty categories.

Despite its significance for public health, this combined specialty did not win full acceptance at the highest academic levels until a relatively late date. While a chair in Vienna was set up in 1869, and one in Paris was founded eight years later, the first chair in this field in Germany was set up in Rostock only in 1904. In the years that followed, the field became increasingly accepted, but more than half of German universities did not have chairs in this combined subject by the outbreak of the World War I.[27] In the postwar period, the situation changed somewhat as a result of intensified public anxiety about syphilis. The state created new jobs for specialists in this field by setting up VD advice centers; by 1931, 264 centers were in operation. The VD Act of 1927 required anyone infected with venereal disease to undergo treatment.[28] As part of the ongoing effort to set up prevention programs for sexually transmitted diseases, dermato-venereology became increasingly prominent in the medical curriculum, and in 1918, the specialty became an independent and obligatory examination subject. In less than a decade, every medical school in Germany had a professor of dermato-venereology.[29]

Despite its belated academic acceptance, practitioners in private practice overwhelmingly dominated the specialty (93 percent in 1937), which had a relatively small elite component.[30] In part this reflected its remarkable growth as a field of practice. In 1903, practitioners in this field constituted about 6 percent of the specialist population in Prussia. As public health programs proliferated, the number of practitioners in this specialty grew dramatically. The proportion of dermato-venereologists among all specialists doubled from 1903 to 1936. In the latter year, the number of dermato-venereologists was larger than the number of surgeons in Berlin and nearly as large as the number of internists (appendix 1).[31] The popularity of this field for doctors would continue into the Nazi era.

Like gynecology in the late nineteenth century, dermato-venereology had a low social status. Because it was a new field, there were few academic and hospital posts relative to the number of practitioners. It also attracted disproportionate numbers of those excluded from or at least marginal to more established specialties; these included women and Jews, who were both significantly overrepresented.[32] Also as in the case of gynecology, its practitioners reacted to intense professional competition by claiming neighboring specialties such as urology. In 1933, just before new regulations made this combination unacceptable, 4 percent of all Prussian specialists were combining urology with dermatology-venereology on the basis, presumably, of the central role of sexual organs in both fields.[33]

In contrast, American venereology seems to have been largely subsumed (and to some degree hidden) by dermatology. There was, for instance, no specific mention of venereology in the specialist abbreviations or in the names of specialty societies recognized by the American Medical Association (AMA) in the *American Medical Directory*, even though it was part of the domains of both dermatology and urology. The constantly changing title of the relevant section of the AMA is testimony to the ambivalence of American specialists toward admitting to links with venereal disease.[34] Many practitioners noted that venereology in the United States was held down by the moral opprobrium connected to the diseases it treated.[35] An analysis in 1925 of the troubled relations between the two fields suggested that American dermatologists were reluctant to identify themselves with syphilology for precisely this reason. Further weakening the links between the two fields, the author proposed, was the association of syphilology in a minority of cases with specialists of the genito-urinary tract.[36] Just before World War I, in fact, an effort to establish an AMA section devoted to "genito-urinary and venereal diseases" failed due to the opposition of both dermatologists and urologists.[37] Nonetheless, military concerns with venereal disease during World War I and the subsequent efforts of leaders of American public health went a long way toward making the field more acceptable.[38] By 1925 the majority of medical schools linked dermatology and venereology in some way.[39] And the *American Medical Directory* combined the two appellations without giving practitioners the option to claim only one, as it did in other such cases. In 1932, the American Board of Dermatology and Syphilology was established to certify specialists in the field.

This combined field remained small in the United States (see appendix 1). Aside from considerations of morality, the lack of any national program of venereal disease prevention and treatment gave practitioners little incentive to specialize in this field. The situation changed only in the mid-1930s. The Social Security Act of 1935 provided the Public Health Service with funds to disburse to the states; more than 10 percent was used to fight syphilis. Three years later Congress passed the National Venereal Disease Control Act, which provided direct federal grants to state boards of health for the purpose of developing measures to combat venereal diseases. The government provided over $15 million for the initial three-year period.[40] These measures had a modest effect on the number of dermatologist-venereologists. In 1923, there were only 361 practitioners in this category; by 1940 the figure was 974, an increase of 170 percent. (The total number of specialists increased during these years by 140 percent.[41]) One might expect that during and after World War II, the needs of the military would have stimulated large numbers of specialists to enter this field. But in actual fact, the proportion of dermato-venereologists among all specialists remained virtually unchanged at about 2.6 percent between 1940 and 1949.[42]

Britain constituted the chief exception to the international tendency to combine the two fields. Here, venereologists as a specialist group had little visibility throughout the nineteenth century. A list of London hospital consultants in 1889[43] included no specific listing for this specialist category. One finds the medical staff of the London Lock Hospital under various categories, chiefly one called "genito-urinary diseases," dominated by urological surgeons; none were listed under the category "diseases of the skin," which boasted many specialist hospitals and wards in general hospitals.[44] Venereology was completely invisible in another directory of London specialists that appeared in the following year.

Nonetheless, venereal disease became increasingly conspicuous after the turn of the century for exactly the same reasons that made it visible elsewhere; it became a social problem that provoked the interest of feminists, advocates of social purity, the social hygiene movement, and Fabian socialists such as George Bernard Shaw. New medical interest in venereal diseases also resulted from the introduction of the Wassermann blood test and Paul Ehrlich's Salvarsan.[45] The report of a royal commission that completed its work in 1916 urged that treatment for syphilis be made more widely available.[46] As a consequence, a venereal medical service was set up in 1916 under the joint jurisdiction of the central government and local authorities. During 1919, over one million patients were seen within the framework of this service. By 1925, 193 clinics had been established.[47]

Venereology as an autonomous specialty domain in Britain grew up around this service. Consequently, it had no particular ties to dermatology; approximately 5 percent of all those who declared themselves as specialists in a medical directory of 1925 identified themselves only as venereologists, without mentioning dermatology (see appendix 2).[48] There were, to be sure, important points of intersection. The Section of Dermatology of the Royal Society of Medicine did not have "venereology" in its title, but numerous papers on syphilis were nonetheless presented. A proposal to change the name of the section to "Dermatology and Syphilology" was introduced but never followed up.[49] There were enough individuals combining the two fields to justify the existence of the British Association of Dermatology and Syphilology and its organ, the *British Journal of Dermatology and Syphilis*, both created in 1917. Nonetheless, there were also enough pure venereologists to give rise to the more limited *British Journal of Venereology*, established in 1925.

Venereology remained a fairly low-status field without its own section in the Royal Society of Medicine. Its practitioners came to it from a wide variety of medical backgrounds, and aside from generalized unhappiness about their low status and poor working conditions in public clinics, they did not develop a strong specialist identity. The BMA's List of Consultants and Specialists of 1938 did not include a separate heading for this specialty; practitioners indicating a special interest in venereology were found among those listed under surgery, obstetrics-gynecology, and dermatology. This is not surprising, given that the national requirement to become a medical officer in a venereal clinic was only 130 hours of training, without the need to pass any examinations. A survey done in 1939 found that only 36 of 259 medical officers in provincial venereal centers, and 11 of 98 in London, were actually specialists in venereal disease.[50]

British dermatologists took some care to distinguish themselves from venereologists. In 1947 the BMA Council approved the recommendation of its Dermatologists Group that doctors in the military be allowed to become specialists in dermatology "as distinct from venereology. The Directors-General of the three fighting Services have accordingly been invited to recognize the general trend to regard dermatology as a separate specialty divorced from venereology. . . . "[51]

In this context, it is hardly surprising that the National Health Service (NHS) upon its inception treated the two fields as completely distinct[52]; existing venereal clinics were simply transferred into the NHS.[53] Even at this late date, venereologists had to fight traditional discrimination against patients suffering from sexually transmitted diseases; the Venereologists Group of the BMA voted in November 1948 to end the traditional prohibition on accepting VD patients in general hospitals.[54] The advent of the NHS seems to have significantly improved the status of British venereologists. Many more were given consultant status despite resistance by hospital medical staff.[55] Nevertheless, the old stigma did not disappear, and as a specialty devoted to a single category of diseases, British venereology proved uniquely vulnerable when antibiotics both lowered the incidence of venereal diseases and made them easy to treat. Its practitioners could not fall back on their dermatological activity, as was the case in other countries. Hospital authorities closed clinics and failed to replace retiring consultants. Not surprisingly, it was one of the few specialties that grew not at all in the decade following the establishment of the National Health Service.[56] A review by the Ministry of Health in 1955 found that only ninety-three consultants and seventy-nine senior hospital medical officers maintained the entire VD service.[57] It remained a "Cinderella service" until the murderous eruption of the AIDS epidemic in the 1980s made it once again central to health policy.[58]

Stomatology Versus Dentistry

Relationships among specialty groups constituted one critical problem that had to be worked out as specialties became regulated and standardized. Another was the association of certain specialties with nonmedical professions functioning in the same sphere. Ophthalmologists thus competed against opticians, and radiologists and electrical specialists struggled against nonmedical technicians. But none of these faced a task as daunting as the one confronting stomatologists, who competed against dentists for the right to treat the mouth and teeth.

Dentistry was traditionally a medical activity. During the eighteenth century, doctors in France were instrumental in transforming the field from one dominated by itinerant tooth pullers into a more sophisticated occupation that included, among other activities, filling cavities, cleaning teeth, producing prosthetic teeth, and orthodontics.[59] Throughout the nineteenth century, in virtually all the major nations, some doctors continued to specialize in the mouth and teeth. They called themselves surgeon-dentists, odontologists, or stomatologists, and, in the German-speaking world, practitioners of *Mund- und Kieferkrankheiten,* to distinguish themselves from mere dentists. But in all countries, such doctors comprised a small minority of dental practitioners.

Almost everywhere during the nineteenth century, efforts were made to raise the status of tooth and mouth care by introducing formal training. Not infrequently, these efforts were characterized by fundamental disagreements: Should dentistry be a medical field open to all doctors, or a medical specialty requiring a specialized degree granted by a medical school *following* the completion of regular medical studies? Or should dental training take place in autonomous institutions and culminate in a degree totally distinct from that of medicine?

This was not a simple issue. Whatever the benefit to doctors of controlling an activity that brought in many patients, did most physicians really want to be confused with individuals practicing what amounted to a manual trade? And if dentists were required to hold medical degrees, might they not choose to practice medicine rather than dentistry, thereby exacerbating the professional overcrowding about which doctors everywhere always complained? Furthermore, doctors who practiced dentistry rarely had much influence within the elite medical circles. In most countries, therefore, organized medical professions lent little support to struggles to medicalize dentistry.

Governments and public health administrations also showed little sympathy for medical dentistry. The notion that doctors with no special training could care for teeth became increasingly improbable as technical innovations were introduced during the course of the nineteenth century. And demanding that those who cared for teeth obtain *both* medical and dental qualifications would have required such a lengthy period of training that few practitioners would comply. Finally, once the dental health of populations became perceived as a public health issue in the twentieth century, the challenge was precisely to train enough practitioners to serve growing national needs. Medical schools in most nations, in contrast, were trying to combat perceived overcrowding in the profession by making medical education increasingly selective. Consequently, the pattern almost everywhere during the twentieth century was that dentistry became an autonomous profession, while care of the mouth and teeth gradually became a marginal part of medicine. Nonetheless, the process was not universal, and its pace and form varied substantially from one country to the next.

At one end of the spectrum we find the United States, where medical dentistry always had a low profile. Here an autonomous dental profession developed early and became linked with some of the nation's many universities; by the twentieth century, dental schools were both independent of medicine and well integrated within universities.[60] American dentistry probably led the world in technical innovations during the nineteenth century and, reversing the more usual trajectory across the Atlantic, European dentists traveled to the United States to see the latest developments at first hand and frequently returned home with the DDS diploma. A medical form of dentistry, "stomatology" existed in the United States, from 1881 on, as one of the fifteen specialty sections of the AMA, and in the early twentieth century its representatives campaigned vigorously for the full medicalization of dentistry.[61] But in 1925 the AMA decided to eliminate this section in order to make room for a new Section of Radiology.[62] During the 1920s and 1930s, stomatologists attempted to reinstate their AMA section and, more generally, to promote stomatology as a medical specialty. But they had little success.[63]

At the other end of the spectrum was stomatology in Austria, which developed earlier and more elaborately than in other nations. Vienna was, to my knowledge, the first medical school in Europe to establish a lectureship in dentistry (in 1821). The second incumbent in the position, Moritz Heider, reached the status of extraordinary professor and also served as a leader in both the German and the Austrian dental associations formed circa 1860. Heider and his successors argued firmly for a dentistry that was an integral part of medicine, and though they were not rewarded with a full university chair—the most visible symbol of such status—they created a vigorous academic world of medical dentistry in Vienna with two small schools in operation at the end of the century. In the twentieth century one victory followed another. In 1898 Julius Scheff was appointed full professor of dentistry at the medical school; in 1903, dentistry became an obligatory subject in the medical curriculum. In 1925, dental surgery became regulated; henceforth, four semesters of study were to be taken at a university institute of dentistry, followed by professional examinations. And in 1930, it was decreed that only physicians with special training were entitled to call themselves dentists.[64]

We can locate Germany and Britain somewhere between these two extreme cases. In both, an autonomous dental profession gradually displaced medical dentistry; nonetheless, medical schools played a key role in dental education, so that stomatologists frequently served as the educational leaders of the profession.

In Germany, the separation of dentistry from medicine was a gradual process. For much of the nineteenth century, under the influence of the Viennese professor, Moritz Heider, German dentistry was considered a medical specialty. However, by the beginning of the twentieth century, the national dental association had moved firmly in favor of separation from medicine.[65] This was also the position of the educational leaders of the dental profession, who admitted the excellence of the Austrian model but nonetheless believed that it could not serve a population whose dental needs were now being covered by the health insurance system.[66]

Dentists (*Zahnärzte*) were explicitly recognized as a category of medical personnel by the Prussian professional regulations of 1825; training and certification were further defined in regulations of 1835 and 1836, and other states quickly followed.[67] But an individual did not require accreditation in order to work on teeth, and many dentists or dental technicians practiced without it. Furthermore, while training for dentists took place in medical schools, it was separated from medical studies and had a lower status. Consequently there were few accredited dentists at midcentury (only 103 in Prussia and about 250 in what was to become the German Empire).[68] Heinrich Albrecht established the first private clinic for tooth maladies in Berlin in 1855. When practical training was made obligatory for dentists in 1866, Albrecht's clinic began playing a major training role.[69]

Crucial for determining future developments was the establishment in 1869 of a dental degree as the culmination of two years of study. This was independent of medicine and was demanded of everyone wishing accreditation as a dentist, including MDs. Henceforth, all dentists, even those with medical training, had an identity that was to some extent distinct. Furthermore, the freedom of medical and dental practice established in 1869 created so much competition with non-accredited practitioners that all university-trained dentists developed a strong interest in reaching agreement about ways to raise educational standards and win a monopoly of practice. As a result, they established one of the earliest specialist associations in Germany.[70] Under such conditions, the number of accredited dentists increased dramatically, from 470 in 1885, to more than 1,000 in 1894, to some

4,000 at the start of the First World War.[71] Meanwhile, some German MDs continued to practice dental medicine, but the field of stomatology became far less secure than it was in Austria, France, Belgium, and Hungary. The number of medical dentists was very low, about 0.5 percent of all dentists in 1910, in both Prussia and the German Empire as a whole.[72] This did not, however, prevent periodic calls for the medicalization of dentistry or the sporadic eruption of sharp conflict between stomatologists and dentists.[73]

The Bremen Guidelines that regulated specialties recognized medicine of the teeth, mouth, and jaws (*Zahn- und Kieferkrankheiten*) as one of the fourteen allowable specialties. But rules required that all candidates for specialty status have dental accreditation, making this field relatively unattractive to doctors. Though the specialty had its own pictogram in the *RMK*'s listing of medical practitioners, few individuals utilized it.[74] During the early 1930s, there were about 160 stomatologists listed in official statistics. It was by far the smallest medical specialty in existence.[75] The fact that it fell under the jurisdiction of both medical and dental professional groups made the status of this specialty very complex and confusing.[76] This situation was resolved only in 1931, when an agreement between the Deutsche Ärztevereinsbund (DÄV) and the association representing dentists limited specialty practice to those MDs with full dental training and, at the same time, restricted both specialization among dentists and the titles that these dentists could assume.[77] Although the dentists' list disappeared from the *RMK*, significant ties, mediated by the MDs who taught in dental programs, continued to exist. The leading national medical journal of the period, the *Deutsche medizinische Wochenschrift*, frequently published articles on dentistry, particularly on the battle between dentists and the dental technicians against whom they competed. These articles usually expressed considerable sympathy for the position of dentists.[78] To be sure, demands to make dentistry a specialty of medicine continued to be raised, but this was not a widely held position.[79]

To some degree the sheer number of dentists was essential to this process insofar as it was impossible for small numbers of stomatologists to plausibly claim to serve the nation's dental needs. From about 2,770 dentists in 1909, the number climbed to over 8,000 in 1924. Even this number was not seen to be sufficient, given growing government concern with dental health.[80] In the late nineteenth and early twentieth centuries, dental work had required a medical referral for insurance coverage. When, in 1911, dental services were incorporated directly into the health insurance system, the insufficient number of dentists forced administrators to utilize unofficial dental practitioners (*Zahntechniker*, whose number was estimated to be about 14,000 in the mid-1920s) for insurance system work.[81] Another essential factor in the eventual predominance of dentists had to do with the changing nature of dental work. While problems such as cavities could be characterized as those of living organs, and hence defined as part of medicine, more and more dental work now had to do with prostheses of one sort or another. This was most definitely not a traditional medical activity. Medical discomfort with it was evident in the argument made by certain supporters of medical dentistry to the effect that doctors should take over the care of all *living* organs of the mouth and jaw, and leave prostheses to mechanical artisans (*Handwerker*). Not surprisingly, such suggestions were not taken very seriously.[82]

Perhaps most determinant was, in the classical manner of "professional" social mobility studies, the introduction of a series of reforms of dental education, culminating in 1919 with the creation of a doctorate of dental science making dentists the titular equals of medical doctors. What is more, this was a diploma granted by medical schools, leaving stomatologists with a continuing role in dental training.[83] Despite the fact that the status of German dentists was improving, freedom of practice for unauthorized competitors continued to exist. Not until 1952 was the practice of dentistry forbidden to anyone without appropriate dental credentials.[84]

The situation in Britain resembled that of Germany, but medical dentistry had a more visible profile and a longer life span. In 1859 a degree of dental surgery, the license in dental surgery (LDS), was established by the Royal College of Surgeons.[85] This diploma was not equivalent to other medical or surgical degrees. Entrance requirements were less stringent, and dentists and medical institutions did not perceive dental surgeons as qualified to practice medicine, although anyone could legally practice either profession. Nonetheless, nothing prevented medical practitioners from getting the LDS, or holders of the latter diploma from taking medical degrees. Some of the leading dental schools, such as the ones attached to the Royal Dental Hospital of London and the Edinburgh Dental Hospital, had a thoroughly medical orientation, restricting their staff to holders of medical credentials and encouraging more ambitious students to acquire such credentials as well.[86] Consequently, dental surgeons constituted a significant segment of all British dentists. In some ways they can be seen as the first trained and certified medical specialists in Britain. And there was always an important branch of the dental reform movement that proposed to take the profession in a resolutely medical direction.[87]

As in Germany, however, the legal freedom of all—including those without any formal credentials—to practice dentistry served as a powerful incentive for credentialed dentists to organize and achieve consensus about educational reform. And since the majority did not have medical qualifications, institutional reform moved strongly in the direction of an autonomous dental profession. In 1878, the Dental Act made it illegal for anyone not registered to call himself "dentist" or "dental surgeon." And only licenciates of the RCS or those engaged in the practice of dental surgery at the time were entitled to be registered. However, the rights of medical practitioners were safeguarded. Unlike everyone else, and despite the fact that the RCS did not authorize the practice, legally qualified medical practitioners were not subject to the prohibition against assuming a dental title without the appropriate dental qualification.[88] In 1879 the British Dental Association was established. The Dentists Act of 1921 prohibited practice by anyone not registered as a qualified dentist (again depending on credentials or active practice at the time the act came into force), but once again allowed any registered medical practitioner to practice dentistry.[89] A Dental Board was established to share responsibility for professional education and ethics with the General Medical Council.[90] In 1922, the number of dentists on the revised dental register more than doubled.[91]

As a result of these measures and the development of various forms of non-medical training and certification for dentists, the proportion of surgeon dentists fell in the twentieth century. According to one report, there were 13,727 registered dentists in 1925, with only 646 having both medical and dental qualifications; 4,801 had only dental qualifications; and 7,296 (60 percent) lacked credentials but qualified for registration by virtue of the Dentists Acts of 1878 or 1921.[92] Members of the RCS who had taken the LDS and chosen to practice dentistry made up a professional elite from whose ranks teachers and hospital consultants were recruited.[93]

As in Germany, the poor dental health of the population came to be seen in the twentieth century as a public health issue, and the idea of establishing a national dental service, parallel to the medical service, gained support. Since the number of medically qualified with good dental training was likely to remain small, the solution to what was perceived as the chief barrier to such a service—insufficient numbers of dentists and poor training—came to be identified with a fully independent dental profession; this was recommended by several reports produced during World War II.[94] Nor did the medical profession attempt to prevent this process. Surgeon dentists did not appear on the list of consultants and specialists that the BMA drew up during the 1930s.[95] Still, medical dentistry was not without supporters. It continued to be championed by the School of the National Dental Hospital during the interwar years. In 1945, the Glasgow Dental School tried to advertise for a dean who was a registered dental practitioner with medical qualifications; the *British Dental Journal* refused to publish the advertisement.[96] And there was opposition during the postwar years to creating a General Dental Council, fully independent of the General Medical Council and emblematic of a fully autonomous profession. This measure was passed only in 1956, as part of the Dentists Act of that year, which gave dentistry the status of a separate profession.[97] Nonetheless, in the interim, the Royal College of Surgeons had established a Faculty of Dental Surgery and a fellowship in dental surgery. Together with the Odontological Museum housed on its premises, this faculty has allowed the RCS to retain a central role in the training of elite dentists even as the latter's status has become increasingly distinct from medicine.[98] The RCS has not, however, been the only institution to treat dental surgery as a medical specialty. From 1947, the National Health Service consistently treated dental surgery as part of its consultant medical service. Among the institutes of postgraduate medical education set up in 1948 to satisfy consultant manpower needs was one devoted to dental surgery.[99]

As in so many other respects, the French situation was unusually complex.[100] Here, as in Belgium and Hungary, stomatology had a strong presence.[101] Dentistry was ignored in the laws organizing French medicine in the early nineteenth century. Political inability to pass any overall reform of the medical profession for most of the century meant that dentistry remained a completely free and unregulated field. It was practiced both by doctors and by many individuals without any credentials. If someone in either group had any specialized training, it was usually through apprenticeship. The obvious solution for raising the status of this occupational group was to introduce formal training with or without a state license. For much of the century, the usual debates about the degree to which dentistry should be a medical profession divided those seeking to introduce educational requirements. By the time medical reform became a realistic possibility in the 1880s, practitioners were divided into three groups, each revolving around a professional society and a newly created school. One organized around the École Dentaire de Paris, founded in 1880, argued for private schools and no formal state system of education and licensing. In practice, it also had a manual orientation focusing on the production of prostheses. A second group, centered around the Institut Odontologique, argued for an autonomous dental diploma granted by the state through the Paris Faculty of Medicine but demanding little medical knowledge. A third group, which formed the Société de Stomatologie de Paris in the late 1880s, argued that dentistry was simply a specialty of medicine and should be practiced only by doctors. In 1892, as part of a generalized reform of the medical profession, dentistry was finally organized and recognized as a profession. Existing dental schools provided training, but it was the Faculty of Medicine that granted a newly established diploma in dental surgery. The law compromised among existing groups by authorizing dental practice for *either* those possessing the new degree in dental surgery *or* doctors of medicine; the latter were not formally required to have any supplementary dental training. This allowed large numbers of doctors to take up the field of stomatology.

Stomatologists constituted a large group within French medicine, comprising 7 percent of all specialists in Paris and in the larger provincial cities in 1935. In 1923, a special corps of stomatologists recruited by special competition (*concours*) was granted a monopoly of dental work in the Parisian hospitals.[102] Despite this strong presence, the place of stomatology in French medicine was not completely secure. It is telling that at least one of the medical directories of Paris (*Medicus*) did not categorize stomatology among the specialties in medicine, but gave it a separate listing. Both dentists and stomatologists in France constituted professional groups large enough to pursue monopolistic aspirations; relations between them were characterized by severe conflict, with the dentists advocating a mandatory dental degree for all practitioners and the stomatologists campaigning to limit practice to holders of the MD diploma. The conflict reached such levels of recrimination, we saw in chapter 8, that it provoked the campaign to introduce specialty certification in France. Stomatology survived these battles, and the introduction of certification in 1947 saw it recognized as a specialist competency. Nonetheless, this victory was accompanied by a major defeat. An article of the newly promulgated Code of Medical Deontology, elaborated by the Ordre des Médecins, placed stomatologists under the jurisdiction of the Ordre des Chirugiens-Dentistes, a situation that years later was still considered a deep affront.[103]

Although they largely abandoned the effort to fully medicalize dentistry, stomatologists and their allies continued to work toward limiting the domain of nonmedical dentistry.[104] The Academy of Medicine in 1966 produced a report recommending that dentists be prohibited from using anesthetics and doing any work beyond the teeth and gums.[105] Dentists continued to struggle successfully against such limits to their practice. Reforms introduced in 1965 normalized the status of dental schools and their personnel, and gave them full university status; laws passed in 1969 and 1971 ended the restrictive definition of allowable dental acts and defined the work of dentists as "the diagnosis and treatment of the teeth, the mouth and the maxillaries."[106] In that year as well, the dental degree became a doctorate in dental surgery, allowing dentists to use the title "doctor." Soon thereafter, they were also accorded the right to prescribe medications.[107] In subsequent years they were permitted to practice in hospitals, though they did not receive the exclusive right to do so.[108]

Today stomatology remains a recognized specialty in France. (There are also significant groups of stomatologists in Italy, Spain, and Portugal.) But the number of practitioners has shrunk slightly since the mid-1980s, during a period when the total number of specialists rose by over 70 percent. In 2000, a little over 1,400 individuals (out of nearly 100,000 specialists) were practicing stomatology.[109] As these persons gradually retire, this field is likely to shrink even further, since in recent years, the number of individuals obtaining the specialty certificate has been minuscule.[110] This most likely reflects the unwillingness of the health administration to support training residencies in this field when dentists are in fact the major health-care providers for the teeth and mouth. In response to such pressures, the specialty is currently in the midst of an identity crisis. It has moved to unite with the tiny field of maxillo-facial surgery that focuses on facial reconstruction, but the process has hardly been smooth or tension-free [111]

Conclusion

Specialization was to a significant degree an international phenomenon. By the 1930s, all four countries we have examined had much the same specialty categories. The distribution of doctors among these categories was also not dissimilar. Women in all four countries tended toward the same low-status specialties. Nonetheless, significant variations from one country to the next remained. Medical gynecology existed, and continues to exist, in France, as does stomatology. Dentistry in the United States has been uniquely cut off from medicine. Venereology, associated historically with dermatology, has not had this relationship in Britain. In the twenty-first century, we shall see, substantial differences remain, despite pressure for international standardization.

General Conclusions

W e have covered an enormous amount of ground in this book. Such scope does not lend itself to an account built around a single determinant or "variable," or to a neat theoretical formulation that ties together everything. We have, rather, confronted many different variables and concepts, operating at diverse levels of social reality and at different moments in time, and embedded in different groups and institutions. A partial list of forces, groups, and institutions that have been discussed in this account of specialization include the following.

First, medical research and education has since the mid-nineteenth century served as a key stimulus for increasingly narrow specialty foci in the academic sphere, which has then had a spillover effect into medical practice. I argue in this book that specialization was transformed from an isolated, individual career choice to a large-scale social phenomenon as a result of the growth of the academic research sector, first in Paris and then throughout the Western world. In the late nineteenth century, specialist practice detached from these elite settings and became increasingly widespread. Nonetheless, the medical education/research sector has continued to play a predominant role in specialty development. The extent to which institutions such as medical schools and hospitals have adopted the research role, and the relationship between such institutions and the rest of the profession, explain a number of variations in the characteristics of national specialty systems.

Second, although I have argued that governments played only a modest and indirect role in the actual introduction of specialty regulation, they have nonetheless played a critical role over the long term in a number of complex ways.

Governments have promoted the research sectors that have constituted a primary locus of specialization. They have frequently created and administered the medical schools, academies, hospitals, and, most recently, research agencies that have allowed the research sector to flourish and produce increasingly specialized knowledge.

Public medical institutions have characteristically dealt with large populations under their jurisdiction by dividing them into smaller, more manageable categories. Not infrequently, these units are organized in some hierarchical pattern. This process is visible in a wide variety of contexts, from the Paris hospitals of the early nineteenth century, or those of London in the twentieth, to the military medical establishments during the two world wars, in which specialization advanced dramatically. Health insurance systems have provided a constant source of pressure to define and standardize specialists.

While there are certainly utilitarian interests at work behind this symbiosis, there is, I would argue, a deeper congruence between the worlds of science and public administration. Both medical scientists and administrators have characteristically dealt with complexity by reducing it to smaller, manageable problems, by dividing in order to conquer. Specialized science is not valued just because it seems productive; it is perceived to be "efficient" in a way that is meaningful to public servants.

What are perceived as "state" interests have consistently led public authorities to stimulate the development of certain areas considered particularly strategic. At various times and in various places this has promoted fields as diverse as obstetrics, rehabilitation medicine, pediatrics, venereology, and ophthalmology; public programs have in some cases created viable specialties.

Finally, and at the most general level, governments influence, sometimes decisively, the parameters of the broader health-care system in which specialties emerge and function. They have made it possible for professional associations to introduce certification or have created public bodies, such as the Ordre des Médecins, with the authority to do so. In more recent times, public financing of medical training and hospitals has had a decisive influence on the development of certain specialties; we shall see in the Epilogue that the spread of family medicine in the United States was directly related to the availability of government monies.

Third, professional strategies to monopolize specific domains have probably been the most thoroughly examined facet of the history of specialization. But just as there are many institutions of research and many kinds of administrative bodies, so medical professions are composed of numerous groups and institutions. There are first of all those representing specialists, individuals who take on a specific professional identity. A wide variety of scientific, technological, and social innovations can provide reasons and opportunities for individuals to focus on narrow fields of knowledge and practice, and to take on new forms of collective identity. Market forces at some point make such choices economically beneficial or at least viable, and specialists form organized groups struggling to control these market forces. They seek acceptance in a variety of institutions: medical schools, hospitals, national medical associations, and, not least, insurance systems. They struggle over the boundaries of their sphere against competing groups. They have sometimes played a leading role in campaigning to regulate and standardize specialties in order to limit competition and protect their spheres of activity. But they have seldom done this alone. They have either depended on (in Germany and France) or come to terms with (in the United States) professionwide associations in order to successfully implement such regulation. The power and nature of national medical associations has been a major variable in the standardization of specialties.

Fourth, the growing faith of the general public in such concepts as "expertise" and "science" has been critical to the success of specialization. Specialists cannot survive unless patients believe that they provide care that is better than that offered by generalists. Furthermore, just as governmental concern with particular issues may stimulate the development of specialties, so public opinion and private philanthropy may at times take a special interest in certain categories of the unfortunate—the blind, sick children, or "cripples"—and support institutions that come to play a key role in specialty formation and consolidation. Public interest need not focus exclusively on types of patients; it can also represent ideological tendencies and fashions. The spread of holistic forms of thinking after World War I, and particularly interest in psychosomatic disease and healing, influenced many specialties and provided psychiatry with a level of prestige that it had not enjoyed previously and arguably has not enjoyed since.

Fifth, mutual influences among nations have played a not inconsiderable role in the spread of specialties. Doctors leave home to study abroad; they emigrate or meet each other at national congresses; and they frequently read medical literature (or accounts thereof) produced in other countries. By the second half of the nineteenth century, huge international congresses divided of necessity into more manageable specialist sections and provided models for national professional meetings. Doctors read foreign journals, and events in one country became the prism through which events in another were understood. In the twentieth century, specialties have established international societies and pressure groups to pursue common aims. As we shall see, collective action by member nations of the European Union has since the 1970s resulted in common regulations for medical specialties that have profoundly influenced the development of health care on that continent.

Although this list is far from exhaustive, it suggests the multifaceted complexity of specialization over the *longue durée*, a complexity to which I have tried to do justice in this book. While a historical narrative of this sort can take any number of forms, I have made national comparison my central framework. National comparison allows us to understand what was international about the development of specialties. But it also reminds us that there was nothing predetermined about the form that specialties would take, and that one should not assume that those forms with which we are most familiar are necessarily "natural." Systems of specialties depended on the institutional conditions that obtained in each country and on the quite different arrangements for specialty training and regulation that were put into place. The process of introducing these systems promoted some degree of international standardization because national authorities and professional leaders looked to conditions abroad and often made similar, but seldom identical, choices about pertinent specialist categories. Nonetheless, variation and difference were not eliminated. As we shall see presently, these continue to be characteristic of systems of specialization and of health care more generally, despite enormous pressure in recent decades to impose standardization.

Epilogue: Specialists and Generalists in the Era of Biomedicine

Creating systems of specialist regulation was a beginning. Soon after, health-care institutions everywhere entered a long period of perpetual and radical transformation. Since the mid-1950s, specialization has become a fundamental characteristic of contemporary medicine, at the core of biomedicine's reliance on technology, fundamental biological research, multicenter clinical trials, and high costs. Despite very different starting points, all four national systems of specialist regulation have thus faced a series of common challenges and dilemmas that seem to be leading them all in similar, though not identical, directions.

1. Perhaps most seriously, all systems have had to confront the continuing multiplication of specialists. This has challenged them to find ways to provide adequate and integrated primary care. Among the strategies that have been available are giving generalists a large and officially sanctioned role in health care; limiting patient access to specialists by introducing mandatory referral; restricting the number of specialists by limiting access to specialist training or reimbursable insurance practice; seeking to valorize and strengthen general practice through improved training or the creation of new specialist categories, such as family medicine, designed for this purpose; and allowing primary care to be shared by existing specialty groups. All four of our countries have tried one combination or another of such strategies.

2. All health-care systems have all had to deal with the explosion of new specialist categories that have emerged continuously since the 1960s. As in the past, many of these new specialties or subspecialties have grown out of innovations produced by the academic research sector (reproductive medicine, medical genetics), while others are a consequence of what are perceived as new social needs (family and adolescent medicine, geriatrics). Whatever their origins, they have seriously strained the old regulatory frameworks.

3. While there may well be too many specialists overall, there are always too few in some fields and in some geographic areas. Virtually all nations have joined the

United Kingdom in attempting to organize some form of workforce planning to assure adequate numbers of specialists where they are needed. The mechanisms created for this purpose have assumed the even more complicated task of planning for future needs.

4. Specialist training continues to evolve as a result of several factors. The constantly increasing volume of knowledge has forced authorities to make training either longer or more intense and effective. Variations in standards of training and practice among different specialties, within different regions of each nation, and, increasingly, among different Western nations have begun to appear increasingly unacceptable as a new kind of managerial ethos has spread across health-care bureaucracies. This has generated enormous pressure for standardization and "harmonization" of specialist categories, training, job descriptions, and even therapeutic practices. All four of our countries have thus moved toward hospital-based specialist training programs culminating in accreditation; variations in training periods have gradually lessened. Such pressure has been especially powerful in Europe, where the EU has produced guidelines that have gradually influenced even recalcitrant national governments and medical professions. Nonetheless, there remain basic contradictions between the imperative to train (and continually retrain) future specialists based on perceived needs and keeping services in hospitals running by using relatively inexpensive personnel-in-training.

5. In recent years, this pressure to standardize has expanded beyond the training of specialists to the practice of medicine itself. As issues such as high costs and legal liability have assumed significant proportions almost everywhere, practice variation has become viewed as a serious problem. Specialties have become key units for the production of formal clinical guidelines in a variety of domains. Nonetheless, specialist groups do not exist in a vacuum, and the development of guidelines now takes place in an exceedingly complex arena including all kinds of medical proponents of "evidence-based medicine," administrators of health insurance systems, ministries of health, economists, and patients' groups.

6. Behind much of the pressure for change is the increasing cost of health care. It is thought by many that money can be saved if variation and bad practice are eliminated. Savings can also ensue if generalists replace many specialists, who, it is believed, are directly responsible for high costs. Not only are they paid more then generalists, but they perform or prescribe some of the most expensive procedures. This reinforces the need to control the spread of specialists and promote generalists as "gatekeepers."

Each of our four countries has been forced to cope with these pressures in the context of its evolving medical and political system. Each has exhibited unique fault lines that generate characteristic problems. Such general factors as overall levels of funding, availability (or not) of health insurance, the existence (or not) of a powerful central state administration, and the conflicting values that characterize political discourse not only have a crucial bearing on the development of specialties, but also have frequently been more important than the specific form of specialist regulation in determining whether the system is perceived to be working well or in need of a major overhaul. In addition, such factors as the declining social status and power of doctors since the heady days of the 1950s and 1960s, as well as the huge influx of women into medicine since the 1980s, have had a major impact on perceptions of specialties.

The United Kingdom and the National Health Service

The National Health Service (NHS) started out in the post-World War II era with a system that rigorously separated primary care from specialist care. Specialists were an elite group, defined by appointment to relatively rare posts as hospital consultants and by far longer training than their counterparts elsewhere. As a result, the British health system has been spared the widespread problem of coping with excessive numbers of specialists. Primary care is said to be far more available in the United Kingdom than in almost any other developed Western nation.[1] However, the need to increase the number of consultants has been a continuing theme of countless commissions, reports, and administrative reforms since the establishment of the NHS. The number of consultants has risen from 10,908 in 1975 to 26,352 in March 2002.[2] And still the figures seem dramatically insufficient. Despite its apparently "rational" bureaucratic structure and division of functions, the British health system appears to be riddled with at least as many chronic problems as those of other nations. The quantity of reports and reform proposals that have appeared in recent years is truly impressive.

The most fundamental reason for recent unrest in the National Health Service has to do with the fact that the British medical system is one of the most poorly funded in the Western world. The gap between the proportion of the gross national product (GNP) spent on health care in the United Kingdom and that spent in the rest of Europe has grown markedly since the 1970s.[3] There is no such thing as a "correct" level of funding, but spending significantly less than neighboring states tends to provoke low morale and a sense of crisis among personnel while exacerbating systemic tensions, notably the competition for resources between the rigidly separated primary and hospital sectors.[4] Most important, since the early 1980s the gap between demand for service and what the system can afford to supply has promoted a managerial ethos that has replaced the traditional deference of NHS administrators toward the consultant elites.[5]

At its inception, the NHS represented a historical compromise; it sought to create a rationalized health-care system run by a national administrative bureaucracy while leaving in place powerful professional institutions, such as the royal colleges and General Medical Council (GMC), dominated by consultant elites with their traditional methods of decision-making based on informal peer groups (unkind critics might call them "old-boy networks"). This combination was inherently unstable.

The rationalizing impulse that led to the NHS could not long tolerate the multiple, quasi-independent centers of power that had been left in place. From 1960 on, the idea of "reorganization" dominated discussions of the NHS.[6] This barely tolerable tension became intolerable as a new managerial ethos spread through the NHS—indeed, throughout the Western world—in response to spiraling health costs. The old informal methods of specialist training and selection came to be seen as impossibly inefficient and anachronistic.

The system of specialist training that developed during the first four decades of the NHS consisted of a complex alphabet soup of institutional acronyms, but its main characteristics can be summed up as follows. Specialist training took place in hospitals. Various different bodies, such as the royal colleges or, later, joint committees of colleges and other organizations, approved specific hospital posts for training purposes in their spheres of jurisdiction. Following completion of general medical studies and a year in a hospital in the post of "house officer," budding specialists applied for training posts and moved through several different hierarchical levels. Characteristic of this progression was the lack of coordination; the sequence depended essentially on what the aspiring specialist could arrange. Complaints about this system have persisted over the years despite repeated reforms. One problem has certainly been the traditional reluctance of committees overseeing training to "lay down rigid prescriptions for the training of specialists" and their worry that "if a scheme is too inflexible it may have the effect of stifling initiative and freedom."[7] The need to ensure flexible services in hospitals has contributed to this attitude.[8]

As well as authorizing training posts, accrediting bodies, such as royal colleges or joint higher training committees, have administered specialist examinations at the midpoint of training that have been a prerequisite for entry into the final training level of senior registrar.[9] They have also provided certificates of accreditation upon completion of all higher training. Many accrediting bodies now actively define the content of specialty training programs. Nonetheless, such accreditation had no legal standing and was for many decades not a mandatory requirement for consultant posts.[10] The Todd Report of 1968 advocated the creation of a specialist register from which advisory appointment committees would have to choose consultants. But only in 1991 did the GMC introduce an "indicative" specialist register that allowed a special suffix to be inserted after the names of those who had completed full specialist training.[11] The European Community, whose directives of 1975 governing recognition of qualifications (EC Directives 75/362 and 75/363) had been ignored in the United Kingdom, at this point threatened proceedings against the British system of specialist accreditation.[12] Among other issues, the British system of specialist training took especially long, an average of twelve years rather than the seven usual elsewhere in Europe, as a result of poor organization and bottlenecks at entry into the highest training grades and consultant posts.

As a result, a working group was set up at the Department of Health under the direction of the chief medical officer, Sir Kenneth Calman. This group decided on the creation of a new certificate of completion of specialist training (CCST), to be granted by the GMC, that would make holders eligible for consultant posts. It was later decided that a formal specialist register would be set up and maintained by the GMC; entry on this register now makes someone eligible for a hospital consultant post. The mechanism for shortening training was to telescope and restructure several existing training grades into a single one, with a view to reducing the average training period to seven years. This reform passed in Parliament in 1996.[13]

The Calman reforms aimed, among other things, to increase consultant numbers and reiterated a long-standing commitment to establish a "new balance" between consultants and trainees, one that would make hospital care "consultant-based." But increasing the number of consultant positions, as has occurred consistently since the 1960s, has not solved the old imbalance because each added consultant increased the need for junior assistants to fulfill service roles in hospitals.[14] This problem has been exacerbated by shortening of the training period, by the insistence that training not be sacrificed to service, and by the progressive reductions in junior doctors' working hours. All these changes have required the creation of an ever-growing number of junior posts to keep hospitals running.[15] The problem has been intensified by enactment into British law of the European Working Time Directive, which further limits the number of hours that doctors in training can work.

One result of this pressure has been the rapid growth of an intermediate level in hospitals, staff grade or associate consultants, which takes some of the pressure off consultants and provides jobs for accredited specialists but which lacks any recognized place in existing career structures. Despite the fact that they are dead-end posts, they make up the fastest-growing part of the hospital workforce. In 1989 there were 819 individuals listed under this category; in 2001, there were 6,355. The Audit Commission Report calls these "the lost tribe of doctors," and a BMA report calls them the "forgotten tribe." There is much pressure to regularize their status.[16]

The creation of a specialist register and more structured training programs, though "revolutionary,"[17] constitutes only a small part of the program of administrative standardization that has been introduced in recent years. Perhaps the most striking instance of this trend is the work of the Audit Commission, which has published several reports since 1995. The first of these reports focused on a wide variety of system weaknesses, but especially the unacceptably variable conditions of consultant practice from one jurisdiction to the next. It argued that all doctors should have detailed job plans setting out working hours, duties, and responsibilities, all determined according to fixed rules. More general written guidelines, it was suggested, should specify the allocation of tasks between doctors and other professions and among different grades of doctors. The trusts managing hospitals were urged to monitor compliance with these job plans.[18] It is hard to imagine a more radical revolution in the informal work style of the British hospital elite. Nonetheless, despite the fact that job plans are now mandatory, the Audit Commission found in 2001 that only 14 percent of trusts managing hospitals had job plans for all their consultants, although most had plans for some of them.[19] One wonders what relationship, if any, exists between these plans (and the forms that are filled out in some office) and realities on the ground.

In any event, consultant specialists complain less about bureaucracy than about overwork. Phrases such as "work-related stress," "rising volume and intensity of workload," and even "psychiatric morbidity" appear regularly in their reports and memoranda.[20] They demand more appropriate (higher) remuneration and more consultant personnel to share their work.[21] While some of the stress they feel may be due to the fact that most engage in private practice as well as NHS work, there may be some basis to such complaints. The United Kingdom has by far the lowest ratio of physicians to population among European nations: in 2000 there were 200 active doctors per 100,000 population. In France and Germany the figure was 330.[22] In the years since the Calman reforms, the main emphasis has been on workforce expansion. The NHS plan published in 2000 calls for no fewer than 7,500 more consultants than at present. Meanwhile, the government has decided that bringing in teams of foreign doctors is the best way to deal with long waiting lists for medical services.[23] Official documents calling for a greater and more direct influence by NHS management over training of doctors are causing no end of worry within the British Medical Association (BMA).[24] Equally striking has been the spread of practice guidelines as part of the drive toward "evidence-based medicine."

Reliance on the NHS hospitals for training has also provoked widespread concern since the 1970s about poorly developed academic research among consultants; both the practical, clinical orientation of training and cuts in university funding are blamed for this situation. More recently, a BMA memorandum argued that doctors are increasingly abandoning academic medicine for standard NHS posts. As a result of such complaints, a tenure-track clinician scientist grade has been introduced, but the BMA argues that more incentives are required to attract qualified individuals to academic medicine.[25] The Royal College of Physicians (RCP) in 2000 proposed a comprehensive plan of training for specialist academics to improve the situation.[26]

A succession of reforms since the establishment of the NHS has sought to raise the status of general practice. Informal training for general practice was replaced during the 1970s with formal "vocational" programs.[27] Particularly since the late 1980s, the development of primary care has been a major political objective. The Fundholder Plan generalized in 1993 gave GPs considerable power to choose secondary services (including access to specialists) for their patients.[28] In recent years the NHS has also sought to increase numbers of GPs, though more modestly than in the case of consultants.[29] But even this goal is proving difficult to attain, thereby forcing authorities to introduce a number of measures to make general practice more attractive. These include flexible work schedules and cash bonuses.[30] Nonetheless, the proportion of GPs among British doctors has been dropping for several decades.[31] The number of newly trained doctors who state that they wish to enter general practice recently hit an all-time low; this is mitigated only partly by the fact that the difficulty of completing specialist training has led a substantial portion of them back to general practice.[32] Because the majority of newly minted GPs are women (58 percent in 1998), who are expected by planners to practice part-time in disproportionate numbers, concerns have been expressed that access to GPs is unlikely to improve substantially.[33] Among the causes cited for existing demographic problems is "low morale among general practitioners, caused largely by feelings of loss of control and being undervalued by government, hospital doctors and patients."[34] These problems, it is thought, will become exacerbated as specialist training becomes shorter, and thus a more attractive career option. As is the case among consultants, recruitment of foreign GPs is being encouraged.[35]

The National Health Service is widely considered to be in crisis. Waiting lists for medical services are long, and the drive for efficiency has brought about a threefold increase in managerial personnel. Morale at all levels is low.[36] Yet another report has recently concluded that "the UK has fallen behind other countries in health outcomes. We have achieved less because we have spent much less and not spent it well. That shows up in significant shortfalls in our capacity to deliver."[37] Efforts to introduce some elements of managed competition into the system have had little apparent effect. The current solution proposed is to spend more, increasing health spending to 11 or 12 percent of the GNP by 2022, and to spend more rationally, following the managerial logic of standardization and regulation. The problems described are certainly very real, but one wonders whether the political centrality of the NHS in British political life and its relative public transparency (as witnessed by all the reports and statistics now on the Internet) do not encourage this sense of crisis. In a highly centralized and politicized health system, many groups pursue their goals by complaining loudly about the widespread inadequacies. The pursuit of even localized objectives seems to demand nothing less than systemic reform.

Continental Europe: Decentralized
Insurance and Health-Care Politics

The systems of specialization established in Germany and France were essentially managed by arms of the organized medical profession that had traditional aims: quality control and limitation of specialist numbers. In both cases, the aims of the profession had to be reconciled with the needs and decisions of a national health insurance system that was notably decentralized.[38] But over the years, as financial pressures have increased, national policy makers have gradually encroached on the traditional powers of medical professions. In both nations, a little more than half of all doctors are specialists, a figure notably higher than in the United Kingdom and due largely to the fact that specialists are not confined to the hospital sphere. In both countries there has also been no sharp division between primary and consultant care. Certain specialties have provided the kind of care given by GPs in the United

Kingdom, and referral from a GP has not in most cases been required in order to receive specialist services. By the end of the 1980s, patients had direct access to 82 percent of all specialties in the Federal Republic of Germany and to 65 percent of those of France.[39]

Both governments have spent relatively generously on their health care system: Germany a little over, and France a little under, 10 percent of their respective GNPs. This may explain the high satisfaction levels with the health system in each country.[40] In recent years, however, they have faced budgetary crises that are leading their governments to similar cost-cutting measures, and their doctors to similar rage and resistance that are frequently coordinated across borders.[41] Financial shortages have particularly impacted specialists because state efforts have aimed to increase access and to lower costs through the promotion of primary care.[42] Resemblances among the two national systems have become accentuated as a consequence of the directives of the EC. These directives are fairly "minimalist," in the words of one commentator,[43] and a French report of 2002 concluded that despite the European directives, "a certain lack of homogeneity in training remains."[44] Nonetheless, the discussions they have provoked have yielded somewhat similar strategies of adaptation in each country. The European Union of Medical Specialists represents over one million specialists throughout Europe; its specialty sections (numbering thirty-six in 2000) have developed programs of training to advance "harmonization."[45] Growing similarities in this domain are only one element in what one scholar has termed "a sort of hybridization of principles of organization" of European health systems.[46] There are now programs to harmonize the production of practice guidelines among the different European nations.[47]

France

The French system of specialist regulation that emerged during the 1950s was complex and cumbersome. There were, first of all, required "certificates" of specialization (CES), granted after completion of programs organized by universities and sanctioned by examinations. Considerable variation existed from one university and specialty to the next. There was in addition the traditional system of elite training, the *internat*, an intensive residency filled through highly competitive examinations. *Internes* who had served most of their terms in specialized wards were granted equivalence to the CES without further training or examination. In some specialties, mainly surgical, the *internat*, rather than the CES, was the single requirement for specialist certification. In addition, special committees for evaluating the capabilities of specialists who did not meet either of these two criteria continued to exist.[48]

By the 1970s this heterogeneous system was seen as increasingly unsatisfactory. First, the number of specialists continued to increase. Between 1967 and 1980 the proportion of specialists among all doctors rose from 32 to 39 percent, and reached 42 percent by 1982.[49] Second, the costs of medical care were beginning to rise, and policy makers saw the problem as due in part to an excessive numbers of specialists. The apparent solution was to increase the proportion of GPs trained by exerting greater control over the training process. Third, the first of the EEC directives on the "harmonization" of specialist programs appeared in 1975. If the French were going to negotiate with other Europeans over the conditions of specialist training, it seemed necessary first to design a single, standardized, national system.

The result was a law first proposed in 1979, passed in 1982, and then implemented gradually from 1985. This created a single, unified specialist diploma, the DES, which was awarded after completion of the hospital *internat*. The latter was expanded by creating new programs for the much larger number of *internes* now being trained. Each training program lasted from three to five years, depending on the specialty. (Over time, the minimum training period was raised to four years.) The system was selective; students took an examination at the national level that ranked them in order of grade. Their rank determined the order in which they chose from available residencies in a region. This meant that some students did not get into the institution or specialty they aspired to, and large numbers were not accepted into any program at all. For those who completed a program, subspecialization was then possible in a number of domains after a further two-year training period.[50]

A number of points about this reform require emphasis. First, the old *internat* had primarily sought to train hospital physicians and surgeons; the new one controlled access to specialties for both private practitioners and the hospital elite. Since the number of training programs in each specialty was now controlled by administrators, it was in theory possible to micromanage the medical population in response to perceived regional needs. The plan was eventually to train about 40 percent of all students in medical specialties and 60 percent in general medicine. However, for most of the 1980s, programs for the old CES continued to exist and larger than usual numbers of medical graduates, knowing that this portal was about to close, entered them to become specialists. As a result, the proportion of specialists rose between 1982 and 1990 from 42 to 49 percent of the medical population. Even after the full introduction of the new system, the number of specialists continued to rise, reaching 51 percent by 2000.[51] Simultaneously, the number of specialties kept rising. By the early twenty-first century there were fifty-seven official specialties and, with subspecialties taken into account, over 100 categories in existence.[52]

The reforms of the 1980s also targeted general practice. In the prereform system, undergraduate medical education followed by a year of practical experience in a hospital determined the right to practice of all doctors. Specialists took *additional* training. This certainly was a cause of inequality, leading to the belief that specialists knew more than generalists. But the two categories were not necessarily considered qualitatively different. It was, for instance, not uncommon for some of those who had gone through the prestigious *internat* to choose general practice rather than a specialty. Specialists might drift back into general practice, and generalists might at some point train for a specialty CES in a local faculty. This situation changed in two fundamental ways following reform.

First, general practice became a field that required special training lasting two years initially, then two and a half (1996), and, more recently, three years. Those who failed specialist examinations could no longer automatically go into general practice, but had to undergo this special training. To some degree, this raised the status of general practitioners by making their training requirements similar to those of specialists. On the other hand, the manner of choosing who became what pretty much destroyed any benefits in status that might have accrued to GPs. The new enlarged *internat* was perceived exclusively as training for specialties; most medical students competed for it in order to keep open their options. Those who were most successful usually chose a specialty program, while those who were ranked too low to become *internes* undertook training for general practice. Specialists, in other words, were "successful" physicians, while GPs were perceived as losers in the competitive struggle for success.[53] It has been calculated by one sociologist that among students with the best grades, 44 percent went into general practice under the old training regime, while under the new system only 28 percent did so.[54] It also seems to have become more difficult for women to enter specialties.[55] This perception of generalists as second-rate has probably contributed as much as significant disparities in income to produce low morale and a perceived sense of crisis among France's GPs. One solution to this crisis proposed regularly since the mid-1990s is recognition of general practice as a full-fledged university discipline. One militant GP group, MG France, has campaigned for a referral system along the lines of the one that exists in the United Kingdom.[56]

During the 1990s, this latter option gathered political support because it seemed a way to control health costs. A step of sorts was taken in 1996 as part of the Juppé reforms, whose primary aim was to control costs by creating separate national "envelopes" for GPs and specialists. Money not spent was to be added to physician incomes within each group, and overspending would be penalized. Simultaneously an experimental program of referral networks was set up, allowing patients to sign up with a generalist who would manage their care; their reward was a higher rate of insurance reimbursement. This program continues to exist, but as of 2000, only 15 percent of generalists had signed up for it.[57]

More significantly, in 1997 general practice was given time in the undergraduate medical curriculum (although its teachers are without the full institutional status enjoyed by specialists), and three years later, training for GPs was extended from two and a half to three years.[58] Most dramatically, it has been decided that general practice will be treated as a full-fledged specialty with its own DES. Starting in June 2004, a single competition will determine assignments to both specialist and upgraded general training programs.[59] This has symbolic significance since highly ranked individuals can in principle opt for general practice. But since fees paid to GPs remain significantly lower than those for specialists, it is not clear whether this formal status of equality with specialists will significantly improve either morale or recruitment.[60] A leading sociologist notes: "These 'victories' for general medicine are part of a compromise by which the public powers accord medical generalists recognition (in terms of revenue and university status) that they have been waiting decades for, in the hope that these [generalists] commit themselves collectively to the structural reform of the health system."[61]

The Juppé reforms created enormous unease within the medical profession. They were viewed with particular trepidation by specialties engaged in primary care, notably pediatricians, who are, according to official statistics, less well paid than even GPs.[62] The specialty had already been dealt a major blow in the preceding years when the government decreased the total number of training posts in the field from 250 per year in 1991 to 110 in 1995.[63] Any referral system would certainly make their professional situation untenable. The attempted reforms, however, provided the spark for an important turnaround in the fortunes of an even more marginal group of primary care givers: medical gynecologists.

The reform of specialty training during the 1980s was not just about numbers and distribution. It was also about standardization. Several specialties that did not have equivalents in the other major European countries were not accorded training programs or DES certificates. Medical gynecology, by now made up predominantly of women and denounced repeatedly by obstetrician-gynecologists, was one of the chief casualties.[64] It did not disappear, however, and continued to be recognized by the health insurance system. Some newcomers joined its ranks after having been trained in obstetrics-gynecology, while small numbers of highly qualified members were recruited through the new subspecialty of reproductive medicine-endocrinology. But for the most part, its practitioners aged. During the 1980s and 1990s, they negotiated quietly with politicians and administrators to win back some form of training and recognition. But by 1997, the Juppé reforms were threatening to substantially cut back on the right of patients to see specialists as primary care physicians; this would have directly affected medical gynecologists, who provided primary care to many women. Consequently, a public campaign erupted in defense of medical gynecology that was led by a coalition of gynecologists and their many women supporters. This in fact became something of a feminist issue in France. The goal was nothing less than recognition of the field as a genuine medical specialty. There were demonstrations, petitions, and public meetings in the Senate. An online petition in support of medical gynecology gathered two million signatures. In 2000, the government proposed a compromise. Obstetrics-gynecology would be divided into two tracks. There would be a common three-year residency in both fields, followed by a more specialized two-year training period in either ObGyn or medical gynecology. This apparent concession, however, was rejected.

During the 2002 election year, defenders of medical gynecology achieved notable political successes. Both the National Assembly and the Senate passed legislation calling for medical gynecology to become an autonomous specialty, and all necessary administrative decrees to this effect were drawn up. In spite of ferocious resistance, training places in this specialty were offered for the first time in the con-

cours d'internat of 2003. But this has been a partial victory at best. Only 20 out of 2,002 posts were reserved for medical gynecology (while 198 were devoted to obstetrics-gynecology), and only a portion of this training must be done in hospital services devoted to this field, meaning that few new wards and professorships in this specialty are likely to be created.[65]

One of the reasons for the opposition to medical gynecology has to do with the perceived shortage of obstetrician-gynecologists. Training is seen as a zero-sum game in which training programs for the former will lead to fewer for the latter. Obstetrician-gynecologists are in fact not the only group perceived to be in demographic difficulty. After years of assuming that there were too many specialists, something like a consensus has emerged in the last few years to the effect that a handful of specialties are already understaffed and that a demographic crisis awaits the entire medical profession within the next two decades as doctors retire. The issue has spawned an impressive number of studies, reports, and debates.[66] There already seems to be a dearth of practitioners in such fields as obstetrics-gynecology, psychiatry, anesthesia, and surgery. As a result of these fears, which some argue are exaggerated, there are now plans to increase the number of medical students generally and to expand the number of training residencies in the most vulnerable specialty fields. Although French political culture makes it impossible to force young doctors to settle in medically disadvantaged areas, most proposals foresee various sorts of incentives to make these regions more attractive. Nonetheless, decisions now will not transform medical demographics for another fourteen years,[67] and there is likely to be a major decline in the density of many specialties between now and then. An official report suggests that it may be necessary to transfer certain responsibilities now assumed by doctors to paramedical occupations, a step the French medical profession has until now resisted. Many of the report's other suggestions have become part of a general debate about the coming doctor shortage.[68]

The most contentious issue in France, as in Germany, has little to do with the overall system of specialties and everything to do with how much doctors are paid. The past few years have seen considerable labor strife and unrest.[69] This is not just about money; it is also about the increasing centralization of power in the hands of the national government and its growing focus on cost-cutting. The French medical profession has gradually lost the little unity and cohesion it once had, and myriad fragmented unions and associations now negotiate with the French health administration.[70] Surprisingly, under these conditions, French doctors have on the whole done rather well economically during the past decades, and they have recently won significant increases in remuneration.[71]

Germany

In post-war East Germany, a radically different system of medical organizations was constructed along highly centralized command and control lines. Specialist associations played an important role in mediating between central authorities and doctors, and were placed in charge of health-care planning, research management, and specialist training.[72] But this system disappeared with the unification of Germany. In West Germany and then united Germany, the basic principles of the Bremen Guidelines of 1924 have survived with remarkable persistence despite numerous reforms. As in so many other domains, the postwar reconstruction of German health care resulted in the restoration of prewar institutional patterns.[73]

The organization of specialties has thus evolved around the existence of a strong medical profession that functions within a relatively fragmented system of multiple sickness insurance funds. The profession's power revolves around two types of organizations whose authority was established during the Weimar and, especially, the Nazi periods:[74] physicians' chambers, organized nationally (with a federal chamber at the summit), which have regulatory power over the practices of members, and an association of insurance doctors that negotiates with insurance boards. These arrangements were reconstituted through passage of a law in 1955 that gave the association of insurance doctors a central role in negotiating with insurance funds and managing payments to doctors.

Medical self-regulation has also been the norm in the specialist domain.[75] The Postgraduate Education Committee of the Federal Chamber of Physicians and the annual assembly of the representatives of local chambers, the *Ärztetag*, have together been responsible for recognition of new specialties and for reforms of structures. Regional chambers have routinely applied the decisions of these national bodies. This relative professional independence, reinforced by the separation of powers between the federal government and the states (*Länder*), has resulted in tight control over the working lives of doctors by official medical bodies.[76] As in other nations, however, the power of the central government is becoming increasingly intrusive.

A distinctive feature of the German system has been the sharp separation between hospital medicine and private practice. Since 1955, hospitals have provided little outpatient care, and their medical staffs may not compete with GPs in primary care. As a result, private practice specialists dominate specialty organizations, and discussions about the status of specialists seldom take hospitals into account.[77] Doctors in private practice are restricted to their particular specialty category, and combinations remain rigorously regulated. In such a system, the practices associated with each specialist category need to be defined and regularly redefined in great detail.

During the years that followed the war, the imposition of national guidelines on the conditions of specialist training continued under the leadership of the organized profession. In 1966 the Essen *Ärztetag* drafted a plan that defined the content of each specialty and set up guidelines for training.[78] In 1968, the Wiesbaden *Ärztetag* introduced comprehensive regulations for graduate and specialty training (*Weiterbildungsordnung*) that set the terms for postgraduate training during the next three decades.[79] Postgraduate training for general practitioners lasting four years was introduced but was not mandatory. Five new specialty categories were recognized.[80] To keep the number of full specialties small, subspecialties were introduced; also introduced were supplementary designations and added qualifications that, unlike subspecialties linked to and following training for specialties, may be acquired by general practitioners and often require only short training periods.[81]

The legal status of the certification process regulated by professional chambers was for many years something of a problem. But in 1972 this situation changed. Reacting to legal challenges, the Constitutional Court ruled that the powers of physician chambers were invalid because they had never been authorized by *Länder* laws. As a result, one *Land* after another passed laws on this matter. These processes frequently involved struggles over control between local governments and medical professions, but invariably the powers of the medical chambers were affirmed.[82] Specialist certification successfully remained within the sphere of professional competence while acquiring legally binding status.[83]

Until the most recent period of reform, most specialties required from four to six years of training. Students had to fend for themselves in a highly competitive market by finding training places within hospitals accredited by the ministries of the various *Länder*; not only were there relatively few such positions (only about 50 percent of candidates could be accommodated), but students were additionally required to perform a certain number of specified procedures in order for their specialist diplomas to be validated.[84] This procedural requirement has been, and remains, a source of controversy among German doctors. It forces students to scramble in order to fulfill their obligations; it is argued as well that this requirement encourages the performance of unnecessary procedures.[85]

As in France, specialists are prohibited from part-time general practice. Furthermore, GPs, who are well represented in physician organizations, have more scope for practice than they do in other countries. A considerable amount of high-tech diagnostic testing takes place in generalists' (as well as specialists') offices rather than in hospitals, where ambulatory care is rare.[86] Nonetheless, the proportion of specialists among doctors in the Federal Republic of Germany has risen inexorably, from 33 percent in the early 1950s to 43 percent in 1965, to 54 percent in 1990. Recent statistics give a figure of over 60 percent of all doctors in private practice. In spite of, or perhaps because of, this growth of the specialist population, there has been considerable resistance to the creation of new specialties by the private practitioners who dominate the medical chambers. While academic medicine in Germany, as elsewhere, has encouraged the development of new fields by recognizing them for the *Habilitation*, the qualification for professorships, German academic medicine as a whole exerts less pressure in this direction because it is more strongly oriented toward patient care than research.[87] Consequently, the number of specialties has increased slowly; by 1956 there were twenty-one, with no subspecialties.[88] In subsequent years, numbers remained small. As of 2001 there were only fifty-one recognized specialties and subspecialties.[89]

The rise in the number of specialists is part of a more general problem peculiar to Germany: an apparent oversupply of doctors. This stems from a constitutional guarantee that qualified students have free access to university and from pressure by the *Länder* to maintain university enrollments. Court decisions as well have forced universities to accept more medical students than planned.[90] Unlike France, Germany did not introduce a radical limitation on the training of medical students. Consequently, it had until fairly recently the second highest medical density in Europe after Italy.[91] Medical density has declined substantially in recent years; attempts are currently under way to cut the number of medical graduates by 20 percent, and there is mandatory retirement at age sixty-eight for insurance practice. One hears increasing warning of upcoming doctor shortages, but this has not yet turned into the kind of widespread anxiety that currently characterizes policy rhetoric in France.[92] Similarly, Germany has an overabundance of hospital beds, twice as many in relation to population as in the United Kingom or the United States.[93] Accompanying such numbers are high costs; Germany devotes a higher proportion of its GNP to health care than most of her European neighbors, while health indicators used to evaluate such matters remain mediocre. This situation became increasingly unacceptable as economic conditions worsened during the 1990s. The symbol of the high cost of health care is the premiums that the insured pay; they have risen from 6 percent (of gross income) in the 1950s to nearly 14 percent in 1998.[94]

In the end, Germany has opted for what is in some ways a radical solution to the demographic situation, one that has been politically unthinkable in France: the introduction of rigorous quotas for insurance medical practice.[95] Since the introduction of the Seehofer reforms of 1993, each geographical unit is assigned a specific number of medical positions of different sorts, depending on its general and medical populations. If these numbers are exceeded, new doctors in the area will not be recognized by the insurance system, which pretty much precludes making a medical living. It has been estimated that the number of geographical units that are open to new doctors has fallen from 40 percent in 1993 to 28 percent in 1997 to 22 percent in 2001. A law passed in 2000 has imposed even more stringent controls on the right of doctors to work within the insurance system.[96] Many young doctors now work exclusively within the hospital sector which is considered inferior to private practice.[97]

As in other nations, efforts to stem the flow of doctors toward specialties have been accompanied by measures to upgrade general practice into something like a specialty. The *Weiterbildungsordnung* of 1968 created a four-year postdoctoral program of special training for generalists. (In that year the federal Health Ministry also reformed the medical curriculum to require all medical students to take training in general practice before receiving their license.) Those taking the diploma are called *Allgemeinärzte* (distinct from *Praktische Ärzte*, who lack postdoctoral training). The generalist diploma was for over two decades not an official requirement for general medical practice. And both academics and professional associations, dominated by specialists in private practice, prevented any real investments in academic general medicine, which was usually taught by part-time lecturers.[98] "Family

(*Hausarzt*) practice" (a term that is roughly equivalent to the term "primary care" in North America) could be entered by doctors without postgraduate qualifications as well as by internists and pediatricians. In 1992, there were a little over 19,000 *Allgemeinärzte* and a little less than 21,000 *Praktische Ärzte*, whose activities were somewhat restricted.[99] Despite the advantages carried by the degree, relatively few graduates chose to become *Allgemeinärzte* because there were insufficient numbers of training programs in hospitals and because patients did not attach much importance to the diploma. The long training period also discouraged potential candidates.[100]

In 1993, training in general practice was made obligatory by law. The title *Allgemeinarzt* was obtained after three years of practical training (one year less than in the previous system), and was made a requirement for insurance practice. Newly trained internists and pediatricians had to choose, from 1996 on, whether they would practice within the context of the insurance system as family physicians or as specialists in their fields.[101] This made some difference to recruitment. As of 2001, the number of *Allgemeinärzte* had risen to 31,803 (making it the largest of the specialty groups, followed by internal medicine), and the number of *Praktische Ärzte* had declined to 12,523. Nonetheless, the combined total of the two groups has changed little since the beginning of the 1990s, while the number and proportion of specialists keeps going up. In both 1996 and 1997, *Ärztetage* decided on the principle that general practice would in the future be reserved for *Allgemeinärzte* and would require five years of training. The status of general practice in relation to specialties was thus supposed to rise and attract larger numbers of young doctors.[102]

During the past few years a series of measures have come into effect to implement and in fact extend these principles. Five years of training in general practice became required of every family practitioner in 1999. *Weiterbildungsordnungen* ratified by *Ärztetage* in 2001 and 2003, and adopted by local chambers, are supposed to completely transform the nature of general family practice during the next few years. As of 2006, specialists such as internists and pediatricians, who are now allowed to choose family medicine rather than their specialty, will be prohibited from doing so. Simultaneously, and despite the fact that the original proposal made by the German medical profession specifically opposed the idea of turning family practitioners into obligatory "gatekeepers" controlling access to all medical services, the reform of 2000 proposes to do just that.[103] Patients will receive financial incentives to consult family physicians first, with the goal of lowering costs.[104] There has understandably been much opposition to this law from specialists,[105] but also from the federal Chamber of Physicians, on the grounds that few candidates will want to spend five years in training for family practice when remuneration remains inferior to that of specialists—who, moreover, have easier access to hospital training programs. Nor do ordinary Germans seem thrilled by the prospect of having to visit a generalist in order to see a specialist, and one can expect significant public opposition when and if this measure is implemented. Nonetheless, both the insurance boards and the federal Ministry of Health are currently investing resources in the training of family practitioners.[106]

In the spring of 2003, the 106th *Ärztetag* in Cologne passed a "master" *Weiterbildungsordnung* (which will be the model for measures introduced in each *Land*) that further transforms the terrain of specialization in Germany. First, all the various specialist categories, subcategories, and appellations have been rationalized in order to reduce their number by about 40 percent and to coordinate training for each with the duties recognized and reimbursed by the insurance system.[107] But perhaps the most radical development has been the "painful compromise" meant to resolve the intense conflict between internists and general physicians that has resulted from the earlier decision to create a single class of family physicians. According to this compromise, general internal medicine will be united with general medicine in a single category associated with, but distinct from, internal subspecialties. After a three-year residency in hospital internal medicine, future specialists will go on to either two years of training in primary care or three years of training in an internal subspecialty. If it is actually implemented, this compromise will mean the end of internal medicine as it has been practiced since the early twentieth century. As one can imagine, many internist and specialist groups cannot reconcile themselves to this change,[108] even as local chambers are beginning to introduce measures to implement it.[109] Compared with such radical measures, the French decision to include general practice in the *concours de l'internat* seems pretty mild.[110]

Since the end of World War II, the German medical profession has been relatively unified and privileged.[111] Nonetheless, the existing regulatory framework has become increasingly constraining as the need to curb spending on health care has become a central political preoccupation. Germans are well aware that they spend more than other Europeans on health care but do not enjoy significantly better health.[112] The result has been a series of structural reforms since about 1990 that make Germany, in the words of one French writer, the "champion" of health-care reform in Europe.[113] Starting in 1986, the government put a cap on spending for medical honoraria within the insurance system. In 1993 the Structural Reform of Health Care restricted growth of health spending to growth in revenue of insurance funds. Also, as we saw, it fixed the number of doctors in each locality to specific population ratios. Finally, it required that overspending of fixed drug budgets be repaid by doctors' associations and the pharmaceutical industry. Since 1996 insurance funds have competed with each other to sign up subscribers. Efforts at administrative control have become increasingly sophisticated, and practice guidelines proliferate and are enforced by insurance authorities.[114]

The result of all these efforts is more and new forms of state intervention, combined with ever more far-reaching controls over doctors by corporatist medical institutions.[115] Still, costs go up and doctors complain and demonstrate about the conditions under which they work. German doctors, in other words, express many of the same complaints as their counterparts in other countries. Since the beginning of the new century, there has emerged a growing consensus that imminent bankruptcy requires draconian measures. During the summer of 2003 the government and opposition parties negotiated an agreement to slash nearly 10 billion

Euros from the health-care budget for 2004, with savings set to rise to 23 billion Euros by 2007. Patients will pay considerably more out of pocket for medical services. On the other hand, the proportion of gross wages collected by insurance funds is expected to fall from 14.4 to 13 percent.[116] Meanwhile, plans for further structural reform continue to advance.

Regulating the Market in the United States

The medical system of the United States is unique. Not only does it famously lack health insurance covering the entire population, while it spends far more on medical care than any other country in the world, but it is distinctive in the degree to which power over the health-care system is decentralized, indeed fragmented. Unlike the other three systems under discussion, American health care lacks a clear center of gravity; power is diffused among many organizations, agencies, and groups. Consequently, except for the issue of health insurance, which surfaces periodically in political debate, medical care is not ordinarily part of "high politics." It tends to get broken down into narrow technical questions dealt with by one or another group of experts.

This is not to say that there is no regulatory logic behind the apparent fragmentation. As in other countries, Michael Moran[117] has shown, there has been movement from a system of regulation controlled by medical elites—in this case, supported by the great philanthropic foundations of American capitalism—to a more open system in which governments, both state and federal, play an important role, as do private insurers and interest groups. Third-party payers, especially, now play a key role in the health-care market. A milestone in this development was the establishment in 1965 of the Medicare program to take charge of the elderly, and Medicaid for the poor and handicapped. Until then, the federal government had little to do with either medical education or health care. The direct administration of these two new programs has given federal and state governments a powerful role in the health-care landscape. The American system, it is true, does not work in the "command and control" manner of its European counterparts, whereby conditions are often dictated (after much negotiation and/or conflict) by state authorities; it functions, rather, in more subtle and even indirect ways as system players use money, power, and influence to modify the health-care market. All of this has had vital implications for the American organization of specialties.

In the United States, the system of certification by specialty boards established during the interwar years has remained substantially unchanged. The result is that specialties dominate the medical landscape. It is fair to say that at this point just about every physician has become a specialist of one sort or another. The number of general practitioners has fallen continuously and precipitously as American medical students have chosen en masse to enter specialties and earn higher incomes. In 1963, GPs made up 28 percent of the active physician population; by 1977 the figure was 13 percent.[118] Since then the figure has continued to decline, so that in the early twenty-first century the traditional GP has almost ceased to exist. She has been replaced by the "primary care specialist," about whom more will be said later. The decline of the GP is real enough by any standards, but also reflects in large measure the peculiar definitions of specialists that have come to predominate. The U.S. figures result from two unique characteristics.

First, there is no legal obligation to obtain specialist certification. Although the number of specialists with no training or certification is probably small,[119] we can be fairly sure that a good number of U.S. doctors who call themselves specialists would not be allowed this status in most other countries.

Second, unlike the situation in our three other countries, the boundaries between general and specialist care are virtually nonexistent. Specialists are permitted to combine their field with general practice. This means (a) that some individuals with only the most tenuous hold on specialist practice call themselves specialists, and (b) that doctors have a powerful incentive to specialize even in overcrowded fields because they can survive economically by combining a specialty with primary care practice.[120]

Despite these caveats, it is clear that these conditions are not just technicalities that result in higher counts of specialists; they actively promote the dominant role of specialization. The possibility of combining specialist with general practice makes this a more desirable career option than it might be otherwise. Almost any would-be specialist group can introduce a certification board, even if this is not recognized officially. (In 2000, there were 137 self-designated boards not recognized by official bodies.[121]) Professional bodies regulating specialties, it should be noted, have not been notably successful at restricting the number of specialist, and especially sub-specialist, categories that they examine and certify.[122] These bodies have been largely controlled by specialists, often leaders of academic medicine. Generalists have thus had little leverage in defending their interests. Competitive pressures that have led specialists elsewhere to limit specialty growth in order to minimize competition do not operate effectively when academic researchers play so prominent a role, because the latter tend to more concerned with the viability of residency programs and service needs of the hospitals in which they work. To the extent that they are involved in research, they have a vested interest in developing new domains that are frequently at the vanguard of scientific advances.

The medical research sector has been largely supported since the 1960s by federal funds. According to Daniel Fox, total research spending in medical schools, adjusted for inflation, grew almost fiftyfold between the postwar years and 1993, with the federal government providing about 75 percent of the funds through the National Institutes of Health (NIH).[123] As a result, new disciplines and domains are constantly emerging in medical schools that have become dependent on research grants.[124] Some of these have practical applications and produce groups of practitioners eager to increase their credibility and access to research funds by becoming recognized as specialists. Consequently, medical schools in the United States play a far more dynamic role in the development of specialties than do their counterparts in the United Kingdom, Germany, or France.[125] Hospitals, uniquely in the United States, operate in a market environment that has encouraged them, like other capitalist enterprises, to embrace technological innovations and hire people capable of using them. This is in addition to their need for residents to provide routine medical services at low cost. The sheer size of the American profession (there were 813,000 American MDs in 2000)[126] quickly produces a critical mass of individuals able to produce the usual accoutrements of specialty aspirations: societies, journals, and demands for academic recognition, jobs, and certification. For much of the twentieth century, nongovernmental third-party insurance providers had little impact on the dominant medical culture of specialization. They continued to pay high fees for specialist care, thereby magnifying the incentives to enter specialties.

In opposition to such forces, there has been, since the mid-twentieth century, consistent concern to limit the number of specialty categories and restrict the flow of doctors into them. Some of this opposition has come from the specialty boards themselves, and especially from the American Board of Medical Specialties (ABMS), which coordinates them; but the latter organization is a coalition of all the involved groups, and thus has enjoyed a limited degree of independent authority. It has made some serious efforts to curb unbridled specialization by, among other means, pushing new groups into subspecialty categories, which has allowed the number of full specialties to remain relatively small. But the spread of subspecialties, although relatively modest until 1985, provoked extensive anxiety about the viability of certain specialties and a unified profession more generally.[127] In recent years, the number of subspecialties has exploded in a burst of new fields, often cutting across established categories and boards. The United States is by far the country with the largest number of recognized specialist categories.[128] And this does not take account of self-designated boards lacking ABMS approval.

Medical institutions have had their most profound impact by transforming general practice into the specialty of family medicine and, more generally, encouraging the development of primary care functions in specialties such as internal medicine and pediatrics. The organizations representing general practice—notably the General Practice Section of the American Medical Association (AMA) (founded 1945) and the American Academy of General Practice (founded 1947)—sought from the 1940s to the mid-1960s to raise the status of their field and to resist the encroachments of specialists into their domain. One of the options they regularly considered, and usually rejected, was transforming general practice into a specialty with its own residency programs.[129] During the 1960s, some pilot two-year training programs in general medicine were set up, but these were not very successful. Pressure to create the new specialty intensified as a result of the continuing fall in the number and status of GPs, and by the mid-1960s, the AMA was taking a strong position in favor of board certification of general practitioners. Three separate reports appeared in 1966 endorsing the idea of a new primary care specialty, though each used different terms to describe it.[130]

These developments were influenced decisively by the shifting political landscape. Until the 1960s, governments had little to do with medical training or access to care. In Michael Moran's wonderful phrase, their interest was "in promoting the supply of technologies which could conquer disease."[131] The setting up in 1965 of Medicare and Medicaid created intense pressures for increased numbers of hospitals and caregivers. As a result, the federal, state, and local governments became directly involved in medical education, providing construction funds, scholarships to medical students, and capitation payments to medical schools. Between 1960 and 1975, the number of entering medical students rose by 85 percent and the physician-population ratio rose from 134/100,000 to 176/100,000.[132] Special programs to provide physicians to underserved areas were introduced.

While government efforts aimed to produce more health-care workers of all types, they devoted special attention to general practitioners, an endangered species that appeared particularly useful for government programs. This increased support for the creation of the new specialty of family medicine, which was formally approved in 1969. The American Board of Family Medicine offered certification in this field after a residency of three years. It was the first board to make certification time-limited (six years) and to require regular recertification. Not to be left behind, the American Board of Internal Medicine established a special certificate in general internal medicine, which occupied much the same structural terrain and which could also be obtained after three years of training. In addition, it established a joint certificate with the American Board of Pediatrics. Federal and state subsidies were granted to medical schools that established training programs in family medicine and (in some states) primary care generally. From 1968 to1980, forty-one states funded family practice training, some establishing community-based medical schools for this purpose. From 1971, the federal government provided funds to hospitals to support training programs in family medicine. A major reform in 1976 extended this aid to medical schools and to programs in general internal medicine and general pediatrics; federal capitation grants to medical schools were tied to the proportion of first-year residents in these three programs.[133] As a result of these and other project grants to schools, the proportion of medical schools with programs in family medicine rose from 47 percent in 1973 to 75 percent in 1984. The number of residents in family practice between these two dates rose from 1,035 to 7,588, making it at the latter date the third largest residency program after internal medicine and general surgery.[134] A little later the government began to subsidize the training of nonphysician primary caregivers, such as nurse practitioners and physician assistants, as yet another strategy to make primary care more available.[135]

One of the more interesting consequences of this new funding was the transformation of the traditional dichotomy between generalists and specialists into the much more flexible distinction between primary and secondary/tertiary care. The notion of primary care certainly existed in the 1950s and 1960s,[136] but it was not a central classificatory category. A PubMed search using the term "primary care" reveals no articles published before 1970.[137] Starting in that year, however, the catalogers of the National Library of Medicine discovered the terms "primary care" and "primary care specialists." There are articles about family medicine, of course, as well as about general internal medicine and pediatrics—and, more surprisingly, obstetrics-gynecology, psychiatry, and several other fields—highlighting the important role they were playing in primary care, now the beneficiary of new federal and state funds. There were many debates about what constituted a primary care specialist; but in the end, it was easier for both funders and statisticians simply to designate as "primary" certain obvious specialties, such as family medicine, general internal medicine, and pediatrics.[138] But nothing kept other, less obvious specialties from inclusion in this category.

After an initial upsurge in recruitment to primary specialties, governments in the 1980s cut back significantly on their support for primary care training programs, which then began having difficulty attracting trainees.[139] The situation changed again in the 1990s, as a result of the spread of managed care organizations that hired more primary physicians in an effort to cut costs; they also restructured fee schedules to make primary care fields more attractive. States established their own programs to promote primary training. As a result, the number of new medical graduates choosing primary care fields (and older specialists recycling themselves as primary caregivers) increased after 1995.[140]

The effects of this activity remain difficult to gauge. Certainly the draconian decline in the number of primary care practitioners that occurred between 1950 and 1970 has been reversed. But results depend to some extent on who is doing the counting. Data collected by the federal Bureau of Health Statistics and available on the Internet suggest a continuing decline in the proportion of primary care physicians to all active physicians, from 37 percent in 1970 to 33 percent in 1985 to 32 percent in 2000. This is not a dramatic fall, but it is a far cry from initial projections estimating that the proportion of primary physicians in 1990 would be 46 percent.[141] While the population of active physicians increased by 136 percent from 1970 to 2000, the number of primary care physicians rose by 106 percent.[142] The AMA, in contrast, calculates that the proportion of primary care physicians in the active physician population has risen very slightly, from 43.8 percent in 1970 to 44.3 percent in 2000.[143] The reason behind this discrepancy is that the AMA counts obstetrician-gynecologists as primary caregivers.

By redefining general medicine as primary care medicine and including more specialties within that definition, one gets statistics that look reasonably impressive. But this procedure hides some real problems. The recruitment to primary care specialties has always been cyclic and, we have seen, dependent on government funding. The largest and most rapidly growing field, internal medicine, is clearly in crisis because it is dominated by subspecialties. (See chapter 10 in this volume.) General internal medicine suffers from something of an identity crisis, having had to hire a public relations firm in 1997 to explain to the public exactly what general internists do and why people should see them.[144] It is not clear that training is fully adapted to the tasks of primary care, and in recent years the number of persons entering internal medicine residencies has dropped. In any case, general internists do not tend to settle in rural areas after they complete training.[145]

Family medicine has achieved all the outer signs of institutional success and is less fragmented than internal medicine; it is also the second largest specialist group in the United States. Nonetheless, it has an ambiguous and relatively low status within medicine.[146] The core of its identity, never very clear, is currently in the midst of a major reformulation.[147] Most seriously, it has not grown as quickly as other primary care fields, and the number of family physicians per population has remained constant for many years at a level far below initial projections. After a sharp rise in the number of residents during the 1990s, recent reports suggest that the number of residents entering training has decreased during the past few years.[148] Since family physicians are far more likely to practice in rural areas than internists and pediatricians, this means that the apparent stability in numbers of primary physicians has done little to redistribute physicians to areas most in need, and is in fact a "root cause of the shortage of rural physicians."[149] Market pressure for more primary physicians to serve as gatekeepers in managed health plans has also eased as providers have responded to public hostility to restrictions on direct patient access to specialists.[150] Although it has been suggested that it may not be necessary to increase the number of primary care physicians because of the explosive growth of nonphysician primary care occupations, it remains troubling to many that primary care, with its undefined and uncoordinated "polyglot of providers,"[151] lacks a formal role within American medicine.

As the number of doctors increased during the 1960s and 1970s, unease about physician shortages gave way to reports predicting a coming overproduction of medical personnel. The most influential, by the Graduate Medical Education National Advisory Committee (GMENAC), was published in 1980; it estimated that by the 1990s the United States would have too many doctors, and too many specialists in particular. Since its creation in 1986, the Council on Graduate Medical Education (COGME) has served as adviser to the government, issuing a steady stream of reports endorsing this view. Concerns about geographical distribution, as well as race, gender, and ethnic composition of the physician workforce, have also become more prominent. Since the mid-1980s there has been something like an orthodox position that fewer doctors should be trained while the balance between primary care physicians and specialists among new graduates should be split about 50/50.[152] Only in the last few years has this consensus been questioned.[153]

Fear of overproduction of doctors led the federal government to end or restrict its direct subsidies to medical faculties and to try to limit the number of foreign MDs.[154] The Clinton reforms were supposed, as part of the total health insurance reform, to create mechanisms for controlling the number of medical personnel. But since their failure, few mechanisms have existed for directly controlling the training of doctors. Consequently, regulation of physician numbers and distribution has been left essentially to market mechanisms and third-party providers seeking to lower costs.[155] A number of individual states have leaped into the breach by introducing specific measures to control the production of health-care workers and increase the number of primary care personnel.[156]

In 1994, COGME, the agency responsible for the medical workforce, recommended the setting up of consortia centered on medical schools to develop a national workforce plan while minimizing "State and Federal government intrusion."[157] This plan was never implemented, and in 1999 a report recommended a permanent and comprehensive system of information collection regarding all aspects of the medical market.[158] The assumption was that one of the chief barriers to effective market self-regulation of specialty choice was lack of public access to appropriate information. Providing accurate information about manpower would, it was thought, allow market mechanisms to appropriately orient doctors' choices of specialties and places of residence. This faith in the economic rationality of fully informed actors seems to lie at the center of current U.S. health workforce policy. There remains no agency with direct regulatory control over health-care professions.

If the fragmentation of jurisdiction within the U.S. system has encouraged a market approach to health manpower needs, as opposed to direct control of training, it has also allowed certain organizations to concentrate on the details of medical education. To a degree that seems quite unusual in comparative perspective, the American medical profession has taken the issue of specialist training to a whole new level. On the ABMS Web site, there are numbers of colloquia and publications related to the nuts-and-bolts aspects of specialist training and examination.[159] And the same is true of other organizations, such as the Council of Medical Specialty Societies.[160] The American medical profession has introduced one genuine innovation into graduate medical education: recertification, an effort to ensure that the knowledge of specialists remains up to date by requiring periodic examinations (usually every six to eight years). Introduced in 1969, recertification was adopted as policy in 1973, and again in 1978, by the American Board of Medical Specialties and its member boards, so that by the 1990s, virtually all boards granted time-limited certificates and about half of all board-certified doctors in the United States hold time-limited specialty certificates.[161] In March 2000, the member boards of ABMS voted to develop their current programs of recertification into programs of "maintenance of certification."[162] This aims to replace snapshot examinations with a continuing process of self-evaluation and retraining that includes not just abstract knowledge but also performance in practice and such skills as communication and "professionalism."[163] Those physicians who condemned recertification as a form of professional overkill that does little to improve health-care outcomes[164] will not be very happy with such programs.

The scope of American efforts in this domain is so extraordinary by international standards that one is forced to seek reasons for it. Certainly American doctors feel under siege, and this can be seen as one response. But European doctors feel at least as much under siege. One explanation may have to do with the fragmented nature of American medicine, which produces an ABMS that does nothing but deal with certification. (Compare the activities of this organization with, say, the Ordre des Médecins in France or the royal colleges in the United Kingdom, responsible for specialty certification but much else besides.) A second explanation has to do with the market orientation of American medicine. In a system controlled by governments or government-controlled insurance funds, certification is essentially an administrative tool that allows authorities to decide who gets paid for what and who can do what. (The goal is often as much about protecting state authorities from criticism as anything else.) But "maintenance of certification" is not about minimum standards, but about seeking, if not perfection, continual self-improvement, a task with no discernible end. There is no such thing as minimum standards in a market environment, because someone can always do something to improve his or her credentials and market share. Patients may choose not to come or, worse, they may come and then sue the doctor for huge sums of money. In such an environment there is no alternative but continual self-improvement.

Europeans (and many Canadians as well) do not know quite what to make of the American system. On the one hand, the degree of social inequality in health-care access is incomprehensible. On the other, American medicine represents a level of technological know-how, scientific achievement, and clinical sophistication that is unique in the world. If Americans seem unable to regulate their impossibly complex system with its many contradictory forces, they have nonetheless developed a number of specialized instruments that are being widely studied, and in some cases imitated, in Europe: turning generalists into primary care specialists; organizing managed care; the use of nonphysician replacement personnel to provide primary care; utilization of competitive market mechanisms to control supply and prices; recertification of specialists. All of the above are being closely watched abroad. If no one in Europe wants to imitate the Americans by abandoning the principles of social solidarity that underlie their health systems, many feel that there are nonetheless "lessons" to be learned from America.[165]

Conclusion

Each country has dealt with the problem of generalist-specialist distribution in different ways. The United Kingdom had created a clearly defined gatekeeping role for GPs while restricting access to both specialist training and specialist posts. The United States has accepted the demise of generalists and created the amorphous category of primary caregiver that includes specific specialties, occasional work by many different sorts of specialists, and reliance on nonphysician practitioners. France has concentrated on controlling access to specialist training by determining nationally the number of training places that are available. It has moved more recently to turning general medicine into a specialty or at least a field with all the trappings of a specialty. Germany, in contrast, has eschewed the effort to control recruitment through training and has instead focused on regulating insurance practice (which in the German context means most private practice) by creating quotas for practitioners in a given geographical unit. It has also tried to turn generalists into specialists, and is now moving determinedly toward the creation of a single category of primary specialists with a broad gatekeeping role. It is too early to tell whether this effort will be successful. Whatever the strategies that have been followed, generalist/primary physicians do not seem to be particularly satisfied or comfortable in their role.

But many specialists seem discontented as well. Patients are voting with their feet and seeking alternative treatments in greater numbers than ever before. Administrators are unhappy with rising costs and variations in practice. Is this discontent attributable to the specialization of medicine? To some degree, perhaps; specialization adds to costs, contributes to the alienation of many patients and doctors, complicates tasks of coordination, and transforms the provision of primary care into a dilemma. But one also suspects that current difficulties extend far beyond any specific form of organization and have to do with the sheer size of the modern medical enterprise (what public enterprises on this scale fully satisfy us?), its public (and therefore politicized) character, and, above all, the multiple, often contradictory tasks that it is expected to perform. Somewhat unrealistically, perhaps, we expect medicine to provide a steady stream of technological miracles, psychological support, and "caring" to suffering patients; easy accessibility for everyone; high-cost care to those suffering from relatively rare conditions; and all of this at a reasonably low price that does not eat up too many of our tax dollars or private savings, and without any serious mistakes by caregivers. No wonder we are dissatisfied with what we actually get. Such exaggerated faith is one of the by-products of the successful division and conquest of medicine by the forces of specialization that advanced precisely because they were so intimately associated with belief in the possibilities of science, expertise, and limitless progress.

Appendices

Appendix 1: Specialists in the US, France, and Germany Compared

	U.S. All 1935	NYC 1935	Boston 1935	Fr. Prov. Cities 1935	Paris 1935	Prussia 1937
Total No. Specialists	50,334[1]	840[2]	513[3]	876[4]	3866[5]	9273
% of All Physicians	31	39	41	52[6](45)	52(45)	28.6
% All Specialists in						
Surgery	26	20	21	21	15	16
Orthopedics	2	3	4	4[3]	2	2
Obstetrics	5	1	1	4	4	NA
Gynecology	3	4	1	7	12	NA
Obgyn	6	8	7	4	4	11
Total	13	13	9	15	20	11
Pediatrics	6	9	9	10	13	8
Ophthalmology	3	5	6	6	5	8
Otolaryngology	4	8	7	7	8	10
Opth/orl	9	2	1	<1	1	NA
Total	16	15	15	14	14	18
Urology	6	6	4	6	8	1
Dermatology	NA	NA	NA	-	2	NA
Venereology	NA	NA	NA	1	1	NA
Derm./vener.	2	4	2	4	4	12
Total	2	4	2	5	7	12
Psychiatry	1	3	2	NA	NA	3
Neurology	<1	2	1	NA	NA	4
Psych/neur	3	3	3	8	6	2
Total	5	7	6	8	6	9

	U.S. All 1935	NYC 1935	Boston 1935	Fr. Prov. Cities 1935	Paris 1935	Prussia 1937
Electricity	NA	NA	NA	1	3	NA
Radiology	4	2	3	4	4	2
Electro-radiol.	NA	NA	NA	5	5	NA
Total	4	2	3	10	11	2
Internal Med.	9	13	14	NA	NA	16
Resp./	NA	NA	NA	4	6	3
Digest./	NA	NA	NA	5	4	NA
Cardio./nutrit .	NA	NA	NA	4	4	NA
Total	NA	NA	NA	13	14	3
Stomatology	NA	NA	NA	7	7	<1
Tuberculosis	2	1	1	1	4	NA
Public Health[7]	2	1	1	3	2	NA
Bacteriology[7]	<1	<1	<1	<1	2	NA
Legal Medicine	NA	NA	NA	0	1	NA
Pathology & Clin. Path	2	1	1	NA	NA	NA

Sources: American Medical Directory 1935; Guide Rosenwald 1935; Wilfried Teicher, (Untersuchungen zur ärztlichen Spezialisierung im Spiegel des Reichmedizinalkalenders am Beispiel Preussens im ersten Drittel des 20. Jahrhunderts (MD Thesis, Johannes Gutenberg-Universität Mainz, 1992), p. 65.

1. Source: *Graduate Medical Education: Report of the Commission on Graduate Medical Education* (1940).

2. Sample based on the first 2000 lisitings for NYC in *AMD*.

3. Sample based on the first 1250 listings for Boston in *AMD*.

4. All provincial specialists in Bordeaux, Lille, Lyon, and Marseille listed in the city listings of *Guide Rosenwald*. In all French listings, individuals with more than one listing are included in each specialty category. Totals thus add up to more than 100 percent. The problem does not arise in the *AMD* which prohibits multiple listings.

5. Sample comprising the first one-third of all Parisian practitioners in *Guide Rosenwald.*

6. Includes those self-identified and those added by editors to specialty lists. Figure in brackets is the percentage when only self-identification is taken into account.

7. Although the category does not exist on specialty lists, individuals identify themselves in this category.

Appendix 2: British Specialists in the Inter-war Years (%)

Specialty	London Doctors (1923)[1]	Who's Who, Britain (1925)[2]	Britain 1938–39	London 1938–39
Specialty as % of Listings	11	40	NA	NA
% of All Specialists[3]				
Medicine	NA	NA	18	22
Surgery	22	20	23	22
Gynecology	9	7		
Obstetrics	5	8	9	8
Ophthalmology	8	9	15	13
Anesthesiology	8	2	5	8
ORL	6	5	10	9
Psychiatry	6	6	2	4
Radiology	3	3	8	5
Pathology	2	4	4	3
Dermatology	5	3	3	3
Orthopedics	NA	NA	4	4
Dent. Surgeons	17	3	NA	NA
Urology	5	2	NA	NA
Venereology	5	3	NA	NA
Neurology	4	5	NA	NA
Pediatrics	3	6	NA	NA
Tropical Med.	3	5	NA	NA
Bacteriology	3	3	NA	NA
Respiratory	3	3	NA	NA
Electricity	2	3	NA	NA
Tuberculosis	2	3	NA	NA
Cardiology	2	2	NA	NA
Public Health	<1	9	NA	NA
Gastric	0	4	NA	NA
Total No. Specialists	263	184	1620	593

Source: The Medical Who's Who, 1925 (London: Grafton, 1925); *London Doctors and Dental Surgeons, 1923–24* (London: Grafton, 1923); Ministry of Health and Department of Health for Scotland, *Report of the Inter-Departmental Committee on the Remuneration of Consultants and Specialists* (London, His Majesty's Stationary Office, 1948).

1. Based on the first 2400 listings.

2. Based on the first 500 listings of individuals living in the British Isles.

3. Individuals with more than one listing are included in each specialty category. Totals thus add up to more than 100 percent.

Notes

Abbreviations

ABMA = *Archives of the British Medical Association*
ANP = Archives Nationales, Paris
ANP/AOM = Archives Nationales, Paris/Archives de l'Ordre des Médecins
ÄVD = Ärztliches Vereinsblatt für Deutschland
BMJ = British Medical Journal
BHM = Bulletin of the History of Medicine
BOM = Bulletin de l'Ordre des Médecins
CMAC = Contemporary Medical Archives Centre. Wellcome Institute
CMd = Concours médical
DÄ = Deutsches Ärzteblatt
DMW = Deutsche medizinische Wochenschrift
JAMA = Journal of the American Medical Association
MdS = Médecin syndicalist
MH =Medical History
MMW= Münchener medizinische Wochenschrift
PMd = Paris médical
PrM = Presse médicale
SHM = Social History of Medicine
TAMA = Transactions of the American Medical Association

Introduction

1. George Rosen, *The Specialization of Medicine with Particular Reference to Ophthalmology* (New York: Froben Press, 1944).

2. Hans-Heinz Eulner, *Die Entwicklung der medizinischen Spezialfächer an den Universitäten des deutschen Sprachgebietes* (Stuttgart: Ferdinand Enke Verlag, 1970).

3. Rosemary Stevens, *Medical Practice in Modern England: The Impact of Specialization and State Medicine* (New Haven, Conn.: Yale University Press, 1966).

4. Rosemary Stevens, *American Medicine and the Public Interest,* updated ed. (Berkeley: University of California Press, 1998; originally published New Haven, Conn.: Yale University Press, 1971).

5. The updated edition of Stevens, *American Medicine;* Alice Juch, *De medisch specialisten in de Nederlandse gezondheidszorg, 1890–1941* (Rotterdam: Erasmus Publishing, 1997);

6. Sydney A. Halpern, *American Pediatrics: The Social Dynamics of Professionalism* (Berkeley: University of California Press, 1988); Glenn Gritzer and Arnold Arluke, *The Making of Rehabilitation: A Political Economy of Medical Specialization, 1890–1980* (Berkeley: University of California Press, 1985).

7. Rosen, *Specialization of Medicine,* p. 15.

8. Rosen, *Specialization of Medicine,* pp. 14–30.

9. George Rosen, *The Structure of American Medical Practice, 1875–1941,* ed. Charles E. Rosenberg (Philadelphia: University of Pennsylvania Press, 1983), especially pp. 81–94.

10. Stevens, *Medical Practice in England* and *American Medicine.*

11. Stevens, *Medical Practice in England,* p. 4.

12. Eulner, *Die Entwicklung;* on specialty practice, Hans-Heinz Eulner, "Das Spezialistentum in der ärztlichen Praxis," in *Der Arzt und der Kranke in der Gesellschaft des 19. Jahrhunderts,* ed. Walter Artelt and Walter Rüegg (Stuttgart: Ferdinand Enke Verlag, 1967), pp. 17–34.

13. Among the books not cited below are W. F. Bynum, C. Lawrence, and V. Nutton, eds., *The Emergence of Modern Cardiology, Medical History,* supp. no. 5 (London: Wellcome Institute for the History of Medicine, 1985); Jan E. Goldstein, *Console and Classify: The French Psychiatric Profession in the Nineteenth Century* (New York: Cambridge University Press, 1987); Russell C. Maulitz and Diana E. Long, eds., *Grand Rounds: One Hundred Years of Internal Medicine* (Philadelphia: University of Pennsylvania Press, 1988); Ornella Moscucci, *The Science of Woman: Gynaecology and Gender in England, 1800–1929* (Cambridge: Cambridge University Press, 1990); Roger Cooter, *Surgery and Society in Peace and War: Orthopaedics and the Organization of Modern Medicine, 1880–1948* (London: Macmillan, 1993); W. Bruce Fye, *American Cardiology: The History of a Specialty and Its College* (Baltimore: Johns Hopkins University Press, 1996); Jack D. Pressman, *Last Resort: Psychosurgery and the Limits of Medicine* (Cambridge: Cambridge University Press, 1998); Heather Monroe Prescott, *A Doctor of Their Own: The History of Adolescent Medicine* (Cambridge, Mass.: Harvard University Press, 1998); Regina Morantz-Sanchez, *Conduct Unbecoming a Woman: Medicine on Trial in Turn-of-the- Century Brooklyn* (New York: Oxford University Press, 1999); Roger Davidson, *Dangerous Liaisons: A Social History of Venereal Disease in Twentieth-Century Scotland, Clio Medica 57* (Amsterdam: Rodopi, 2000); Patrice Pinell, *The Fight Against Cancer: France 1890–1940,* trans. David Madell (London: Routledge, 2002).

14. Everett Hughes, *Men and Their Work* (Glencoe, Ill.: Free Press, 1958).

15. Elliot Freidson, *Profession of Medicine: A Study of the Sociology of Applied Knowledge* (New York: Dodd, Mead, 1970), and *Professional Dominance: The Social Structure of Medical Care* (New York: Atherton Press, 1970).

16. Magali Sarfatti Larson, *The Rise of Professionalism: A Sociological Analysis* (Berkeley: University of California Press, 1977).

17. Andrew Abbott, *The System of Professions: An Essay on the Division of Expert Labor* (Chicago: University of Chicago Press, 1988).

18. On historians of professions, see John C. Burnham, *How the Idea of Profession Changed the Writing of Medical History* (London: Wellcome Institute for the History of Medicine, 1998).

19. See especially the classic brief article by Rue Bucher and Anselme Strauss, "Professions in Process," *American Journal of Sociology*, 66 (1961), 325–34.

20. Abbott, *System of Professions*; Gritzer and Arluke, *Making of Rehabilitation*.

21. Halpern, *American Pediatrics*.

22. William Ray Arney, *Power and the Profession of Obstetrics* (Chicago: University of Chicago Press, 1982); Sarah Nettleton, *Power, Pain and Dentistry* (Buckingham, U.K., and Philadelphia: Open University Press, 1992), and "Inventing Mouths: Disciplinary Power and Dentistry," in *Reassessing Foucault: Power, Medicine and the Body*, ed. Colin Jones and Roy Porter (London and New York: Routledge, 1994), pp. 73–90; Elizabeth Lunbeck, *The Psychiatric Persuasion: Knowledge, Gender, and Power in Modern America* (Princeton, N.J.: Princeton University Press, 1994).

23. Isabelle Baszanger, *Inventing Pain Medicine: From the Laboratory to the Clinic* (New Brunswick, N.J.: Rutgers University Press, 1998).

24. Jeffrey P. Baker, *The Machine in the Nursery: Incubator Technology and the Origins of Newborn Intensive Care* (Baltimore: Johns Hopkins University Press, 1996); Keith Wailoo, *Drawing Blood: Technology and Disease Identity in Twentieth-Century America* (Baltimore: Johns Hopkins University Press, 1997).

25. Marion Döhler, "Comparing National Patterns of Medical Specialization: A Contribution to the Theory of Professions," *Social Science Information*, 32 (1993), 185–231; Arnold J. Heidenheimer, "Organized Medicine and Physician Specialization in Scandinavia and West Germany," *West European Politics*, 3 (1980), 373–87; William Leeming, "Professionalization Theory, Medical Specialists and the Concept of National Patterns of Specialization," *Social Science Information*, 40 (2001), 455–85.

26. "Specialties," in this book, refers to clinical specialties as opposed to pure laboratory specialties.

27. Paul Ghalioungui, "Early Specialization in Ancient Egyptian Medicine and Its Possible Relation to an Archetypal Image of the Human Organism," *MH*, 13 (1969), 383–86. For other examples, see Rosen, *Specialization of Medicine*, ch. 2.

28. Galen, *On the Parts of Medicine . . .* , ed. K. Kalbfleisch, trans. Malcolm Lyons (Berlin: Akademie-Verlag, 1969), pp. 27–28. I am grateful to Vivian Nutton for calling this source to my attention.

29. R. Steven Turner, "The Great Transition and the Social Patterns of German Science," *Minerva*, 25 (1987), 56–76.

30. This paragraph is based on Lorraine Daston, "The Academies and the Unity of Knowledge: The Disciplining of the Disciplines," *Difference: A Journal of Feminist Cultural Studies*, 10 (1998), 67–86. For a rather different interpretation, see Rudolf Stichweh, *Zur Enstehung des modernen Systems wissenschaftlicher Disziplinen: Physik in Deutschland, 1740–1890* (Frankfurt: Suhrkamp, 1984).

31. Toby Gelfand, "The Origins of a Modern Concept of Medical Specialization: John Morgan's Discourse of 1765," *BHM*, 50 (1976), 511–35.

32. Carl August Wunderlich, *Wien und Paris: Ein Beitrag zur Geschichte und Beurteilung den gegenwärtigen Heilkunde in Deutschland und Frankreich* (Stuttgart: Ebner & Seubert, 1841; new ed., Bern: H. Huber, 1974), p.120.

33. Thomas Neville Bonner, *Becoming a Physician: Medical Education in Great Britain, France, Germany, and the United States, 1750–1945* (Oxford: Oxford University Press, 1995).

34. Among many other sources, see Bonner, *Becoming a Physician*.

35. John Prentiss Lord, "Factors in the Advancement of Orthopedic Surgery," *JAMA*, 89 (1927), 653.

36. See especially Roger Cooter and Steve Sturdy, "Of War, Medicine and Modernity: Introduction," in *War, Medicine and Modernity*, ed. Roger Cooter, Mark Harrison, and Steve Sturdy (Stroud, U.K.: Sutton, 1998), p. 2.

37. On medical holism, see the essays in Christopher Lawrence and George Weisz, eds., *Greater Than the Parts: Holism in Biomedicine, 1920–1950* (New York: Oxford University Press, 1998), particularly Jack D. Pressman, "Human Understanding: Psychosomatic Medicine and the Mission of the Rockefeller Foundation," pp. 189–208.

38. "Association Professionnelle des Médecins," *BMJ* (1935), 2, supp., 220. All translations from French and German are my own.

Chapter 1

1. Matthew Ramsey, "The Conception of Specialization in Eighteenth- and Nineteenth-Century French Surgery," in *History of Ideas in Surgery: Proceedings of the 17th International Symposium on the Comparative History of Medicine*, ed. Yosio Kawakita et al. (Tokyo: Ishiyaku Euro-America, 1997), pp. 69–117. Also see Matthew Ramsey, *Professional and Popular Medicine in France 1770–1830: The Social World of Medical Practice* (Cambridge: Cambridge University Press, 1988); and Roger King, *The Making of the Dentiste, c. 1650–1760* (Aldershot, U.K.: Ashgate, 1998), pp. 34–48.

2. Toby Gelfand, *Professionalizing Modern Medicine: Paris Surgeons and Medical Science and Institutions in the Eighteenth Century* (Westport, Conn.: Greenwood Press, 1980). Also see King, *Making of the Dentiste*, ch. 4.

3. Ramsey, "Conception of Specialization," p. 79.

4. Laurence Brockliss and Colin Jones, *The Medical World of Early Modern France* (Oxford: Clarendon Press, and New York: Oxford University Press, 1997), p. 62. For what follows, see pp. 542, 611.

5. Zina Weygand, *Les causes de la cécité et les soins oculaires en France au début du XIXe siècle, 1800–1815* (Vanves: Centre Technique National d'Études et de Recherches sur les Handicaps et les Inadaptations (Evry: Diffusion Presses Univ de France, 1989), p. 35; Helen Corlett, "'No Small Uncertainty': Eye Treatments in Eighteenth-Century England and France," *MH*, 42 (1998), 221.

6. Brockliss and Jones, *Medical World*, p. 559.

7. King, *Making of the Dentiste*, pp. 156–71.

8. King, *Making of the Dentiste*, pp. 88–90 and, more generally pp. 7–126.

9. King, *Making of the Dentiste*, pp. 100–16.

10. King, *Making of the Dentiste*, pp. 181–89.

11. Ramsey, "Conception of Specialization," p. 79.

12. *État de médecine, chirurgie et pharmacie en Europe pour l'année 1776* (Paris: Didot Jeune, 1776), pp. 78–94.

13. King, *Making of the Dentiste*, p. 212; Perre Baron, "'Dental Experts' in Lyon at the End of the Eighteenth Century," and Pierre Laudet, "Two Dental Experts from Toulouse: The Delgas," in *Dental Practice in Europe at the End of the Eighteenth Century: Transactions of the Liverpool Meeting, October 1993*, ed. Christine Hillam (Liverpool: 1993), pp. 27–34 and 44–49, respectively.

14. For other examples, see Corlett, "'No Small Uncertainty,'" pp. 226–27.

15. For some examples, see Gelfand, *Professionalizing Modern Medicine*, p. 153.

16. On Gilibert, see Samuel Kotteck, "'Citizens! Do You Want Children's Doctors?' An Early Vindication of 'Paediatric' Specialists,'" *MH*, 35 (1991), 103–16.

17. Jean-Emmanuel Gilibert, *L'anarchie médicinale, ou la médecine considérée comme nuisible à la société*, 3 vols., 2nd ed. (Paris: no publisher 1776; originally published Neuchâtel, 1772). The two essays are in vol. 3, pp. 220–48 and 249–87, respectively.

18. Kottek, "'Citizens! Do You Want Children's Doctors?'" pp. 104–5.

19. Ramsey, "Conception of Specialization," pp. 81–82; George Weisz, "Mapping Medical Specialization in Paris in the Nineteenth and Twentieth Centuries," *SHM*, 7 (1994), 177–211.

20. For more specific figures, see Weisz, "Mapping Medical Specialization"; and Ramsey, "Conception of Specialization," pp. 82–83.

21. L. Hubert, *Almanach général des médecins pour la ville de Paris* (Paris: Gabon, 1830; 1st ed., 1827).

22. Hubert, *Almanach général*, p. 101.

23. On obstetrical training during the eighteenth century, see Jacques Gélis, *La sage-femme ou le médecin: Une nouvelle conception de la vie* (Paris: Fayard, 1988); and Paul Delaunay, *La Maternité de Paris* (Paris: Pousset, 1909).

24. The Faculty of Paris in fact had two such chairs, a clinical chair and a theoretical chair that combined *accouchement* with diseases of women and children.

25. For the case of one oculist's long-term quest for state favor, see Jan E. Goldstein, *Console and Classify: The French Psychiatric Profession in the Nineteenth Century* (New York: Cambridge University Press, 1987), pp. 60–62.

26. Erwin Ackerknecht, *Medicine at the Paris Hospital, 1794–1848* (Baltimore: Johns Hopkins University Press, 1967), pp. 163–80; Goldstein, *Console and Classify*, pp. 55–63.

27. For instance, in the May 1844 issue, Duval's book on foot and leg deformities was reviewed by Dr. Dalasiauve of the Bicêtre Hospital. The issue of December 1840 contained a special section made up of case histories from Parisian hospitals. On Broussais's influence, see *Revue des spécialités et innovations médicales et chirurgicales*, 1 (1839), 1.

28. S. Furnari, "Introduction," *L'esculape: Journal des spécialités médico-chirurgicales*, 1 (1839), 1–2; *Revue des spécialités et innovations médicales et chirurgicales*, 1 (1839), 1–5.

29. On the significance of these encyclopedias for Paris medicine, see George Weisz, "Reconstructing Paris Medicine," *BHM*, 75 (2001), 105–19; and for more detail about their editorial boards, see Weisz, "The Development of Medical Specialization in Nineteenth-Century Paris," in *French Medical Culture in the Nineteenth Century, Clio Medica*, 25, ed. Ann F. La Berge and Mordechai Feingold (Amsterdam and Atlanta: Rodopi, 1994), pp. 149–88. To my knowledge, no comparable works appeared in Lon-

don. Several did appear in Germany, but the largest was far smaller than the average Parisian publication. I am grateful to Michael Stolberg for providing me with a list of comparable German medical publications.

30. "Accoucheur," in *Dictionnaire des sciences médicales*, vol. 1 (Paris: Crapart, 1812), p. 101.

31. Antoine Dugès, "Accouchement," in *Dictionnaire de médecine et de chirurgie pratique*, vol. 1 (Paris: Gabon, 1829), p. 124.

32. M.-J. Raige Delorme, "Oculiste," in *Dictionnaire de médecine*, vol. 15 (Paris: Béchet Jeune, 1826), pp. 216–17.

33. J. N. Marjolin, "Dentiste," in *Dictionnaire de médecine*, vol. 6 (Paris: Béchet Jeune, 1823), pp. 478–79.

34. This is noted in Ackerknecht, *Medicine at the Paris Hospital*, p. 162. We discuss this preface below.

35. M.-J. Raige Delorme, *Dictionnaire de médecine*, 2nd ed., vol. 21 (Paris: Béchet Jeune, 1840), p. 189.

36. J. F. Oudet, *Dictionnaire de médecine*, 2nd ed., vol. 21, p. 236.

37. A. Velpeau, "Ophthalmologie," in *Dictionnaire de médecine*, 2nd ed., vol. 22 (Paris: Béchet Jeune, 1840), pp. 195–96.

38. John Harley Warner, *Against the Spirit of System: The French Impulse in Nineteenth-Century American Medicine* (Princeton, N.J.: Princeton University Press, 1998), pp. 293–94.

39. Adolf Muehry, *Observations on the Comparative State of Medicine in France, England, and Germany*, trans. Edward G. Davis (Philadelphia: A. Waldie, 1838).

40. Carl Wunderlich, *Wien und Paris: Ein Beitrag zur Geschichte und Beurteilung den gegenwärtigen Heilkunde in Deutschland und Frankreich* (Stuttgart: Ebner & Seubert 1841; new ed., Bern: H. Huber, 1974), p. 35. The translation of the quote is by Ackerknecht, *Medicine at the Paris Hospital*, p. 163.

41. Hubert, *Almanach général*, pp. 61–65.

42. Henri Meding, *Paris médical: Vade-mecum des médecins étrangers dans Paris*, 2 vols. (Paris: Baillière, 1852), vol. 2, pp. 353–62.

43. C. Sachaile de la Barre, *Les médecins de Paris jugés par leurs oeuvres* (Paris: 1845), discussed in Ackerknecht, *Medicine at the Paris Hospital*, p. 163.

44. *Almanach général de médecine et pharmacie pour la France, l'Algérie et les colonies* (Paris: L'Union Médicale, 1852).

45. On urban population growth during this period, see Paul M. Hohenberg and Lynn Hollen Lees, *The Making of Urban Europe: 1000–1950* (Cambridge, Mass.: Harvard University Press, 1985), table 7.2; and Paul Bairoch et al., *La population des villes européenes de 800–1850* (Geneva: Centre d'Histoire Économique Internationale and Droz, 1988), p. 283.

46. See my account of Rosen's work in the Introduction.

47. Ackerknecht, *Medicine at the Paris Hospital*, pp. 163–64.

48. On these matters, see Goldstein, *Console and Classify*.

49. Rosen, *Specialization of Medicine*, p. 29.

50. Gilibert, *L'anarchie médicinale*, p. 220.

51. Toby Gelfand, "The Origins of a Modern Concept of Medical Specialization: John Morgan's Discourse of 1765," *BHM*, 50 (1976), 511–35. Also see Goldstein, *Console and Classify*, pp. 56–60.

52. Gilibert, *L'anarchie médicinale*, pp. 221–23, especially p. 222.

53. Gilibert, *L'anarchie médicinale*, p. 225.

54. Gilibert, *L'anarchie médicinale*, pp. 222–29.

55. Gilibert, *L'anarchie médicinale*, p. 233.

56. Gilibert, *L'anarchie médicinale*, pp. 233–34, 243.

57. Gilibert, *L'anarchie médicinale*, p. 230.

58. Gilibert, *L'anarchie médicinale*, pp. 230–31.

59. Joseph Ben-David, *The Scientist's Role in Society: A Comparative Study* (Chicago: University of Chicago Press, 1984; 1st ed., 1971), p. 89. Also see Rudolf Stichweh, *Études sur la genèse du système scientifique moderne*, trans. Fabienne Blaise (Lille: Presses Universitaires de Lille, 1991), p. 113.

60. George Weisz, *The Medical Mandarins: The French Academy of Medicine in the Nineteenth and Early Twentieth Centuries* (New York and Oxford: Oxford University Press, 1995). The classic study of Paris medicine during the first half of the nineteenth century is Ackerknecht, *Medicine at the Paris Hospital*. A theoretical analysis of its intellectual origins is Michel Foucault, *The Birth of the Clinic: An Archaeology of Medical Perception*, trans. A. M. Sheridan Smith (London: Tavistock, 1973). Also relevant to its origins is the final section of Gelfand, *Professionalizing Modern Medicine*. Other significant works include John E. Lesch, *Science and Medicine in France: The Emergence of Experimental Physiology, 1790–1855* (Cambridge, Mass.: Harvard University Press, 1984); Jean-François Braunstein, *Broussais et le matérialisme: Médecine et philosophie au XIXe siècle* (Paris: Méridiens Klincksieck, 1986); Russell C. Maulitz, *Morbid Appearances: The Anatomy of Pathology in the Early Nineteenth Century* (Cambridge: Cambridge University Press, 1987); Othmar Keel, *L'avènement de la médecine clinique moderne en Europe, 1750–1815: Politiques, institutions et savoirs* (Montreal: Presses de l'Université de Montréal, 2001). The most recent comprehesive reevaluation of this subject is the essays in Caroline Hannaway and Ann La Berge, eds., *Constructing Paris Medicine, Clio Medica 50* (Amsterdam and Atlanta: Rodopi, 1998). I review this last work in my "Reconstructing Paris Medicine," *BHM*, 75 (2001), 105–19.

61. Louis Peisse, *La médecine et les médecins: Philosophie, doctrines, institutions, critiques, mœurs, et biographies médicales*, 2 vols. (Paris: Baillière, 1857), vol. 1, p. 310.

62. Lorraine Daston, "The Academies and the Unity of Knowledge: The Disciplining of the Disciplines," *Difference: A Journal of Feminist Cultural Studies*, 10 (1998), 67–86. Also see Roger Hahn, *The Anatomy of a Scientific Institution: The Paris Academy of Sciences, 1666–1803* (Berkeley: University of California Press, 1971), pp. 10–12.

63. The disciplines covered on these editorial boards are discussed in Weisz, "Development of Medical Specialization."

64. Peisse, *La médecine*, vol. 1, pp. 311, 313.

65. For more detail, see Weisz, *Medical Mandarins*, ch. 1.

66. Danièle Ghesquier, "A Gallic Affair: The Case of the Missing Itch Mite in French Medicine in the Early Nineteenth Century," *MH*, 43 (1999), 32. Also see Charles Coury and Mireille Wiriot, "'Unter den Linden' ou la naissance de la dermatologie française," in *Medizingeschichte in unserer Zeit: Festgabe für Edith Heischkel-Artelt und Walter Artelt zum 65. Geburtstag*, ed. Hans-Heinz Eulner et al. (Stuttgart: Ferdinand Enke Verlag, 1971), pp. 233–40.

67. Susan P. Conner, "The Pox in Eighteenth-Century France," in *The Secret Malady: Venereal Disease in Eighteenth-Century Britain and France*, ed. Linda Merians (Lexington: University Press of Kentucky, 1996), p. 27.

68. Jacques Tenon, *Mémoires sur les hôpitaux de Paris*, xl, cited in Goldstein, *Console and Classify*, p. 60.

69. For the case of the maternity hospital, see Scarlett Beauvalet-Boutouyrie, *Naître à l'hôpital au XIXe siècle* (Paris: Belin, 1999), pp. 42–43.

70. Max Neuburger, *Das alte medizinische Wien in zeitgenössischen Schilderungen* (Vienna and Leipzig: Moritz Perles, 1921), pp. 63–72.

71. Dora B. Weiner, *The Citizen-Patient in Revolutionary and Imperial Paris* (Baltimore and London: Johns Hopkins University Press, 1993), p. 145.

72. On the St. Louis Hospital see Ghesquier, "Gallic Affair," p. 32.

73. Beauvalet-Boutouyrie, *Naître à l'hôpital*, pp. 59–70.

74. Weiner, *Citizen-Patient*, p. 184.

75. The best discussion of the system and its operations is Weiner, *Citizen-Patient*, pp. 133–90.

76. *Rapport fait au Conseil Général des Hospices, par un de ses membres, sur l'état des hôpitaux . . . depuis le 1er janvier 1804 jusqu'au 1er janvier 1814* (Paris: Imprimerie de Madame Huzard, 1816), p. 5.

77. *Rapport . . . au Conseil Général des Hospices*, p. 7.

78. Ramsey, "Conception of Specialization," p. 85.

79. Peisse, *La médecine*, vol. 1, pp. 307–8.

80. Goldstein, *Console and Classify*, pp. 60–62.

81. Alex Dracobly, "Ethics and Experimentation on Human Subjects in Mid-Nineteenth-Century France: The Story of the 1859 Syphilis Experiments," *BHM*, 77 (2003), 337–66.

82. Philippe Pinel, *La médecine clinique rendue plus précise et plus exacte par l'application de l'analyse* (Paris: Brosson, 1802), quoted with translation in Weiner, *Citizen-Patient*, p.164.

83. Ghesquier, "Gallic Affair," pp. 33–36.

84. For instance, at midcentury there were five physicians and two surgeons working at the St. Louis; there were three venereologists at the Midi (for men) and another three at the Lourcine (for women). There were seven doctors at the Enfants Malades and another two at Enfants Trouvés. On the staffs of special hospitals, see Meding, *Paris médical*, pp. 80–106; Ghesquier, "Gallic Affair," p. 42; Kathryn Norberg, "From Courtesan to Prostitute: Mercenary Sex and Venereal Disease, 1730–1802," in *The Secret Malady: Venereal Disease in Eighteenth-Century Britain and France*, ed. Linda Merians (Lexington: University Press of Kentucky, 1996), p. 45.

85. Gavarret, speaking at the meeting of the faculty assembly, Paris Faculty of Medicine, February 10, 1859, in ANP, AJ 16 6251, p. 233.

86. Despite his identification with hospital orthopedics in the 1840s, F. Malgaigne proved to be a dogged opponent of specialization.

87. In psychiatry, these included J.E.D. Esquirol, who opened a private mental hospital in Ivry, and Jules Falret, whose private asylum was in Vanves. Jules Guérin had a private orthopedic clinic, as did Bouvier. Julius Sichel, an ophthalmologist from Vienna, established a private clinic in Paris in 1832. See Wunderlich, *Wien und Paris*,

p. 102; Ackerknecht, *Medicine at the Paris Hospital*, p.179; and Weiner, *Citizen-Patient*, p. 163.

88. Weiner, *Citizen-Patient*, p. 187.

89. In Hubert, *Almanach général*.

90. Peisse, *La médecine*, vol. 1, p. 316.

91. Wunderlich, *Wien und Paris*, p. 36.

92. M.-J. Raige Delorme, "Preface," in *Dictionnaire de médecine*, 2nd ed., vol. 1 (Paris: Béchet Jeune, 1832), pp. xvii–xviii and xix–xx; quote is on p. xx. For one response to such views, see Peisse, *La médecine*, vol. 1, pp. 315–16.

93. ANP, AJ16 6251, meeting of the faculty assembly, February 10, 1859.

94. The presentation of this report is in ANP, AJ16 6251, March 17, 1859, p. 229. What seems to be an incomplete version of this report is in AJ16 6310.

95. Discussion of this issue went on for three meeting of the faculty. ANP, AJ16 6251, March 17, 24, and 28, 1859, pp. 229–55.

96. Gavarret, ANP, AJ16 6251, p. 233.

97. ANP, AJ16 6251, April 28, 1859, pp. 253–55.

98. ANP, AJ16 6251, April 17, 1859, p. 229.

99. ANP, AJ16 6253, January 23, 1862, pp. 6–7.

100. ANP, AJ16 6253, April 24, 1862, p. 411.

101. There is no mention of this reform in the minutes of the faculty, suggesting that Rayer avoided consulting his colleagues on this matter.

102. George Weisz, *The Emergence of Modern Universities in France, 1863–1914* (Princeton, N.J.: Princeton University Press, 1983).

103. Goldstein, *Console and Classify*, pp. 346–48; Jacques Poirier, "La Faculté de Médecine face à la montée du spécialisme," *Communications*, 54 (1992), 209–27, especially 214.

104. Émile Martin, *Les spécialistes: Réponse au discours académique du Docteur Coste, directeur de l'École de Médecine de Marseille* (Marseilles: A. Arnaud, 1868).

105. For a more detailed discussion of early specialist journals, see Weisz, "Development of Medical Specialization."

106. Weisz, *Emergence of Modern Universities*, chs. 1–3.

107. The clearest expression of these concerns is Léon LeFort, *Rapport sur la création de chaires cliniques spéciales à la Faculté de Médecine*, pp. 4–5. read to the Faculty April 18, 1878, in ANP, AJ16 6310. The conclusions were voted unanimously. Also see the comments by Hardy to the faculty assembly January 6, 1876, ANP, AJ16 6257.

108. See, for instance, the faculty discussions of December 30, 1875, and January 6, 1876, ANP, AJ16 6357. Poirier, "La Faculté," pp. 214–18, gives a good account of these discussions.

109. LeFort, *Rapport*, pp. 4–5.

110. LeFort, *Rapport*, p. 7.

111. This judgment was developed as early as 1868. See Martin, *Les spécialistes*, p. 13.

112. Most medical directories at that time treated them as separate fields. Nonetheless, the earliest journals in the field combined the two specialties. See the discussion of these two fields in chapter 11.

113. LeFort, *Rapport*, p. 13.

114. ANP, AJ16 6259, January 16, 1879, p.187.

115. ANP, AJ16 1081; Paul Legendre, *Du Quartier Latin à l'Académie (Réminiscences)* (Paris: Maloine, 1930).

116. This point is well made by Christian Bonah, *Instruire, guérir, servir: Formation et pratique médicales en France et en Allemagne* (Strasbourg: Presses Universitaires de Strasbourg, 2000), p. 87.

117. Paul Legendre, in discussing his experiences as a medical student during this period, describes many of those he worked under in hospitals as specialists. Legendre, *Du Quartier Latin.*

118. Nadine Lefaucher, "La résistible création des accoucheurs des hôpitaux," *Sociologie de travail,* 30 (1988), 323–52; and Jeffrey P. Baker, *The Machine in the Nursery: Incubator Technology and the Origins of Newborn Intensive Care* (Baltimore: Johns Hopkins University Press, 1996), p. 34.

119. The alienists discussed here served in the major Parisian hospitals, the Salpêtrière and the Bicêtre. Those in smaller departmental asylums were part of a different administration that was also evolving; regulations drawn up at about the same time introduced special competitions for asylum interns. Somewhat later, junior asylum physicians also came to be chosen by special competitions.

120. *Bulletin de l'Académie de Médecine,* 17 (1887), 592–645, and 19 (1888), 155–469. The Academy supported this proposal but with no consequences. A decade later, another proposal by Fournier was unsuccessful. *Bulletin de l'Académie de Médecine,* 42 (1899), 533, 577.

121. What follows is based on Paul Brouardel, "Création des services pour le traitement des maladies spéciales dans les hôpitaux," in Conseil de Surveillance de l'Assistance Publique, session 1897–1898, pp. 931–48. This is located in the archives of the Assistance Publique. Also see P. Pfister, "Le phénomène de spécialisation médicale au 19e siècle" (doctoral thesis in medicine, Université de Paris-Créteil, 1976), p. 38

122. XIIIième Congrès International de Médecine, Paris, 1900, *Paris médical: Assistance et enseignement* (Paris: Masson, 1900), p. 222.

123. For the year 1871–72, the *Almanach général de médecine* listed 101 self-identified specialists, including 32 homeopaths.

124. A. Chéreau, "Spécialités médicales," in *Dictionnaire encyclopédique des sciences médicales,* vol. 10 (Paris: Asselin et Masson, 1881), pp. 797–98.

Chapter 2

1. On the links between professional fragmentation, political conflicts, and intellectual controversies in comparative anatomy during this period, see Adrian J. Desmond, *The Politics of Evolution: Morphology, Medicine, and Reform in Radical London* (Chicago: University of Chicago Press, 1989), especially chs. 1 and 3. On medical politics more generally, see Ivan Waddington, *The Medical Profession in the Industrial Revolution* (Dublin: Gill and Macmillan, 1984).

2. Susan Lawrence has calculated that in 1800 there were twenty-two physicians and twenty-two surgeons, as well seven assistants, at the seven London hospitals. From 1800 to1819, only thirty-five physicians were appointed. Susan C. Lawrence, *Charitable Knowledge: Hospital Pupils and Practitioners in Eighteenth-Century London* (Cambridge: Cambridge University Press, 1996), pp. 351–52. Also see Thomas Neville Bonner, *Amer-*

ican Doctors and German Universities: A Chapter in International Intellectual Relations, 1870–1914 (Lincoln: University of Nebraska Press: 1963), pp. 93, 101.

3. Desmond, *Politics of Evolution*, ch. 1.

4. Lawrence, *Charitable Knowledge*, suggests that the leaders of the independent research community that had emerged in London after about 1750 seem by the turn of the century to have been largely co-opted by the royal colleges.

5. On the views of early nineteenth-century American doctors in London, see John Harley Warner, "American Doctors in London During the Age of Paris Medicine," in *The History of Medical Education in Britain*, ed. Vivian Nutton and Roy Porter (Amsterdam and Atlanta: Rodopi, 1995), pp. 342–65.

6. John Harley Warner, *Against the Spirit of System: The French Impulse in Nineteenth-Century American Medicine* (Princeton, N.J.: Princeton University Press, 1998), pp. 72–73, 195–200.

7. Lorraine Daston, "The Academies and the Unity of Knowledge: The Disciplining of the Disciplines," *Difference: A Journal of Feminist Cultural Studies*, 10 (1998), 67–86, especially 71.

8. The phrase is borrowed from Dorothy Ross, "Professionalism and the Transformation of American Social Thought," *Journal of Economic History*, 38 (1978), 497.

9. M. Jeanne Peterson, *The Medical Profession in Mid-Victorian London* (Berkeley: University of California Press, 1978), pp. 2–3, 124, 141–43, 166–67.

10. This was the Provincial Medical and Surgical Association. Its inspiration was the British Association for the Advancement of Science. Peter Bartrip, *Themselves Writ Large: The British Medical Association, 1832–1966* (London: BMJ Publishing Group, 1996), pp. 5–6, 10.

11. Peterson, *Medical Profession*, pp. 2–73. Also see Christopher Lawrence, "Incommunicable Knowledge: Science, Technology and the Clinical Art in Britain 1850–1914," *Journal of Contemporary History*, 20 (1985) 503–20.

12. W. F. Bynum, "Treating the Wages of Sin: Venereal Disease and Specialism in Eighteenth-Century Britain," in *Medical Fringe and Medical Orthodoxy, 1750–1850*, ed. W. F. Bynum and Roy Porter (London: Croom Helm, 1987), pp. 5–28.

13. On bonesetters and orthopedists, see Roger Cooter, "Bones of Contention? Orthodox Medicine and the Mystery of the Bonesetter's Craft," in *Medical Fringe and Medical Orthodoxy, 1750–1850*, ed. W. F. Bynum and Roy Porter (London: Croom Helm, 1987), pp. 153–83.

14. Adrian Wilson, *The Making of Man-Midwifery: Childbirth in England 1660–1770* (London: UCL Press, 1995).

15. Wilson, *Making of Man-Midwifery*, pp. 200–1.

16. Peterson, *Medical Profession*, p. 260; Irvine Loudon, *Medical Care and the General Practitioner, 1750–1850* (Oxford: Clarendon Press, 1986), pp. 189–90; David Innes Williams, *The London Lock: A Charitable Hospital for Venereal Disease, 1746–1952* (London: Royal Society of Medicine, 1995), pp. 13–14; Donna T. Andrew, *Philanthropy and Police: London Charity in the Eighteenth Century* (Princeton, N.J.: Princeton University Press, 1989); Kevin P. Siena, *Venereal Disease, Hospitals and the Urban Poor: London's "Foul Wards," 1600–1800* (Rochester, N.Y.: University of Rochester Press, 2004).

17. On specialist entrepreneurship, see Lindsay Granshaw, "'Fame and Fortune by Means of Bricks and Mortar': The Medical Profession and Specialist Hospitals in Britain,

1800–1948," in *The Hospital in History*, ed. Lindsay Granshaw and Roy Porter (London and New York: Routledge, 1989), pp.199–220; Peterson, *Medical Profession*, pp. 244–82; and Elizabeth M. R. Lomax, *Small and Special: The Development of Hospitals for Children in Victorian Britain*, MH, supp. no. 16 (London: Wellcome Institute for the History of Medicine, 1996). Of 144 hospitals founded in the nineteenth century, 83 percent were founded by doctors with lay support. The remaining 17 percent were primarily inspired by laypersons. Charles Newman, "The Rise of Specialism and Post-Graduate Education," in *The Evolution of Medical Education in Britain*, ed. F.N.L. Poynter (London: Pittman Medical Publishing, 1966), p.172.

18. Good examples are Frederick Salmon, discussed in Granshaw, "Fame and Fortune," p. 205, and Charles West, in Lomax, *Small and Special*, pp. 24–27.

19. Godelieve van Heteren, "Students Facing Boundaries: The Shift of Nineteenth-Century British Student Travel to German Universities and the Flexible Boundaries of a Medical Education System," in *The History of Medical Education in Britain*, ed. Vivian Nutton and Roy Porter (Amsterdam and Atlanta: Rodopi, 1995), pp. 302–3, mentions three individuals in the early nineteenth century who after study in Germany became specialists, two in orthopedics and one in ophthalmic surgery.

20. Lomax, *Small and Special*, pp. 24, 27; John V. Pickstone, *Medicine and Industrial Society: A History of Hospital Development in Manchester and Its Region, 1752–1946* (Manchester: Manchester University Press, 1985), p. 119.

21. For several examples, see Lomax, *Small and Special*, p. 21.

22. For examples from two women's hospitals, see Ornella Moscucci, *The Science of Woman: Gynaecology and Gender in England, 1800–1929* (Cambridge: Cambridge University Press, 1990), pp. 82–84, 96.

23. Granshaw, "Fame and Fortune," p. 200, and *St. Mark's Hospital, London: A Social History of a Specialist Hospital* (London: King Edward's Hospital Fund for London, 1985), pp. 26–29, pretty much discount scientific interests in the rise of specialist hospitals and emphasize motives of social mobility as well as the logic of philanthropy. In the cases she puts forward, publication is usually treated as a strategy for social mobility. An earlier work by Jeanne Peterson also emphasizes issues of mobility but acknowledges briefly that new scientific interests may also have been at work. For one of many examples of specialty hospitals that generated serious medical publications directed at doctors, see Bynum, "Treating the Wages of Sin," p. 24.

24. Lomax, *Small and Special*, pp. 155–57. Despite this and many other factors that kept pediatrics from emerging as a strong specialty, Lomax provides abundant evidence that children's hospitals were a locus of considerable knowledge production.

25. Peterson, *Medical Profession*, pp. 362–63; Granshaw, "Fame and Fortune," p. 204.

26. Luke Davidson, "'Identities Ascertained': British Ophthalmology in the First Half of the Nineteenth Century," *SHM*, 9 (1996), 313–33, especially 314–16.

27. One of the first specialty congresses, the Ophthalmological Congress, took place in 1857, at which time three general hospitals had appointed ophthalmic surgeons. One of the first specialist journals, *The Ophthalmic Hospitals Reports*, came out of Moorfields. In 1880, the Ophthalmic Society of the United Kingdom was formed, and a section devoted to the subject was organized for the first time at the BMA meeting.

28. Steve Sturdy and Roger Cooter, "Science, Scientific Management, and the Transformation of Medicine in Britain *c.* 1870–1950," *History of Science,* 36 (1998), 421–66, especially 426.

29. Zachary Cope, *The Royal College of Surgeons of England: A History* (London: Blond, 1959), p. 72.

30. "To the Right Honorable Sir George Grey, Bart. Her Majesty's Principal Secretary of State for the Home Department, 23 April 1850." This is an uncataloged printed pamphlet in the RCS archives that was the College's response to calls for the establishment of a Royal College of General Practitioners.

31. *London and Provincial Medical Directory, 1847* (London: Churchill, 1847). For a brief but illuminating quantitative analysis of the professional information in this volume (which does not discuss specialties), see Loudon, *Medical Care and the General Practitioner,* pp. 224–27, and "Two Thousand Medical Men in 1847," *Bulletin of the Society of the History of Medicine,* 33 (1983), 4–8.

32. David Innes Williams, "The Obstetrical Society of 1825" *MH,* 42 (1998), 235–45.

33. *London and Provincial Medical Directory, 1851,* (London: Churchill, 1851) p. vi.

34. This subject is discussed in greater detail in chapter 5 of this volume.

35. Peterson, *Medical Profession,* pp. 262–63; Roger Cooter, *Surgery and Society in Peace and War: Orthopaedics and the Organization of Modern Medicine, 1880–1948* (London: Macmillan, 1993), pp. 13–17. On the case of Manchester, see Pickstone, *Medicine and Industrial Society,* pp. 100, 113–22. Also see Richard Kershaw, *Special Hospitals: Their Origin, Development, and Relationship to Medical Education, Their Economic Aspects and Relative Freedom from Abuse* (London: Pulman, 1909), pp. 61–72, for a complete list of hospitals created from 1801 to 1899.

36. The government also offered occasional financial support. *BMJ* (1863), 1, 369, reported on funds voted by Parliament for several special hospitals. Also see Keir Waddington, *Charity and the London Hospitals, 1850–1898* (Woodbridge, UK: Boydell Press in association with the Royal Historical Society, 2000).

37. Peterson, *Medical Profession,* p. 264.

38. *The Lancet* (1851), 1, 137.

39. "London: Saturday, October 22, 1852," *The Lancet* (1852), 1, 382.

40. "London: Saturday, October 22, 1852," p. 382.

41. "London: Saturday, October 22, 1852," p. 382.

42. "London: Saturday, October 22, 1852," p. 383.

43. "London: Saturday, October 22, 1852," p. 383.

44. "Specialism," *The Lancet* (1857), 2, 635.

45. "London: Saturday, December 25, 1858," *The Lancet* (1858), 2, 658–59.

46. "London: Saturday, December 26, 1857," *The Lancet* (1857), 2, 650; "London: Saturday, July 14, 1860," *The Lancet* (1860), 1, 40.

47. "Special Hospitals," *The Lancet* (1860), 2, 97.

48. "Special Hospitals," *The Lancet* (1860), 2, 574–75.

49. Keith Waddington, "Finance, Philanthropy and the Hospital: Metropolitan Hospitals 1850–1898," Ph.D. Thesis, University College, London, 1995, pp.163–64, suggests that special hospitals were actually more successful at attracting philanthropic support than were general hospitals.

50. Benjamin C. Brodie, "Sir Benjamin Brodie on Special Hospitals," letter of July 16, 1860, in *The Lancet* (1860), 2, 92. See also "London: Saturday, August 6, 1864," *The Lancet* (1864), 2, 159.

51. See, for instance, the letter from Walter Rivington, "A Plea for Special Hospitals," *BMJ* (1863), 1, 31.

52. *The Lancet* (1859), 2, 624.

53. For instance, "Special Hospitals: Letter from Dr. Henry Savage," *The Lancet* (1858), 2, 47–48.

54. Henry I. Bowditch, "Minority Report," *TAMA*,17(1866), 511–12; this is reprinted in Charles E. Rosenberg, ed., *The Origins of Specialization in American Medicine* (New York: Garland, 1989), pp. 29–30. This is discussed in chapter 4 of this volume.

55. "London: Saturday, September 1, 1860," *The Lancet* (1860), 2, 216–17.

56. Guy's opened an ophthalmic department in 1824, an electrotherapy department in 1833, and an obstetric department in 1842; but it does not seem to have created another department—for the throat—until 1885.

57. "London: Saturday, February 6, 1869," *The Lancet* (1869), 2, 197.

58. "London: Saturday, February 6, 1869," p. 195.

59. "London: Saturday, July 14, 1860," *The Lancet* (1860), 2, 40–41; "London: Saturday, September, 1, 1860," *The Lancet* (1860), 2, 216–17. This idea was taken up by his successor in "London: Saturday, August 6, 1864," *The Lancet*, (1864), 2, 159–60.

60. "London: Saturday, July 14, 1860," *The Lancet* (1860), 2, 40–41; "London: Saturday, July 21, 1860," *The Lancet* (1860), 2, 65–66; "London: Saturday, September, 1, 1860," *The Lancet* (1860), 2, 216–17. For similar views by Wakley's successor, see "London: Saturday, August 6, 1864," *The Lancet* (1864), 2, 159–60.

61. For examples, see Peterson, *Medical Profession*, pp. 276–77.

62. "Specialism," *The Lancet* (1866), 2, 732.

63. Brian Abel-Smith, *The Hospitals, 1800–1948: A Study in Social Administration in England and Wales* (London: Heinemann, 1964), p.159. This is based on a report of the *Hospital Gazette.*

64. Peterson, *Medical Profession*, p. 248.

65. T. McCall Anderson, "The Progress of Dermatology During the Last Quarter Century," *BMJ* (1879), 2, 239–40. Obstetricans were particularly unhappy that they were not permitted to do gynecological surgery. Clemont Godson, "Address, Section of Obstetrical Medicine, Annual Meeting BMA, 1884," *BMJ* (1884), 2, 232–33.

66. My comments are based on communications from Keir Waddington and Elsbeth Heaman. I am grateful to both for sharing their opinions with me. For an extended discussion of these hospitals, see Waddington, *Charity and the London Hospitals,* and *Medical Education at St. Bartholomew's Hospital, 1123–1995* (Woodbridge, U.K., and Rochester, N.Y.: Boydell Press, 2003); E. A. Heaman, *St Mary's: The History of a London Teaching Hospital* (Montreal: McGill-Queen's University Press, 2003).

67. "London: Saturday, February 6, 1869," *The Lancet* (1869), 1, 196–97.

68. "The Ethics of Specialism," *The Lancet* (1866), 2, 777. Shortly before, he had defended specialization as a necessity of medical progress. *The Lancet* (1866), 2, 552.

69. Cooter, *Surgery and Society*, p. 28.

70. George Hunter, "The Place of Specialism in General Practice, with Reference to Diseases of the Eye, Ear, and Throat," *Edinburgh Medical Journal*, 31 (1885), 429–34, 521–

26, and "The Place of Specialism in General Practice, with Reference to Diseases of the Eye, Ear, and Naso-Pharynx," *Edinburgh Medical Journal*, 33 (1888), 905–12, 997–1009.

71. Sturdy and Cooter, "Science, Scientific Management," pp. 427–28.

72. Granshaw, "Fame and Fortune," p. 212. Such movement is also evident from posts listed in medical directories. See George Weisz, "Medical Directories and Medical Specialization in France, Britain and the United States," *BHM*, 71 (1997), 23–68.

73. "London: Saturday, October 2, 1875," *The Lancet* (1875), 2, 495; J. Russel Reynolds, "An Address on Specialism in Medicine," *The Lancet* (1881), 2, 655–58. One could also set good specialism that sought to benefit mankind and the profession against a bad, self-interested and commercial form of specialism. "Legitimate and Illegitimate Specialization," *BMJ* (1891), 2, 112.

74. "London: Saturday, May 13, 1876," *The Lancet* (1876), 1, 712–13. A year later the journal endorsed a proposal to combine several special hospitals into a "polyclinique" that could be used for teaching purposes. "A United Special Hospital," *The Lancet* (1877), 1, 885–86.

75. Geoffery Rivet, *The Development of the London Hospital System* (London: King Edward Hospital Fund, 1986), p. 49.

76. Peterson, *Medical Profession*, p.191.

77. This was Robert Brudenell Carter, *List of Lecturers and Lectures at the Royal College of Surgeons of England, 1810–1900, compiled by Victor Plarr* (London: Taylor and Francis, 1900), p. 11. The original announcement was in "London: June 24, 1876," *The Lancet* (1876), 1, 930–31.

78. Archives of the Royal College of Surgeons, Minutes of the Council, vol. 11, Mar. 11, 1869, pp. 538–39; May 13, 1869, pp. 549–51; Aug. 12, 1869, p.578. When he retired from it after ten years, James Paget was instrumental in transforming it, with Wilson's agreement, into a professorship in pathology. Minutes of the Council, vol. 12, June 12, 1879, pp. 638–40.

79. "Wilson, Sir William James Erasmus (1809–1884)," in Victor Plarr, *Lives of the Fellows of the Royal College of Surgeons of England* (Bristol: Royal College of Surgeons, 1930) pp. 534–35; Rosemary Stevens, *Medical Practice in Modern England: The Impact of Specialization and State Medicine* (New Haven, Conn.: Yale University Press, 1966), p. 28.

80. Cope, *Royal College of Surgeons*, p. 73.

81. "London: Saturday, June 24, 1876," *The Lancet* (1876), 1, 931. Also see *The Lancet* (1890), 2, 253; and John St. Swithin Wilders, "An Addresss . . . Section of Laryngology and Rhinology . . . BMA . . . 1890," *BMJ* (1890), 2, 376–77.

82. Sturdy and Cooter, "Science, Scientific Management," p. 429.

83. "Specialism," *The Lancet* (1905), 1, 727.

84. Minutes of the Arrangements Committee, in BMA Archives, Minutes of Council and Subcommittees, 1888–89, p.1165.

85. Sturdy and Cooter, "Science, Scientific Management," pp. 429–30.

86. "The Obstetrician-Physician or Surgeon?" *The Lancet* (1902), 1, 979, as well as 1138, 1211–12, and 1270; Geoffrey Chamberlain, *Victor Bonney: The Gynaecological Surgeon of the Twentieth Century* (New York and London: Parthenon, 2000).

87. "The Relation of the Anaesthetists to the Patient and to the Surgeon," *The Lancet* (1903), 2, 1442–43, discussion, 1464; also 1683–85 and 1756–57; "The Professional Status of the Anaesthetists," *The Lancet* (1908), 2, 1805–06.

88. "Specialism," *The Lancet* (1905), 1, 727.

89. Peterson, *Medical Profession*, p. 269; Lomax, *Small and Special*, pp.153–55.

90. "General Council of Medical Education and Registration," *BMJ* (1890), 1, 1305.

91. Peterson, *Medical Profession*, p. 266.

92. "The Multiplication of Specialty Societies," *The Lancet* (1893), 1, 373.

93. Maurice Davidson, *The Royal Society of Medicine: The Realization of an Ideal, 1805–1955* (London: Royal Society of Medicine, 1955), pp. 31–32.

94. Peterson, *Medical Profession*, pp. 267, 270–71.

95. *The Specialist*, 1 (1880–81) and 2 (1881–82). It was edited by Herbert Junius Hardwick, who described himself as physician at the Public Hospital for Skin Diseases and at the Ear and Throat Hospital, both in Sheffield.

96. This was called *Medical Specialists and Their Work* and was criticized in "Medical Specialists," *BMJ* (1891), 2, 1244, as well as in *The Lancet* (1889), 1, 89.

97. This was W.P.W. Phillimore, ed., *The Dictionary of Medical Specialists: Being a Classified List of London Practitioners Who Chiefly Attend to Special Departments of Medicine and Surgery* (London: Chas. J. Clark, 1889). The second publication was C. Bracebridge Allen, *London Medical Specialists* (London: Ward and Lock, 1890).

98. Robert Pinker, *English Hospital Statistics, 1861–1938* (London: Heinemann, 1966), p. 57.

99. Pinker, *English Hospital Statistics*, p. 61.

100. Calculated from Phillimore, *Dictionary of Medical Specialists.*

101. On Manchester, see Pickstone, *Medicine and Industrial Society*, pp. 190–93.

102. "The Development of Specialism," *BMJ* (1908), 1, 946–47.

103. Archives of Saint Mary's Hospital, MS/AD 5/3, 82a. Elsbeth Heaman kindly provided me with this quote.

104. "The Development of Specialism," *BMJ* (1908), 1, 947.

105. "Development of Specialism," p. 946.

106. Stevens, *Medical Practice in England*, p. 3, calculates that in 1939 there was one specialist for every six or seven GPs.

107. Phillimore, *Dictionary of Medical Specialists*, defines specialists as those having hospital affiliation. Bracebridge Allen, *London Medical Specialists*, does not, but most of the specialists he lists, have hospital posts. An exception is pediatrics.

108. Anne Digby, *The Evolution of British General Practice, 1850–1948* (Oxford: Oxford University Press, 1999), p. 294.

109. This is discussed in detail in Weisz, "Medical Directories and Medical Specialization," especially pp. 62–64.

110. Stevens, *Medical Practice in England*, pp. 32–33.

111. *International Directory of Laryngologists and Otologists*, ed. Richard Lake (London: Rebman Publishing, 1899; 2nd ed., 1961), preface to 2nd ed.

112. Lawrence, "Incommunicable Knowledge," 503–20. For a good example, see "London: Saturday, October 22, 1881," *The Lancet* (1881), 2, 720.

113. This is discussed by Cooter, *Surgery and Society*, pp. 46–52.

114. Peterson, *Medical Profession*, p. 278; Stevens, *Medical Practice in England*, p. 29.

115. D. Argyll Robertson, "Address to the Section of Ophthalmology," *BMJ* (1898), 2, 308–9. For examples in pediatrics, see Lomax, *Small and Special*, p. 155.

116. Felix Semon, "English and German Education: A Parallel," *BMJ* (1907), 2, 1198. Also see "The Profession of Medicine," *BMJ* (1905), 2, 473. The situation was little changed in 1918, although the syllabus for the University of London included material in otorhinolaryngology and skin diseases. It also included a three-month clerkship in obstetrics and gynecology and another three months in a special department. George Newman, *Some Notes of Medical Education in England* (London: His Majesty's Stationery Office, 1918), pp. 24, 71.

117. "Post-graduate Study," *BMJ* (1905), 2, 514.

118. "Post-graduate Study," p. 514.

119. *The Lancet* (1905), 1, 1020–21, gives an account of the views of Sir William Church and Sir Frederick Treves at the initial planning meeting.

120. *The Lancet* (1907), 1, 1719. Also see Royal Society of Medicine, *Record of the Events and Work Which Led to the Formation of That Society by the Amalgamation . . .* (London: Adlard, 1914); Penelope Hunting, *The History of the Royal Society of Medicine* (London: Royal Society of Medicine Press, 2001), pp. 170–76.

121. David Innes Williams, "RSM 1907: The Acceptance of Specialization," *Journal of the Royal Society of Medicine*, 93 (2000), 642–45.

122. G. N. Clark, *A History of the Royal College of Physicians of London*, 3 vols. (Oxford: Clarendon Press for the Royal College of Physicians, 1964–72), vol. 3 (by A. M. Cooke), p. 885.

123. Clark (Cooke), *History of the Royal College of Physicians*, pp. 885–86.

124. "Annual Meeting," *BMJ* (1861), 1, 124–28; "Historical Sketch of the British Medical Association," *BMJ* (1882), 1, 847–64.

125. Recent books on the BMA, such as Bartrip, *Themselves Writ Large*, have nothing to say about the institution's response to specialization.

126. In 1906 the Ethical Committee of the BMA decided that doctors should not furnish photographs or biographical information to directories. *BMJ* (1906), 1, 1567.

127. For instance, John St. Swithin Wilders, "An Addresss . . . Section of Laryngology and Rhinology . . . BMA . . . 1890."

128. *History of the British Medical Association* (London: the Association, 1982), vol. 1, comp. Ernest Muirhead Little, p. 320 (originally published 1932); vol. 2, ed. E. Grey-Turner and F. M. Sutherland, pp. 68, 170–71, 272, 317.

129. When the *British Medical Directory*, before World War I, decided that entries could list only three previous hospital appointments, the measure raised a storm because the career history of hospital appointments was recognized to be a key indicator of specialist competence. "The Medical Directory for 1914," *BMJ* (1913), 2, 352, 436, 776.

Chapter 3

1. Mary Lindemann, *Health and Healing in Eighteenth-Century Germany* (Baltimore and London: Johns Hopkins University Press, 1996), pp.145–64; Sabine Sander, *Handwerkschirurgen: Sozialgeschichte einer verdrängten Berufsgruppe* (Göttingen: Vandenhoeck & Ruprecht, 1989), pp. 55–66.

2. Lindemann, *Health and Healing*, p. 151.

3. Rainer Nabielek, "Zur Entwicklung der Augenheilkunde in Berlin 1800–1850," in *Die Medizin an der Berliner Universität und an der Charité zwischen 1810 und 1850*, ed.

Peter Schneck and Hans-Uwe Lammel (Husum: Matthiesen Verlag, 1995), p.168, claims that there were no surgical specialists of the eye in the mid-eighteenth century.

4. Wilfried Teicher, "Untersuchungen zur ärztlichen Spezialisierung im Spiegel des Reichsmedizinalkalenders am Beispiel Preußens im ersten Drittel des 20. Jahrhunderts" (M.D. thesis, Johannes-Gutenberg-Universität Mainz, 1992), p. 22; Jürgen Schlumbohm, "'The Pregnant Women Are Here for the Sake of the Teaching Institution': The Lying-in Hospital of Göttingen University, 1751-c. 1830," *SHM*, 14 (2001), 59–78, especially 60–61.

5. Sander, *Handwerkschirurgen*, pp. 61, 76, and 296, n. 39.

6. Quoted in Hermann Lampe, *Die Entwicklung und Differenzierung von Fachabteilungen auf den Versammlungen von 1823 bis 1913: Bibliographie zur Erfassung der Sektionsvortäge mit einer Darstellung der Entstehung der Sektionen und ihrer Problematik* (Hildesheim: Verlag Dr. H. A. Gerstenberg, 1975), p. 2.

7. Claudia Huerkamp, *Der Aufstieg der Ärzte im 19. Jahrhundert: Vom gelehrten Stand zum professionellen Experten; Das Beispiel Preußens* (Göttingen: Vandenhoeck & Ruprecht, 1985), and "The Making of the Modern Medical Profession, 1800–1914: Prussian Doctors in the Nineteenth Century," in *German Professions, 1800–1950*, ed. Geoffrey Cocks and Konrad H. Jarausch (New York and Oxford: Oxford University Press, 1990), pp. 66–84, at p. 68.

8. Thomas Neville Bonner, *Becoming a Physician: Medical Education in Great Britain, France, Germany, and the United States, 1750–1945* (Oxford: Oxford University Press, 1995), p. 93.

9. Huerkamp, "Making of the Modern Medical Profession," p. 68.

10. Bonner, *Becoming a Physician*, pp. 187–88.

11. Manfred Stürtzbecher, "Allgemeine und Spezialkrankenhäuser, insbesondere Privatkrankenanstalten im 19. Jahrhundert in Berlin," in *Studien zur Krankenhausgeschichte im 19. Jahrhundert im Hinblick auf die Entwicklung in Deutschland*, ed. Hans Schadewaldt (Göttingen: Vandenhoeck & Ruprecht, 1976), pp. 105–6.

12. Johanna Bleker, "To Benefit the Poor and Advance Medical Science: Hospitals and Hospital Care in Germany, 1820–1870," in *Medicine and Modernity: Public Health and Medical Care in Nineteenth- and Twentieth-Century Germany*, ed. Manfred Berg and Geoffrey Cocks (Cambridge: Cambridge University Press, 1997), pp. 17–33, at p. 24.

13. Hans-Heinz Eulner, "Das Spezialistentum in der ärztlichen Praxis," in *Der Arzt und der Kranke in der Gesellschaft des 19. Jahrhunderts*, ed. Walter Artelt and Walter Rüegg (Stuttgart: Ferdinand Enke Verlag, 1967), p. 20; Huerkamp, *Aufstieg der Ärzte*, p. 93.

14. Bonner, *Becoming a Physician*, p. 160. Hans-Heinz Eulner, *Die Entwicklung der medizinischen Spezialfächer an den Universitäten des deutschen Sprachgebietes* (Stuttgart: Ferdinand Enke Verlag, 1970), at the end of each chapter devoted to a specialty adds lists of events relevant to that specialty, including courses offered during these early years.

15. Eulner, "Spezialistentum in der ärztlichen Praxis," p. 21.

16. Volker Hess, "Raum und Disziplin: Klinische Wissenschaft im Krankenhaus," *Berichte zur Wissenschaftsgeschichte*, 23 (2000), 317–29.

17. Peter Schneck, "Die Anfänge der Krankenwärterausbildung an der Charité durch Johann Friedrich Dieffenbach (1792–1847) und Carl Emil Gedike (1797–1867)," in *Die Medizin an der Berliner Universität und an der Charité zwischen 1810 und*

1850, ed. Peter Schneck and Hans-Uwe Lammel (Husum: Matthiesen Verlag, 1995), p. 180; Nabieklek, "Entwicklung der Augenheilkunde," p. 175.

18. Isabelle von Bueltzingsloewen, *Machines à instruire, machines à guérir: Les hôpitaux universitaires et la médicalisation de la société allemande, 1730–1850* (Lyons: Presses Univeritaires de Lyons, 1997), p. 210.

19. A university clinic was established in 1838 but was not very successful. Johanna Bleker, " . . . der einzig wahre Weg, brauchbare Männer zu bilden"—Der medizinisch-klinische Unterricht an der Berliner Universität, 1810–1850," in *Die Medizin an der Berliner Universität und an der Charité zwischen 1810 und 1850*, ed. Peter Schneck und Hans-Uwe Lammel (Husum: Matthiesen Verlag, 1995). On conflicts between universities and hospitals, see Bleker, "To Benefit the Poor," pp. 24–25.

20. R. Steven Turner, "The Great Transition and the Social Patterns of German Science," *Minerva*, 25 (1987), 56–76, especially 62–56.

21. Lorraine Daston, "The Academies and the Unity of Knowledge: The Disciplining of the Disciplines," *Difference: A Journal of Feminist Cultural Studies*, 10 (1998), 67–86, at 72. On early university reform, see Charles McClelland, *State, Society, and University in Germany, 1700–1914* (Cambridge: Cambridge University Press, 1980); Turner, "The Great Transition"; Gert Schubring, ed., *"Einsamkeit und Freiheit" neu besichtigt: Universitätsreformen und Disziplinenbildung in Preußen als Modell für Wissenschaftspolitik im Europa des 19. Jahrhunderts* (Stuttgart: Franz Steiner Verlag, 1991).

22. Timothy Lenoir, *The Strategy of Life: Teleology and Mechanics in Nineteenth-Century German Biology* (Chicago: University of Chicago Press, 1989; 1st ed., 1982).

23. Lampe, *Entwicklung und Differenzierung*, pp. 1–22.

24. For the argument that the ideals of humanist *Bildung* were in fact compatible with disciplinary specialization, see Rudolf Stichweh, *Études sur la genèse du système scientifique moderne*, trans. Fabienne Blaise (Lille: Presses Universitaires de Lille, 1991), pp. 111–30.

25. Theodor Billroth, *The Medical Sciences in the German Universities: A Study in the History of Civilization*, trans. and with an introduction by William H. Welch (New York: Macmillan, 1924), p. 30.

26. Erna Lesky, *The Vienna Medical School of the Nineteenth Century*, trans. L. Williams and I. S. Levij (Baltimore: Johns Hopkins University Press, 1976), p. 39.

27. Lesky, *Vienna Medical School*, p. 205.

28. Lesky, *Vienna Medical School*, p. 52.

29. Von Bueltzingsloewen, *Machines à instruire*, pp. 102–3.

30. Elizabeth M. R. Lomax, *Small and Special: The Development of Hospitals for Children in Victorian Britain*, Medical History, supp. no. 16 (London: Wellcome Institute for the History of Medicine, 1996), p. 15; Lesky, *Vienna Medical School*, pp. 40–41.

31. Nabielek, "Entwicklung der Augenheilkunde," pp. 167–77; Eulner, *Entwicklung der medizinischen Spezialfächer*, p. 345.

32. Lesky, *Vienna Medical School*, pp. 60–62; Helmut Wyklicky and Manfred Skopec, "The Development of Clinical Instruction in Vienna," in *History of Medical Education: Proceedings of the 6th International Symposium on the Comparative History of Medicine—East and West*, ed. Teizo Ogawa (Tokyo: Taniguchi Foundation, 1983), pp. 146–47.

33. Godelieve van Heteren, "Students Facing Boundaries: The Shift of Nineteenth-Century British Student Travel to German Universities and the Flexible Boundaries of a

Medical Education System," in *The History of Medical Education in Britain*, ed. Vivian Nutton and Roy Porter (Amsterdam and Atlanta: Rodopi, 1995), pp. 280–340 especially p. 305.

34. Wilhelm Herzig, *Das medicinische Wien: Wegweiser für Aerzte and Naturforscher, vorzugsweise für Fremde* (Vienna: Braumüller & Seidel, 1844), p. 210.

35. Carl Wunderlich, *Wien und Paris: Ein Beitrag zur Geschichte und Beurteilung der gegenwärtigen Heilkunde in Deutschland und Frankreich* (Stuttgart: Ebner & Seubert, 1841; new ed., Bern: H. Huber, 1974). See chapter 1 in this volume.

36. Surgery was not as well represented in German universities as in Paris. Eulner, *Entwicklung der medizinischen Spezialfächer*, pp. 320–21; Billroth, *Medical Sciences in German Universities*, p. 33. Even in the 1930s, though medical faculties had many lower-level surgical personnel, they continued to have relatively few full professorships in surgery. Johannes Müller, *Statistische Untersuchungen über Vorlesungen und Dozenten der medizinischen Fakultäten der deutschen Universitäten in den Jahren 1927 bis 1931–32* (Berlin: Struppe & Winckler, 1933), pp. 98–99.

37. Eulner, "Spezialistentum in der ärztlichen Praxis," pp. 20–21.

38. Lesky, *Vienna Medical School*, pp. 16–18, 96–98.

39. In what follows, I base myself on the accounts in Lesky, *Vienna Medical School*; and Leopold Schönbauer, *Das medizinische Wien: Geschichte, Werden, Würdigung*, 2nd ed. (Vienna: Urban & Schwarzenberg, 1947), pp. 206–300.

40. Lesky, *Vienna Medical School*, p. 160; Schönbauer, *Das Medizinische Wien*, p. 267.

41. Based on Lesky, *Vienna Medical School*, pp. 99, 102, 206; Schönbauer, *Das Medizinische Wien*, p. 265; Eulner, *Entwicklung der medizinischen Spezialfächer*, p. 223. Eighteen lecturers were appointed in 1848 and 1849.

42. Lesky, *Vienna Medical School*, p. 104.

43. Lesky, *Vienna Medical School*, p. 36; Schönbauer, *Das Medizinische Wien*, p. 267.

44. Lesky, *Vienna Medical School*, p. 102; Schönbauer, *Das Medizinische Wien*, p. 244–50, 268.

45. Herzig, *Das medicinische Wien*, pp. 374–82.

46. Van Heteren, "Students Facing Boundaries," p. 310.

47. "Note from *Wien Med.Wochen*," *BMJ* (1864), 2, 371, mentions several oculists and a laryngologist.

48. "Specialist, einer, der einem besondern Fach der Wissenschaft sich ausschließlich widmet, z.B. Specialarzt. . . . " Eulner, "Spezialistentum in der ärztlichen Praxis," pp. 17–18.

49. Eulner, *Entwicklung der medizinischen Spezialfächer*, pp. 258–59.

50. George Rosen, *The Specialization of Medicine with Particular Reference to Ophthalmology* (New York, Froben Press, 1944), discussed in the introduction and chapter 1, above. Also see Eulner, "Spezialistentum in der ärztlichen Praxis," p. 20.

51. R. Steven Turner: "The Growth of Professorial Research in Prussia, 1818 to 1848—Causes and Context," *Historical Studies in the Physical Sciences*, 3 (1971), 137–82; "University Reformers and Professorial Scholarship in Germany, 1769–1806," in *The University in Society*, ed. Lawrence Stone, 2 vols. (Princeton, N.J.: Princeton University Press, 1974), vol. 2, pp. 495–531;"The Great Transition," pp. 56–76; and "German Science, German Universities: Historiographical Perspectives from the 1980s," in *"Einsamkeit und Freiheit" neu besichtigt: Universitätsreformen und Disziplinenbildung in*

Preußen als Modell für Wissenschaftspolitik im Europa des 19. Jahrhunderts, ed. Gert Schubring (Stuttgart: Franz Steiner Verlag, 1991), pp. 24–36. Also see Rudolf Stichweh, *Zur Entstehung des modernen Systems wissenschaftlicher Disziplinen: Physik in Deutschland, 1740–1890* (Frankfurt: Suhrkamp, 1984).

52. On German universities, see McClelland, *State, Society, and University;* Christian Bonah, *Instruire, guérir, servir: Formation et pratique médicales en France et en Allemagne* (Strasbourg: Presses Universitaires de Strasbourg, 2000); Christophe Charle, ed., *Les universités germaniques XIXe–XXe siècle* (Paris: Service d'Histoire de l'Éducation INRP, 1994).

53. Ludwig Traube, "Ueber Special-Kliniken," *Medicinische Reform,* 1 (1848), 16–19, 23–25, 31–33. Reprinted Hildesheim and New York: Georg Olms Verlag, 1975. Reprint, facsimile edition of journal.

54. Traube, "Ueber Special-Kliniken," p. 32.

55. Traube, "Ueber Special-Kliniken," p. 33.

56. Huerkamp, *Aufstieg der Ärzte;* Dominik Gross, *Die Aufhebung des Wundarztberufs: Ursachen, Begleitumstände, und Auswirkungen am Beispiel des Königreichs Württemberg, 1806–1918* (Stuttgart: Franz Steiner Verlag, 1999); Bonah, *Instruire, guérir, servir,* pp. 163, 166–68.

57. Bonah, *Instruire, guérir, servir,* pp.164, 171.

58. For illustrations provided by the careers of Jacob Henle and others, see Arleen Marcia Tuchman, *Science, Medicine and the State in Germany: The Case of Baden, 1815–1871* (New York and Oxford: Oxford University Press, 1993), pp. 54–68.

59. Tuchman, *Science, Medicine, and the State,* p. 75. Also see Peter Borscheid, *Naturwissenschaft, Staat und Industrie in Baden (1848–1914)* (Stuttgart: Klett, 1976).

60. Timothy Lenoir, "Laboratories, Medicine and Public Life in Germany 1830–1849: Ideological Roots of the Institutional Revolution," in *The Laboratory Revolution in Medicine,* ed. Andrew Cunningham and Perry Williams (Cambridge: Cambridge University Press, 1992), pp. 14–71.

61. For instance, Otto Körner, *Die Arbeitsteilung in der Heilkunde* (Wiesbaden: Verlag von J.F. Bergmann, 1909), p. 10.

62. Lampe, *Entwicklung und Differenzierung,* pp. 26, 82–121.

63. In many cases, the creation of a section preceded by a few years the establishment of an independent specialist society.

64. Paul Börner, *Das Medicinalwesen Deutschlands im Jahre 1883: Separatabdruck von Dr. Paul Börner's Reichs-Medicinal-Kalender, II. Theil, 1884* (Berlin: Verlag von Theodor Fischer, 1884), pp. 295–96.

65. Eulner, *Entwicklung der medizinischen Spezialfächer,* provides chronologies throughout.

66. This was the procedure followed by Albrecht von Graefe in Berlin and Alfred Karl Graefe in Halle. Wolfram Kaiser and Arina Völker, "Zur Entwicklung klinischer Spezialdisziplinen an der Universität Halle," *Wissenschaftliche Zeitschrift der Wilhelm-Pieck-Universität Rostock,* 32 (1983), Gesellschaftswissenschaftliche Reihe, Heft 9, 66–70.

67. Bonah, *Instruire, guérir, servir,* pp. 112–17; Eulner, *Entwicklung der medizinischen Spezialfächer,* throughout. Also see Lesky, *Vienna Medical School;* Wyklicky and Skopec, "Development of Clinical Instruction in Vienna,"; Billroth, *Medical Sciences in German Universities,* p. 35; and Kaiser and Völker, "Entwicklung klinischer Spezialdisziplinen," pp. 67–68.

68. Stürtzbecher, "Allgemeine und Spezialkrankenhäuser," p. 116.

69. Bonah, *Instruire, guérir, servir,* pp. 170–71, discusses the movement to transform municipal hospitals into university institutions.

70. Michael H. Kater, "Professionalization and Socialization of Physicians in Wilhelmine and Weimar Germany," *Journal of Contemporary History,* 20 (1985), 677–701, especially 680–81.

71. Kaiser and Völker, "Entwicklung klinischer Spezialdisziplinen."

72. On courses in the fundamental sciences, many of which had existed in France since the beginning of the century, see Bonah, *Instruire, guérir, servir,* pp. 109–17. The German emphasis on basic sciences has been noted by Bonner, *Becoming a Physician.*

73. Bonah, *Instruire, guérir, servir,* pp. 113–17.

74. Bonah, *Instruire, guérir, servir,* p. 227; McClelland, *State, Society and University,* p. 280.

75. Friedrich Paulsen, *The German Universities and University Study,* trans. Frank Thilly and William Elwang (New York: Longmans, Green, 1906), p. 219.

76. Arthur Hartmann, "Die medicinische Ausbildung in Specialfächern," *ÄVD,* 21 (1892), 64.

77. Report in *ÄVD,* 6 (1879), 10.

78. Börner, *Medicinalwesen Deutschlands 1883,* pp. 295–96, 314–15.

79. Billroth, *Medical Sciences in German Universities,* pp. 74–76. On Billroth, see Karel B. Absolon, *The Belle Epoque of Surgery: The Life and Times of Theodor Billroth* (Rockville, Md.: Kabel Publishers, 1995).

80. Börner, *Medicinalwesen Deutschlands 1883,* pp. 295–96.

81. The figures were 23.6 hours weekly versus 41.5 hours weekly. Heinrich Quinke, "Über ärztliche Spezialitäten und Spezialärzte," *MMW,* 53 (1906), 1263.

82. Otto Winkelmann, "Die privaten Krankenanstalten und die Medizin des 19. Jahrhunderts," in *Medizingeschichte in unserer Zeit: Festgabe für Edith Heischkel-Artelt und Walter Artelt zum 65. Geburtstag,* ed. Hans-Heinz Eulner et al. (Stuttgart: Ferdinand Enke Verlag, 1971), pp. 369–83; Stürtzbecher, "Allgemeine und Spezialkrankenhäuser," p.112. Dentistry is included here thanks to a personal communication from Ulrich Tröhler.

83. Winkelman, "Die privaten Krankenanstalten," p. 373.

84. Stürtzbecher, "Allgemeine und Spezialkrankenhäuser," p.112; Winkelmann, "Die privaten Krankenanstalten," p. 381.

85. Heinrich Riedl, "Die Auseinandersetzungen um die Spezialisierung in der Medizin von 1862 bis 1925" (M.D. thesis, Faculty of Medicine, Technische Universität München, 1981), p. 9.

86. Other cases included Hauner in Munich, pediatrics; Heine in Wurtzburg, pediatrics; and Georg Beer in Vienna, ophthalmology. Teicher, "Untersuchungen zur ärztlichen Spezialisierung," p. 14.

87. Winkelmann, "Die privaten Krankenanstalten," pp. 381–82.

88. Teicher, "Untersuchungen zur ärztlichen Spezialisierung," p. 70.

89. Bonah, *Instruire, guérir, servir,* pp. 459–72.

90. Huerkamp, *Aufstieg der Ärzte,* pp. 108–9; Bonah, *Instruire, guérir, servir,* p. 288.

91. Eulner, *Entwicklung der medizinischen Spezialfächer,* throughout; Riedl, "Auseinandersetzungen um die Spezialisierung," p. 8.

92. For example, the report of a speech by Prof. V. Tröltsch arguing that the wide-spread nature of ear maladies justified a placed on the *Prüfung*. *ÄVD*, 6 (1879), 10; Albert Neisser, "Die Dermatologie und Syphilologie in dem Entwurf der Prüfungsordnung," *DMW*, 22 (1896), 685–86.

93. Huerkamp, "Making of the Modern Medical Profession," p. 69; Eulner, *Die Entwicklung der medizinischen Spezialfächer*, p. 181.

94. Huerkamp, "Making of the Modern Medical Profession," p. 69; Riedl, "Auseinandersetzungen um die Spezialisierung," p. 84; J. Schwalbe, "Standesangelegenheiten," *DMW*, 28 (1902), 16–17.

95. The best sources of information on these matters are the lists that Eulner, *Entwicklung der medizinischen Spezialfächer*, appends to his chapters on individual specialties. The ones mentioned here are on pp. 281 (psychiatry), 255 (dermatology/venereology), 294 (gynecology), and 346 (ophthalmology). On the history of the major specialty journals in Germany, see Vitolf Laube, "Die deutschen Referatenblätter der medizinischen Spezialfächer im 19. und frühen 20. Jahrhundert" (M.D. thesis, Johann-Wolfgang-Goethe-Universität zu Frankfurt-am-Main, 1954).

96. Eulner, *Entwicklung der medizinischen Spezialfächer*, p. 255.

97. Pierre Huard and M. J. Imbault-Huart, "L'enseignement libre de la médecine à Paris au XIXe siècle," *Revue d'histoire des sciences*, 37 (1974), 45–62.

98. Paul Börner's directory, *Medicinalwesen Deutschlands 1883*, included listings of these other German-language universities, pp. 312–18.

99. Whereas in 1919 there were 176 professors and 251 middle- and junior-level personnel in France, a year later there were 292 professors and 863 middle- and junior-level personnel in just the twenty medical schools of Germany. Bonah, *Instruire, guérir, servir*, pp. 84–85.

100. Joseph Ben-David, *The Scientist's Role in Society: A Comparative Study* (Chicago: University of Chicago Press, 1984; 1st ed., 1971).

101. Albert Neisser, "Über den Nutzen und Notwendigkeit von Spezialkliniken für haut- und venerische Kranke," *Klinisches Jahrbuch*, 2 (1890), 197, cited in Eulner, *Entwicklung der medizinischen Spezialfächer*, p. 224. Also see Neisser, "Dermatologie und Syphilologie," 685–86.

102. Eulner, "Spezialistentum in der ärztlichen Praxis " p. 23.

103. Lesky, *Vienna Medical School*, p. 208.

104. Eulner, *Entwicklung der medizinischen Spezialfächer*, p. 261.

105. Heinrich Rohlfs, "Über den Sozialismus in der Medizin," *Deutsche Klinik*, 14 (1861–62), 94–95, cited in Riedl, "Auseinandersetzungen um die Spezialisierung," pp.11, 58.

106. *Die Verbreitung des Heilpersonals, der pharmazeutischen Anstalten und des pharmazeutischen Personals im Deutschen Reiche, nach dem amtlichen Erhebungen vom 1. April 1887, bearbeitet im Kaiserlichen Gesundheitsamte* (Berlin: Verlag von Julius Springer, 1889).

107. Huerkamp, *Aufstieg der Ärzte*, p. 180.

108. Börner, *Medicinalwesen Deutschlands 1883*.

109. *Berlin-Verzeichniss der Einwohner nach ihren Beschäftigungen und Gewerben, 1883*. Berlin Stadt-Bibliothek (City Library), Berlin Einwohner Verzeichniss microfilm collection, 1883/9/20.

110. Annette Drees, *Die Ärzte auf dem Weg zu Prestige und Wohlstand: Sozialgeschichte der württembergischen Ärzte im 19. Jahrhundert* (Münster: F. Coppenrath Verlag, 1988), pp. 172–77.

111. Georg Heimann, "Deutschlands Spezialärzte," *DMW*, 27 (1901), 377. The three above-mentioned cities had a ratio of specialists to all doctors of 1:3 or less. The ratio in Berlin was 1:6.4.

112. *BMJ* (1906), 1, 752.

113. Teicher, "Untersuchungen zur ärztlichen Spezialisierung," p. 48.

114. Konrad H. Jarausch, "The German Professions in History and Theory," in *German Professions, 1800–1950*, ed. Geoffrey Cocks and Konrad H. Jarausch (New York and Oxford: Oxford University Press, 1990), pp. 9–24, especially p. 12, where he speaks of "the often-derided German propensity to join associations (*Vereinsmeierei*)." For an examination of medical associations during this period, see Hedwig Herold-Schmidt, "Ärztliche Interessenvertretung im Kaiserreich, 1871–1914," in *Geschichte der deutschen Ärzteschaft*, ed. Robert Jütte (Cologne: Deutscher Ärzte-Verlag, 1997), pp. 43–96.

115. Huerkamp, "Making of the Modern Medical Profession," p. 79.

116. Hagen Steinhoff, "Die Einwirkung der Deutschen Ärztetage seit ihrem Beginn 1873 auf die Entstehung, das Werden and Wachsen des ärztlichen Berufsrechts, insbesondere der ärztlichen Berufsordnungen" (M.D. thesis, University of Düsseldorf, 1974); Huerkamp, *Aufstieg der Ärzte*, p. 182; and especially Riedl, "Auseinandersetzungen um die Spezialisierung." Throughout.

117. Jarausch, "The German Professions," p. 15. In 1878 such freedom was introduced for the legal profession as well.

118. Huerkamp, "Making of the Modern Medical Profession," pp. 77–79; McClelland, *State, Society and University*, p. 78.

119. Huerkamp, "Making of the Modern Medical Profession," p. 78; Bruno Glaserfeld, "Die Reform der preußischen Aerztekammern und Ehrengerichete," *DMW*, 49 (1923), 1161–63. Several years later, disciplinary honors courts were established as well.

120. Paul Weindling, "Bourgeois Values, Doctors, and the State: The Professionalization of Medicine in Germany, 1848–1933," in *The German Bourgeoisie: Essays on the Social History of the German Middle Class from the Late Eighteenth to the Early Twentieth Century*, ed. David Blackbourn and Richard J. Evans (London and New York: Routledge, 1990), pp. 198–223, especially p. 204; Huerkamp, "Making of the Modern Medical Profession," p. 75; McClelland, *State, Society and University*, p. 136.

121. Eulner, "Spezialistentum in der ärztlichen Praxis," p. 26; Riedl, "Auseinandersetzungen um die Spezialisierung," pp. 29, 39.

122. For instance, the draft questions for debate about the reform of medical training that were prepared for the *Ärztetag* of 1891 included one on the role of specialty clinics. "Organisation des medecinischen Unterrichts," *ÄVD*, 20 (1891), 161.

Chapter 4

1. John Harley Warner, *The Therapeutic Perspective: Medical Practice, Knowledge, and Identity in America, 1820–1855* (Cambridge, Mass.: Harvard University Press, 1986), pp. 11–12.

2. On the most important medical biographies of the nineteenth century, see "American Medical Biography: A Review of the Seven Books on the Subject," *Medical Review of Reviews*, 24 (1918), pp. 1–15. This essay appeared at the front of Howard Atwood Kelly, *Cyclopedia of American Medical Biography* (Philadelphia and London: W.B. Saunders, 1912), vol. 1.

3. Stephen W. Williams, *American Medical Biography: Or Memoirs of Eminent Physicians* (Greenfield, Mass.: L. Merriam & Co., 1845).

4. Williams, *American Medical Biography*, p. 31.

5. Williams, *American Medical Biography*, p. 274.

6. Williams, *American Medical Biography*, p. 17.

7. Williams, *American Medical Biography*, p. 28.

8. Williams, *American Medical Biography*, pp. 583–84, 588.

9. John Morgan, *A Discourse upon the Institution of Medical Schools in America* (Philadelphia: William Bradford, 1765; repr. Baltimore: Johns Hopkins Press, 1937).

10. Abraham Flexner's introduction to the 1937 reprint of Morgan, pp. iii–vi, treats it as an example of specialization. Harold Speert, *Obstetrics and Gynecology in America: A History* (Chicago: American College of Obstetricians and Gynecologists, 1980), p. 85, is even more emphatic on this point.

11. James Jackson, letter of September 17, 1813, in Countway Library, Harvard University, H MS C81.

12. Amalie M. Kass, *Midwifery and Medicine in Boston: Walter Channing M.D., 1786–1876* (Boston: Northeastern University Press, 2002).

13. Samuel David Gross, ed., *Lives of Eminent Physicians and Surgeons of the Nineteenth Century* (Philadelphia: Lindsay and Blakiston, 1861).

14. Gross, *Lives of Eminent Physicians*, p. 343.

15. Gross, *Lives of Eminent Physicians*, p. 514.

16. Gross, *Lives of Eminent Physicians*, p. 628.

17. Gross, *Lives of Eminent Physicians*, p. 821.

18. Gross, *Lives of Eminent Physicians*, pp. 534–35.

19. William Atkinson, ed., *Physicians and Surgeons of the United States* (Philadelphia: Charles Robson, 1878), p. 3.

20. For a brief and useful outline of these developments, see Howard A. Kelly, "History of Obstetrics," in his *Cyclopedia of American Medical Biography*, vol. 1, pp. liv–lvii.

21. Among the permanent committees set up in 1848 was the Committee on Obstetrics. *The Reports of the Committee on Medical Literature* from 1849 included a section on midwifery, and diseases of women and children. *TAMA*, 2 (1849), 371–419.

22. *Medical Directory of Philadelphia, Pennsylvania, Delaware and the Southern Half of New Jersey* (Philadelphia: P. Blakiston, 1885).

23. Deborah Kuhn McGregor, *From Midwives to Medicine: The Birth of American Gynecology* (New Brunswick, N.J.: Rutgers University Press, 1998), especially ch. 3. The account in Regina Morantz-Sanchez, *Conduct Unbecoming a Woman* (New York: Oxford University Press, 1999), also emphasizes the importance of innovation, particularly of the surgical variety, in legitimating the professional identity of gynecologists. This is done less explicitly by Frederick N. Dyer in his *Champion of Women and the Unborn: Horatio Storer, M.D.* (Canton, Mass.: Science History Publications, 1999).

24. Kelly, *Cyclopedia of American Medical Biography*, vol. 1, p. 322.

25. Harry Friedenwald, "Ophthalmology," in Kelly, *Cyclopedia of American Medical Biography*, vol. 1, p. lxii. See also William Campbell Posey and Samuel Horton Brown, *The Wills Hospital of Philadelphia: The Influence of European and British Ophthalmology upon It* (Philadelphia: J.B. Lippincott, 1931), p. 14.

26. For instance, the early New York ophthalmologist Henry Noyes had studied in London with Astley Cooper and Abernathy. Henry D. Noyes, "Account of the Origin and First Meeting of the American Ophthalmological Society, 1864," National Library of Medicine, Archives, Ms. G10, box 1.

27. Posey and Brown, *Wills Hospital*, p. 18.

28. *New York Evening Post*, Mar. 13, 1821, in Noyes, "Account . . . American Ophthalmological Society."

29. In Posey and Brown, *Wills Hospital*, p. 61.

30. Thomas Neville Bonner, *American Doctors and German Universities: A Chapter in International Relations* (Lincoln: University of Nebraska Press, 1963), pp. 89–90.

31. On asylum superintendents during this period, see Constance M. McGovern, *Masters of Madness: Social Origins of the American Psychiatric Profession* (Hanover, N.H.: University Press of New England, 1985); and Charles E. Rosenberg, *The Trial of the Assassin Guiteau: Psychiatry and Law in the Gilded Age* (Chicago: University of Chicago Press, 1968), ch. 3.

32. Morris Vogel, *The Invention of the Modern Hospital: Boston, 1870–1930* (Chicago: University of Chicago Press, 1980), p. 85.

33. Vogel, *Invention of the Modern Hospital*, pp. 88–92.

34. William H. Mahoney, "Benevolent Hospitals in Metropolitan Boston," *Publications of the American Statistical Association*, 13 (1912–1913), pp. 420, 423. I am grateful to Harry Marks for bringing this source to my attention.

35. *The Philadelphia Medical Register and Directory, 1868* (Philadelphia: Collins, 1868).

36. *Philadelphia Medical Register 1868;* Thomas J. Morton, *The History of Pennsylvania Hospital 1751–1895*, rev. ed. (Philadelphia: Times Printing House, 1897), pp. 201–2.

37. *Philadelphia Medical Register, 1868*, p. 75.

38. Isaac Hays seems to have been active in both institutions. College of Physicians and Surgeons of Philadelphia, Minute Books, and Pennsylvania Infirmary for the Eye and Ear, 10a/98, Mss. 6/0008 Wills Hospital (uncataloged).

39. *Philadelphia Medical Register, 1868*, p. 77. Also see Samuel Risley, "The Wills Hospital," in *Founders' Week Memorial Volume*, ed. Frederick P. Henry (Philadelphia: [F. A. Davis], 1909), pp. 763–70; and Posey and Brown, *Wills Hospital*, p. 63.

40. Charles Sinkler, "The Philadelphia Orthopaedic Hospital and Infirmary for Nervous Disease," in *Founders' Week Memorial Volume*, ed. Frederick P. Henry (Philadelphia: [F. A. Davis], 1909), pp. 794–801.

41. *Philadelphia Medical Register, 1868*, pp. 129–30.

42. "Editorial: The Asserted Decadence of Philadelphia as a Medical Centre," *Philadelphia Medical Times*, 5 (1874–75), 134–35.

43. *The Philadelphia Medical Register and Directory, 1885* (Philadelphia: Collins, 1885), pp. 95–99.

44. *Philadelphia Medical Register and Directory, 1885*, pp. 100–3.

45. Stephen J. Peitzman, "'Thoroughly Practical': America's Polyclinic Medical Schools," *BHM*, 54 (1980), 166–87.

46. Peitzman, "'Thoroughly Practical,'" pp. 178–79.

47. *Philadelphia Medical Register and Directory, 1885*, p. 113.

48. R. Max Goepp, "The Philadelphia Polyclinic and College for Graduates in Medicine," in *Founders' Week Memorial Volume*, ed. Frederick P. Henry (Philadelphia: [F. A. Davis], 1909).

49. His biography is in the computerized catalog of manuscripts in the College of Physicians and Surgeons of Philadelphia (CPP).

50. *Medical Directory of Philadelphia, 1884.*

51. Whitfield J. Bell, *The College of Physicians of Philadelphia: A Bicentennial History* (Canton, Mass.: Science History Publications, 1987), pp. 187–89; W. B. McDaniel, "Recognition of the Specialties in the 'Organic Law' of the College of Physicians of Philadelphia," unpublished ms., CPP, cage 210a4.

52. Francis H. Brown, *The Medical Register for New England* (Boston: Cupples Upham, 1884), pp. 125–32.

53. George Rosen, *The Structure of American Medical Practice, 1875–1941*, ed. Charles E. Rosenberg (Philadelphia: University of Pennsylvania Press, 1983), pp. 18–19.

54. Thomas Neville Bonner, *Medicine in Chicago, 1850–1950: A Chapter in the Social and Scientific Development of a City*, 2nd ed. (Urbana: University of Illinois Press, 1991), pp. 66–67.

55. For the case of the Chicago GP James Herrick, see Rosen, *Structure of American Practice*, pp. 27–28.

56. "Report of a Special Committee on the Measures Suggested in the Report on Medical Literature for 1849," *TAMA*, 3 (1850), 203.

57. S. D. Gross, "Report on the Causes Which Impede the Progress of American Medical Literature," *TAMA*, 9 (1856), 359.

58. R. J. Breckinridge et al., "Committee on Medical Literature," *TAMA*, 9 (1856), 383.

59. The proportion of the urban population increased from 11 percent of total population in 1840 to 20 percent in 1860 to 40 percent in 1900. Meanwhile, the overall population rose during these years by nearly 150 percent. Rosemary Stevens, *American Medicine and the Public Interest*, updated ed. (Berkeley: University of California Press, 1998). The number of hospitals grew from 178 in 1873 to 4,978 in 1923. Charles Rosenberg, *The Care of Strangers: The Rise of America's Hospital System* (New York: Basic Books, 1987), p. 341.

60. Bonnie E. Blustein, "Linking Science to the Pursuit of Efficiency in the Reformation of the Army Medical Corps During the Civil War," in *Major Problems in the History of American Medicine and Public Health: Documents and Essays*, ed. John Harley Warner and Janet A. Tighe (Boston and New York: Houghton Mifflin, 2001), p. 191.

61. Kenneth M. Ludmerer, *Learning to Heal: The Development of American Medical Education* (New York: Basic Books, 1985), chs. 1–4; Thomas S. Huddle, "Competition and Reform at the Medical Department of the University of Pennsylvania, 1847–1877," *Journal of the History of Medicine and Allied Sciences*, 51 (1996), 251–92, and "Looking Backward: The 1871 Reforms at Harvard Medical School Reconsidered," *BHM*, 65 (1991), 340–65.

62. Warner, *Therapeutic Perspective*, pp. 37–40.

63. Alfred Stillé et al., "Committee on Medical Literature," *TAMA*, 3 (1850), 186.There were eight medical journals in 1828 and fifty-four in 1876. Ludmerer, *Learning to Heal*, p. 65.

64. John S. Billings, "Literature and Institutions," in Edward H. Clark et al., *A Century of American Medicine, 1776–1876* (Philadelphia: Henry C. Lea, 1876), pp. 290–366.

65. John P. Harrison, "Report of the Committee on Medical Literature," *TAMA*, 2 (1849), 418. For continuing AMA efforts in this direction, see Huddle, "Looking Backward," p. 361.

66. John Harley Warner, *Against the Spirit of System: The French Impulse in Nineteenth-Century American Medicine* (Princeton, N.J.: Princeton University Press, 1998), p. 294.

67. Bonner, *American Doctors*, p. 23, estimates that some 15,000 individuals went there from 1870 to 1914.

68. For some good examples, see Warner, *Against the Spirit of System*, pp. 307–12, 334.

69. The classic study of German influence on specialization in the United States is Bonner, *American Doctors*, especially ch. 3. For a local example of the influence of German-trained practitioners after midcentrury, see Leo J. O'Hara, *An Emerging Profession: Philadelphia Doctors, 1860–1900* (New York and London: Garland, 1989), pp. 96–99.

70. This was certainly true in the case of the Philadelphia dermatologist Louis Duhring, who was on the resident staff of the Philadelphia Almshouse when he decided to complete his studies in Vienna. O'Hara, *Emerging Profession*, pp. 98–99. For the case of Horatio Storer, see Dyer, *Champion of Women*, pp. 71–73.

71. Blustein, "Linking Science to . . . Efficiency," p. 201.

72. The term is borrowed from Burton J. Bledstein, *The Culture of Professionalism: The Middle Class and the Development of Higher Education in America* (New York: Norton, 1976); see also Warner, *Against the Spirit of System*, p. 337.

73. "Clarence Blake, a Young Boston Physician Studying in Europe, Finds in Clinical Specialization the Path to a New Scientific Medicine, 1869," in *Major Problems in the History of American Medicine and Public Health: Documents and Essays*, ed. John Harley Warner and Janet A. Tighe (Boston and New York: Houghton Mifflin, 2001), p. 202

74. These phrases appear in "Clarence Blake," pp. 201, 202, and 203, respectively.

75. "Clarence Blake," p. 204.

76. "Clarence Blake," p. 203.

77. "Clarence Blake," p. 202.

78. Rosenberg, *Care of Strangers*, pp.166–68.

79. "Leading Article: Medical Education Abroad," *Philadelphia Medical Times*, 2 (1871–72), 30–32.

80. Rosenberg, *Care of Strangers*, pp. 171–72.

81. Henry M. Hurd, "The Proper Division of the Services of the Hospital," *JAMA*, 59 (1912), 1677.

82. On children's hospitals, for example, and the careers of the first generation of pediatricians, see Sydney A. Halpern, *American Pediatrics: The Social Dynamics of Professionalism* (Berkeley: University of California Press, 1988), pp. 40–47.

83. Billings, "Literature and Institutions," pp. 363–64.

84. See, for example, "The Presidential Address of William O. Baldwin," *TAMA*, 20 (1869), 75, pointing out the discrepancy between the nearly thirty professorships in Paris and Berlin and the eight to ten found in even the best American medical schools. The report of the AMA's Committee on Medical Education in 1871 was explicit in recommending the teaching of certain specialties. "Report of the AMA's Committee on Medical Education," *TAMA*, 22 (1871), 139.

85. "Report of the Committee on Medical Education," *TAMA*, 16 (1865), 596. Also see later reports of this committee in *TAMA*, 19 (1868), 108–9, and 22 (1871), 113. For resolutions by individuals regarding specific disciplines, see *TAMA*, 21 (1870), 51 (mental disorders) and 64 (gynecology).

86. Ludmerer, *Learning to Heal*, pp. 38–42. An illustration of this symbiotic relationship is the role of Harvard University President Charles Eliot in imposing reform on the medical faculty. Ludmerer, *Learning to Heal*, pp. 48–52.

87. Bonnie Ellen Blustein, "New York Neurologists and the Specialization of American Medicine," *BHM*, 53 (1979), 170–83, at 173. Also see C. G. Goetz and E. J. Pappert, "Early American Professorships in Neurology," *Annals of Neurology*, 40 (1996), 258–63; Louis Duhring, "The Rise of American Dermatology," in *The Origins of Specialization in American Medicine: An Anthology of Sources*, ed. Charles E. Rosenberg (New York: Garland, 1989), pp. 101–2; and Milo Buel Ward, "Chairman's Address, Section on Obstetrics and Diseases of Women," *JAMA*, 28 (1897), 930.

88. Halpern, *American Pediatrics*, pp. 44–45.

89. The first argument is made in Kenneth M. Ludmerer, "Reform at Harvard Medical School," *BHM*, 55 (1981) pp. 343–70, and *Learning to Heal*, pp. 48–52; the second is made in Huddle, "Looking Backward," pp. 340–65.

90. Dyer, *Champion of Women*, p. 380.

91. At the University of Pennsylvania in 1890, there were eleven professors or clinical professors of medical specialties (excluding surgery) and thirteen lecturers or instructors (William B. Atkinson, *The Medical and Dental Register-Directory and Intelligencer of Pennsylvania and Delaware*, [Philadelphia: G Keil, 1890] pp. 51–52). The College of Physicians and Surgeons of Chicago in 1884 had twelve specialist professors and five lecturers (*The Medical Directory of Chicago, 1884*). Postgraduate institutions that organized resources within a city could boast even more staff. The New York Post-Graduate Medical School and Hospital in 1887 had sixteen professors in clinical specialties (advertisement in the *Medical Directory of the City of New York*, [New York: Medical Society of the county of New York, 1887]), while in 1892 that of Chicago had fourteen (*Medical and Surgical Register of the United States* [Detroit: R. L. Polk, 1892], advertisement, p.1221). To put these figures in perspective: at the the University of Berlin in 1889, there were four regular and thirteen adjunct professors in the clinical specialties. Paul Börner, *Reichs-Medicinal-Kalender für Deutschland auf das Jahr 1890* (Leipzig: Verlag von Georg Thieme, 1889).

92. Rosenberg, *Care of Strangers*, pp.169–73; Stevens, *American Medicine*, p. 47; Rosen, *Structure of American Practice*, pp. 46–47

93. Halpern, *American Pediatrics*, pp. 46–47, 51–53.

94. This incident is briefly discussed in Donald E. Konald, *A History of Medical Ethics, 1847–1912* (Madison: State History Society of Wisconsin, 1962), pp. 36–37. In my

view, his version of events overstates the degree of hostility to specialization within the AMA.

95. *TAMA*, 15 (1864), 52.

96. *TAMA*, 16 (1865), 45–46.

97. These were not published, but the contents of both reports are summarized in Dyer, *Champion of Women*, pp. 198–201.

98. Worthington Hooker and James Kennedy, "Report of the Committee of Medical Ethics on Specialties," *TAMA*, 17 (1866), 501–11; reprinted in Rosenberg, *Origins of Specialization*, pp. 21–29.

99. Henry I. Bowditch, "Minority Report," *TAMA*, 17 (1866), 511–12; reprinted in Rosenberg, *Origins of Specialization*, pp. 29–30. Pagination below is from Rosenberg.

100. Rosenberg, *Origins of Specialization*, p. 30.

101. Rosenberg, *Origins of Specialization*, p. 30.

102. Rosenberg, *Origins of Specialization*, p. 34.

103. *TAMA*, 17 (1866), 39.

104. "Presidential Address of D. Humphreys Storer," *TAMA*, 17 (1866), 55–65.

105. "Presidential Address . . . Storer," p. 65.

106. "Presidential Address of Henry F. Askew," *TAMA*, 18 (1867), 66–71.

107. "Presidential Address . . . Askew," p. 69.

108. *TAMA*, 19 (1868), 35.

109. E. Loyd [*sic*] Howard and Christopher Johnston, "Report of the Committee on Specialists and on the Propriety of Specialist Advertising," *TAMA*, 20 (1869), 111–13.

110. Howard and Johnston, "Report . . . Advertising," pp. 111–12.

111. Howard and Johnston, "Report . . . Advertising," pp. 112–13.

112. *TAMA*, 20 (1869), 28.

113. *TAMA*, 21 (1870), 39, contains a motion from the Gynecological Society of Boston to rescind this resolution.

114. *TAMA*, 25 (1874), 31.

115. Editorial, *JAMA*, 1 (1883), 512.

116. *Medical Directory of Philadelphia, Pennsylvania, Delaware and the Southern Half of New Jersey.*

117. This is the argument in Konald, *History of Medical Ethics*, p. 37.

118. These were Anatomy and Physiology, Chemistry and Materia Medica, Practical Medicine and Obstetrics, Surgery, Meteorology, Medical Topography and Epidemic Diseases, Medical Jurisprudence, and Hygiene. "History of the Sections of the American Medical Association," *JAMA* 38 (1902), 1504–15; Morris Fishbein, "The Scientific Sections of the American Medical Association," in *A History of the American Medical Association, 1847 to 1947*, ed. Morris Fishbein (Philadelphia and London: W.B. Saunders, 1947), p. 1092.

119. "Address of N. S. Davis, President of the Association," *TAMA*, 16 (1865), 74.

120. William G. Rothstein, *American Physicians in the Nineteenth Century: From Sects to Science* (Baltimore: Johns Hopkins University Press, 1972), p. 199.

121. McGovern, *Masters of Madness*, pp. 87–88.

122. H. R. Storer, "Report of the Delegate to the Association of Superintendents of Asylums for the Insane, for 1865," *TAMA*, 17 (1866), 406.

123. Charles A. Lee, "Report on Insanity," and John P. Chapin, "Report on Provision for the Chronic Insane," *TAMA*, 19 (1868), 161–88 and 191–201, respectively.

124. Storer, "Report of the Delegate," p. 398. The Association of Superintendents remained aloof from the AMA, although it did begin sending delegates to the annual meeting (McGovern, *Masters of Madness*, p. 88). The explanation for its refusal to associate with the AMA is in "Communication from the Association of Superintendents of Insane Asylums," *TAMA*, 22 (1871), 101–3.

125. See, for instance, the quote by N. S. Davis cited in Rothstein, *American Physicians*, p. 213.

126. According to figures given by Morris Fishbein and presented in Rothstein, *American Physicians*, p. 212, from 1850 to 1859, six general practitioners served as meeting president; from 1880 to 1889, the figure was four; and from 1890 to 1899, the figure was only two.

127. These were Practice of Medicine; Obstetrics and Diseases of Women; Surgery and Anatomy; Hygiene and Sanitary Science; Ophthalmology; Diseases of Children; Stomatology; Neurology and Mental Diseases; Cutaneous Medicine and Surgery; Laryngology and Otology; Materia Medica, Pharmacology, and Therapeutics; Physiology; Pathology and Bacteriology. On the sections see "History of the Sections of the American Medical Association."

128. In 1894, James F. Hibbard estimated that except for three or four sections, genuine specialists comprised only about one-tenth of the membership; the rest were GPs with specialist interests. James F. Hibbard, "President's Address, 1894," *JAMA*, 22 (1894), 860.

129. John Harley Warner: "Ideals of Science and Their Discontents in Late Nineteenth-Century Medicine," *Isis*, 82 (1991), 464–75, and "The 1880s Rebellion Against the AMA Code of Ethics: 'Scientific Democracy' and the Dissolution of Orthodoxy," in *The American Medical Ethics Revolution*, ed. Robert Baker et al. (Baltimore: John Hopkins University Press, 1999), pp. 52–69.

130. On the history of this society, see A. McGehee Harvey, *The Association of American Physicians, 1886–1986: A Century of Progress in Medical Science* (Baltimore: The Association, 1986).

131. Konald, *History of Medical Ethics*, pp. 39–40; Warner, "The 1880s Rebellion."

132. "An Important Question," *JAMA*, 11 (1888), 741–42.

133. "The Number and Variety of Medical Societies," *JAMA*, 11 (1888), 777–78.

134. "Minutes," *Transactions of the Congress of American Physicians and Surgeons*, 1 (1888), xxv–xxvi. Also see Rothstein, *American Physicians*, pp. 214–16.

135. Leartus Conner: "Other Methods of Promoting the Development of the Sections," *JAMA*, 17 (1891), 297–98; "The Publication of Section Work," ibid., 453–54; and "Constitution of Bylaws," *JAMA*, 20 (1893), 370, 427–28; Konald, *History of Medical Ethics*, pp. 40–41.

136. Stevens, *American Medicine*, p. 54.

137. E. Fletcher Ingals, "Address of the Chairman, Section of Laryngology and Otology," *JAMA*, 23 (1894), 445; C. A. Wheaton, "Address of the Chairman, Section of Surgery and Anatomy," *JAMA*, 26 (1896), 1049–50.

138. "The Association of Military Surgeons of the United States," *JAMA*, 26 (1896), 881.

139. Lewis H. Taylor, "Work of the Section on Ophthalmology," *JAMA*, 46 (1906), 1897–98.

140. See *JAMA*, 45 (1906), 256, 276, 283, for the unsuccessful request for section status by specialists in electrotherapeutics; and "Report of the Committee on Sections," *JAMA*, 84 (1925), 1736–39, supporting the addition of radiology as a section, the elimination of stomatology, and recommending against granting this status to physiotherapy. On AMA opposition to a specialty of andrology, see Stevens, *American Medicine*, p. 54.

141. Hugh Patrick, "Neurology and Medical Jurisprudence," *JAMA*, 36 (1900), 202–4.

142. Quoted in Blustein, "New York Neurologists," pp. 173–74.

143. John V. Shoemaker, "An Address in Medicine to the Medical Society of Pennsylvania," *JAMA*, 7 (1886), 57.

144. Dudley S. Reynolds, "The Present Status of the Medical Profession," *JAMA*, 20 (1893), 619.

145. *JAMA*, 22 (1894), 508; N. S. Davis, "Proposed Revision of the Code of Ethics," *JAMA*, 20 (1893), 556–58.

146. Rosemary A. Stevens, "The Challenge of Specialism: Negotiating the American Medical Association's Code of Ethics in the Early 1900s," in *The American Medical Ethics Revolution*, ed. Robert Baker et al. (Baltimore: John Hopkins University Press, 1999), pp. 70–90.

Chapter 5

1. Just after the AMA lifted its ban on specialist self-identification, *Pettigrew's New England Professional Directory* (Boston: Garden Press, 1904) included specialist information in its alphabetical listing. In Boston, 21 percent of those listed mentioned specialties.

2. These figures are analyzed in greater detail in George Weisz, "Medical Directories and Medical Specialization in France, Britain and the United States," *BHM*, 71 (1997), 23–68.

3. In Prussia the proportion of physicians with hospital posts rose from 16 percent in 1903 to 24 percent in 1937 (Wilfried Teicher, "Untersuchungen zur ärztlichen Spezialisierung im Spiegel des Reichsmedizinalkalenders am Beispiel Preußens im ersten Drittel des 20. Jahrhunderts" [MD thesis, Johannes-Gutenberg-Universität, Mainz, 1992], p. 65). In Paris, where the proportion of academic and hospital physicians was already quite high, it rose slightly, from 20 to 22 percent between 1905 and 1935 (George Weisz, "Mapping Medical Specialization in Paris in the Nineteenth and Twentieth Centuries," *SHM*, 7 [1994], 177–211, at 202). In the United States, hospital affiliation is not a significant indicator of academic or elite status because it was so widely available. According to one AMA survey in 1930, over two-thirds of all American doctors had such affiliation ("Hospital Service in the United States," *JAMA*, 94 [1930], 992–94).

4. These figures are from Paul Weindling, "Bourgeois Values, Doctors and the State: The Professionalization of Medicine in Germany, 1848–1933," in *The German Bourgeoisie: Essays on the Social History of the German Middle Class from the Late Eighteenth to the Early Twentieth Century*, ed. David Blackbourn and Richard J. Evans (London and New York: Routledge, 1991), pp. 198–223, especially pp. 211–12; George Weisz, *The*

Emergence of Modern Universities in France, 1863–1914 (Princeton, N.J.: Princeton University Press, 1983), p. 363; George Rosen, *The Structure of American Medical Practice, 1875–1941*, ed. Charles E. Rosenberg (Philadelphia: University of Pennsylvania Press, 1983), pp. 14–15; and Rosemary Stevens, *American Medicine and the Public Interest*, updated ed. (Berkeley: University of California Press, 1998), p. 421.

5. A study of doctors in Detroit in 1929 found that GPs spent 43 percent of their time, partial specialists 31 percent of their time, and specialists only 13 percent of their time on home visits. Nathan Sinai and Alden B. Mills, *A Study of Physicians and Dentists in Detroit: 1929* (Washington, D.C.: Committee on the Costs of Medical Care, 1931).

6. See Sinai and Mills, *Study of Physicians*, p. 30. Sinai and Mills found that full-time specialists in Detroit earned a mean net income of $7,805 while GPs earned a mean of $4,750. Similar data are especially abundant for American doctors. See also Rosen, *Structure of American Medical Practice*, pp. 35, 87–88; and R. G. Leland, "Income from Medical Practice," *JAMA*, 96 (1931), 1683–91, at 1686–87.

7. Louis I. Dublin and Mortimer Spiegelman, "Mortality of Medical Specialists, 1938–1942," *JAMA*, 137 (1948), 1519–24. The reasons cited for this disparity included the possibility that physicians who undertook rigorous postgraduate training tended to be healthier to start with, attained higher income levels, had more favorable conditions of work, and, since they lived predominantly in urban areas, had better medical care.

8. For example, George Heimann, "Deutschlands Spezialärzte," *DMW*, 27 (1901), 377.

9. Rosen, *Structure of American Medical Practice*, p. 32.

10. *Tout-Paris: Annuaire de la société parisienne, 1921* (Paris: A. La Fare, 1921), pp. 724–35.

11. Dr. Henius, "Spezialärzte für das Naturheilverfahren," *DMW*, 27 (1901), 826–27.

12. On almanacs, see Geneviève Bollème, *Les almanachs populaires aux XVIIe et XVIIIe siècles: Essai d'histoire sociale* (Paris: Mouton, 1969); Bernard Capp, *English Almanacs 1500–1800: Astrology and the Popular Press* (Ithaca, N.Y.: Cornell University Press, 1979); Marion Barber Stowell, *Early American Almanacs: The Colonial Weekday Bible* (New York: Burt Franklin, 1977); and Ronald Gosselin, *Les almanachs républicains: Traditions révolutionnaires et culture politique des masses populaires de Paris (1840–1851)* (Paris: Éditions L'Harmattan; Quebec: Presses de l'Université Laval, 1992). On medieval *computus* manuscripts, see Faith Wallis, "Images of Order in the Medieval *Computus*," in *Ideas of Order in the Middle Ages*, ed. Warren Ginsberg, Acta 15 (Binghamton, N.Y.: Binghamton Center for Medieval and Early Renaissance Studies, 1990), pp. 45–68; and "The Church, the World and the Time: Prolegomena to a History of the Medieval *Computus*," in *Normes et pouvoir à la fin du moyen âge*, ed. Marie-Claude Déprez-Masson (Montreal: CERES, 1989), pp. 15–29.

13. On British directories, see P. J. Atkins, *The Directories of London, 1677–1977* (London: Mansell, 1990); Gareth Shaw and Allison Tipper, *British Directories: A Bibliography and Guide to Directories Published in England and Wales (1850–1950) and Scotland (1773–1950)* (Leicester: Leicester University Press, 1989); and Jane E. Norton, *Guide to the National and Provincial Directories of England and Wales, Excluding London, Published Before 1856* (London: Offices of the Royal Historical Society, 1950). On French directo-

ries, see John Grand-Carteret, *Les almanachs français (1600–1895)*, 2nd ed. (Geneva: Slatkine Reprints, 1968); and *Catalogue de l'histoire de France*, sec. 3, *Annuaires* (Paris: Bibliothèque Nationale, 1968), part 1, ch. 4, pp. 591–701. On American directories, see Dorothea N. Spear, *Bibliography of American Directories Through 1860* (Worcester, Mass.: American Antiquarian Society, 1961). On German directories and agendas, see Werner Heegewaldt and Peter P. Rohrlach, *Berliner Adreßbücher und Adreßenverzeichnisse, 1704– 1945: Eine annotierte Bibliographie mit Standortnachweis für die "ungeteilte" Stadt* (Berlin: Helmut Scherer Verlag, 1990); Maria Gräfin Lanckoronska and Arthur Rüman, *Geschichte der deutschen Taschenbücher und Almanache aus der klassisch-romantischen Zeit* (Munich: Ernst Heimeran Verlag, 1954), particularly ch. 11; and York-Gothart Mix, ed., *Almanach- und Taschenbuchkultur des 18. und 19. Jahrhunderts* (Wiesbaden: Harrassowitz Verlag, 1996).

14. *État de la médecine, chirurgie et pharmacie, en Europe, pour l'année 1776* (Paris: P.-F. Didot, 1776); *État de la médecine, chirurgie et pharmacie, en Europe, et principalement en France, pour l'année 1777* (Paris: Thiboust, 1777); *The Medical Register for the Year 1779*, ed. Samuel Foart Simmons (London: John Murray, 1779), further volumes of which appeared in 1780 and 1783.

15. Christian Gruner, ed., *Almanach für Aerzte und Nicht-Aerzte* (Jena: Cuno, 1783– 88, 1791–96).

16. L. Hubert, *Almanach général de médecine pour la ville de Paris* (Paris: Gabon, 1827, 1830). The other directory, *Almanach médical pour l'année . . .* (Paris: Chez Liore/Chez C. Farcy), appeared annually from 1824 to 1827.

17. Dr. Félix Roubaud, *Annuaire médical et pharmaceutique de la France* (Paris: Baillière, 1849).

18. Data about the various publications is from Archives Nationales de Paris (hereafter ANP), Registry of Publications, Ministry of the Interior, F18* II 27, 1840, entries nos. 5379, 6665; F18* II 35, 1849, entry no. 273; F18* II 40, 1850, entries nos. 10160, 10294; and F18* II 40, 1851, entry no. 782. This material is discussed in greater detail in Weisz, "Medical Directories."

19. The full title was *Annuaire médical et pharmaceutique du Dr. Félix Roubaud et Almanach général de médecine et de pharmacie réunis* (Paris: Agence de Publications Médicales et Scientifiques, 1886–1913). I will refer to this unified publication as the *Annuaire Roubaud*.

20. ANP, Registry of Publications, Ministry of the Interior, F18* III 235, 1909, entry no. 560. This was a notable improvement from the situation in 1890–91, when it printed 2,300 copies, the same number as the *Guide Rosenwald;* two other medical directories had printings of 2,000 and 1,000, respectively, while the successful general business directory *Didot-Bottin* had a printing of 20,000. ANP, Registry of Publications, Ministry of the Interior, F18* III 199, 1890, entries no. 7014, 7047; and 1891, entries no. 99, 364–65.

21. *Guide Rosenwald: Annuaire de statistique médicale et pharmaceutique* (Paris: L. Rosenwald, 1887–).

22. "The London and Provincial Medical Directory," *London Journal of Medicine* (1851), 3, 923.

23. This episode is discussed in detail in Weisz, "Medical Directories."

24. "The American Medical Directory," *JAMA*, 47 (1906), 1196.

25. "Minutes of the Ninth Annual Meeting," *TAMA*, 9 (1856), 41.

26. "Minutes of Annual Meeting" *TAMA*, 19 (1868), 33–35; Gross's comments are in ibid, p. 66.

27. *TAMA*, 19 (1869), 20; *TAMA*, 21 (1870), 49

28. Samuel W. Butler, M.D., *The Medical Register and Directory of the United States* (Philadelphia: Office of *Medical and Surgical Reporter*, 1874), p. 8.

29. *Medical and Surgical Register of the United States* (Detroit: R. L. Polk, 1890), p. 19.

30. *Medical and Surgical Register*, advertisement opposite p. 881.

31. "The Organization of the Medical Profession," *JAMA*, 38 (1902), 25.

32. "An American Medical Directory," *JAMA*, 47 (1906), 1196–97.

33. "Biographical Card Index and Directory," *JAMA*, 45 (1905), 1575; "Official Minutes—House of Delegates," JAMA, 45 (1905), 269, 277.

34. *JAMA*, 41 (1903), 739.

35. "American Medical Directory," *Proceedings of the House of Delegates of the AMA* (1925), 11. The same publication in 1929 reported that the 10th ed. had sold 8,200 copies as of December 1928, with a net loss of $98.24. *Proceedings of the House of Delegates of the AMA* (1929), 5.

36. On Schwalbe, see W.U. Eckart, "'Ein Temperament griff hier zur Feder'—Julius Schwalbe und DMW, 1894–1930," *DMW*, 124 (1999), 1539–40.

37. "Dr. Paul Börner (30. Aug. 1885) und seine Bedeutung für die deutsche med. Presse," *ÄVD*, 14 (1885), 298–302.

38. In 1927 the publication became associated with the Hartmannbund, the trade union of the medical profession and, at the same time, the official source for all professional statistics. Freidrich Prinzing, "Die Aerzte Deutschlands im Jahre 1928," *DMW*, 55 (1929), 280.

39. Teicher, "Untersuchungen zur ärztlichen Spezialisierung," p. 5.

40. John Shrady, ed., *The Medical Register of the City of New York and Vicinity, 1868–69* (New York: New York Medico-Historical Society, 1868).

41. Discussed in Weisz, "Medical Directories."

42. These figures are from the pages of advertisements in *The Medical Directory* of 1913. The major directories devoted to "fashionable"society cost only 5 shillings during this same period. Atkins, *Directories of London*, p. 53.

43. This information is taken from the advertisements in the 1900 volume of *Medical and Surgical Register*.

44. Note in *MMW*, 77 (1930), 444. I am grateful to my colleague Thomas Schlich for advising me on the monetary significance of this figure.

45. "British Medical Association: Current Notes: Classified Directories," supp. to *BMJ* (1922), 2, 193, 209.

46. "Le Guide Rosenwald: Historique," *Guide Rosenwald* (1987) (the centenary ed.), unpaginated essay at the front of the volume.

47. *Guide médical et pharmaceutique de Paris* (Paris: Source de Paradis, 1901).

48. This was the *Annuaire médical belge (Congo Belge et Grand-Duché de Luxembourg)* (Brussels: Cie. Fermière de Vichy et Office Belge de Publicité Médicale et Scientifique, 1898–1946).

49. The cost of an annual subscription to *The Lancet* was 42 shillings.

50. *Presse médicale*, 46 (1938), 463.

51. Notice in *ÄVD*, 31 (1902), 22.

52. For examples, see Rosemary Stevens, *American Medicine*, pp. 44–46. Also see the reports of 1866 on this issue by the AMA's Committee on Medical Ethics on Specialties, in *The Origins of Specialization in American Medicine: An Anthology of Sources*, ed. Charles E. Rosenberg (New York: Garland, 1989), pp. 19–30.

53. Shrady, *Medical Register of the City of New York*, p. 373.

54. *Das Medicinalwesen Deutschlands im Jahre 1883: Separatabdruck von Dr. Paul Börner's Reichs-Medicinal-Kalender, II. Theil 1884* (Berlin: Verlag von Theodor Fischer, 1884).

55. *Berlin-Verzeichnis der Einwohner nach ihren Beschäftigungen und Gewerben, 1883*, Berlin Stadt-Bibliothek (City Library), Berlin Einwohner Verzeichnis microfilm collection, 1883/9/20.

56. *Annuaire des familles, ou Almanach de Paris* (Paris: Courrier de Famille, 1859).

57. C. Bracebridge Allen, *London Medical Specialists* (London: Ward and Lock, 1890), unpaginated preface.

58. *New York Medical Practitioners Engaged in Special Branches* (New York: Eugene R. Trott, 1899), p. iii.

59. *New York Medical Practitioners*, p. iii. On earlier medical hostility to specialization, see Rosenberg, *Origins of Specialization*.

60. Bracebridge Allen, *London Medical Specialists*, unpaginated preface.

61. This was *Medical Specialists and Their Work by a London Physician*, discussed in "Medical Specialists," *BMJ* (1891), 2, 1244.

62. W. P. W. Phillimore, ed., *The Dictionary of Medical Specialists: Being a Classified List of London Practitioners Who Chiefly Attend to Special Departments of Medicine and Surgery* (London: Chas. J. Clark, 1889).

63. *Annuaire des spécialités médicales et pharmaceutiques* (Paris: P. Bouland, 1880–86).

64. Although most Parisian directories also included general lists of medical practitioners in the provinces (in which information about specialties was included), they did not contain separate specialist lists of provincial practitioners.

65. Weisz, "Mapping Medical Specialization," pp. 180–84.

66. *The Standard Medical Directory of North America* (Chicago: Engelhard, 1903), p. 697.

67. "Vorrede," in *Reichs-Medizinal-Kalender für Deutschland auf das Jahr 1901, Theil II*, ed. Julius Schwalbe (Leipzig: Fischer & Wittig (1900), p. iii.

68. "Vorrede," p. iv.

69. Although these criteria were not explicitly mentioned in the *Directory* until after World War I, they seem to have been in effect from the very beginning. See Frank V. Cargill, "The American Medical Directory," in *A History of the American Medical Association, 1847 to 1947*, ed. Morris Fishbein (Philadelphia: W.B. Saunders, 1947), pp. 1170–79, especially p. 1175.

70. "British Medical Association: Current Notes: Classified Directories," supp. to *BMJ* (1922), 2, 193.

71. Supp. to *BMJ* (1922), 2, 201, 209. There was, however, little enthusiasm for the new directory. The *British Medical Journal*, in reviewing the publication, described it briefly, with virtually no comment. "Notes on Books," *BMJ* (1923), 1, 526.

72. *London Doctors and Dental Surgeons, 1923–24* (London: Grafton, 1923), p. vi. On the activities of the BMA's Ethics Committee with respect to medical advertising during

this period, see Andrew A. G. Morrice, "'The Medical Pundits': Doctors and Indirect Advertising in the Lay Press, 1922–1927," *MH*, 38 (1994), 255–80.

73. *The Medical Who's Who, 1925* (London: Gration, 1925), pp. vi–viii.

74. *Medical Who's Who, 1925*, p. viii.

75. "Directories, Question of Doctors' Names Appearing in," CMAC, D.231, box 178.

Chapter 6

1. Arnold J. Heidenheimer, "Organized Medicine and Physician Specialization in Scandinavia and West Germany," *West European Politics*, 3 (1980), 373–87, at 378.

2. Christian Bonah, *Instruire, guérir, servir: Formation et pratique médicales en France et en Allemagne* (Strasbourg: Presses Universitaires de Strasbourg, 2000), p. 148.

3. Wolfram Kaiser and Arina Völker, "Zur Entwicklung klinischer Spezialdisziplinen an der Universität Halle," *Wissenschaftliche Zeitschrift der Wilhelm-Pieck-Universität Rostock*, 32 (1983), Gesellschaftswissenschaftliche Reihe, Heft 9, 66–70.

4. Johannes Müller, *Statistische Untersuchungen über Vorlesungen und Dozenten der medizinischen Fakultäten der deutschen Universitäten in den Jahren 1927 bis 1931–32* (Berlin: Struppe & Winckler, 1933), summary table, p. 145.

5. Müller, *Statistische Untersuchungen*; C. Benda, "Reformbestrebungen der Privatdozenten," *DMW*, 45 (1919), 214–15, 244–46.

6. Manfred Stürtzbecher, "Allgemeine und Spezialkrankenhäuser, insbesondere Privatkrankenanstalten im 19. Jahrhundert in Berlin," in *Studien zur Krankenhausgeschichte im 19. Jahrhundert im Hinblick auf die Entwicklung in Deutschland*, ed. Hans Schadewaldt (Göttingen: Vandenhoeck & Ruprecht, 1976), p. 116. For the situation two decades earlier, see "Eine Denkschrift, die Reform des städischen Medizinalwesens in Berlin," *ÄVD*, 32 (1903), 225.

7. This subject is ubiquitous in medical journals in the decades preceding and following the First World War. It was a major issue at both the Eisenach *Ärztetag* of 1919 and the Karlsruhe *Ärztetag* of 1921.

8. Prof. Dr. Hilgermann, "Zur Neugestaltung des medizinischen Studiums," *DMW*, 45 (1919), 22–23.

9. Paul Horn, "Zur Reform der ärztlichen Prüfungsordnung und des Unterrichts in der Versicherungsmedizin," *DMW*, 45 (1919), 1112–13.

10. Erich Meyer, "Zur Reform des medizinischen Unterrichts," *DMW*, 45 (1919), 693, 695.

11. Claus Schilling, "Die Zukunft der deutschen Kolonial- und Auslandsärzte," *DMW*, 45 (1919), 1365–66. On the ideological context of colonial medicine, see Wolfgang U. Eckart, *Medizin und Kolonialimperialismus: Deutschland 1884–1945* (Paderborn: Ferdinand Schöning, 1997), ch. 5; and Stefan Wulf, *Das Hamburger Tropeninstitut, 1919 bis 1945: Auswärtige Kulturpolitik und Kolonialrevisionismus nach Versailles* (Berlin: D. Reimer, 1994), ch. 1.

12. Prof. Schieck, "Zur Neuordnung des medizinischen Studiums," *DMW*, 49 (1923), 452–53; Bernhard Fischer-Wasels, "Verbesserung der ärztlichen Ausbildung und der ärztlichen Prüfungsvorschriften," *DMW*, 56 (1930), 587.

13. In 1929, cities with from 30,000 to 60,000 inhabitants had substantially the same proportion of specialists among all doctors as did those with more than 100,000

(a little over 40 percent). In towns with from 10,000 to 20,000 inhabitants, the proportion of specialists was still over 25 percent. (Dr. [Friedrich] Prinzing, "Die Fachärzte in kleinen Städten," *DMW*, 55 [1929], 1185–86). Also see Dr. Hadrich, "Die Zahl der Allgemeinpraktiker und Fachärzte in den deutschen Groß- und Mittelstädten im Jahre 1934," *DÄ*, 64 (1934), 528–34.

14. In Austria such degrees existed until 1869. "Verhandlungen des XX. deutschen Aerztetages zu Leipzig, im 27. und 28. Juni 1892: (Referent Dr. Stimmel)" *ÄVD*, 21 (1892), 422.

15. Claudia Huerkamp, "The Making of the Modern Medical Profession, 1800–1914: Prussian Doctors in the Nineteenth Century," in *German Professions, 1800–1950*, ed. Geoffrey Cocks and Konrad H. Jarausch (New York and Oxford: Oxford University Press, 1990), p. 79.

16. For an overview of professional issues during this period, see Hedwig Herold-Schmidt, "Ärztliche Interessenvertretung im Kaiserreich, 1871–1914," in *Geschichte der deutschen Ärzteschaft*, ed. Robert Jütte (Cologne: Ärzte-Verlag, 1997), pp. 43–97.

17. See, for example, Hüllmann, "Ueber das moderne Specialistenthum," *ÄVD*, 19 (1890), 20; Arthur Hartmann, "Die medicinische Ausbildung in Specialfächern," *ÄVD*, 21 (1892), 61; Dr. Bloch, "Zur Specialistenfrage," *ÄVD*, 21 (1892), 214.

18. Albert Neisser, "Die Dermatologie und Syphilologie in dem Entwurf der Prüfungsordnung," *DMW*, 22 (1896), 685; Hartmann, "Medicinische Ausbildung," p. 64.

19. Heinrich Riedl, "Die Auseinandersetzungen um die Spezialisierung in der Medizin von 1862 bis 1925" (MD thesis, Fakultät für Medizin, Technischen Universität München, 1981), p. 21.

20. Otto Körner, *Die Arbeitsteilung in der Heilkunde* (Wiesbaden: Verlag von J. F. Bergmann, 1909), p. 7.

21. Hüllmann, "Das moderne Specialistenthum," p. 21.

22. Dr. Chandon, "Das Manchesterthum in der ärztlichen Praxis," *ÄVD*, 15 (1886), 358; Hüllmann, "Das moderne Specialistenthum," p. 22.

23. Hüllmann, "Das moderne Specialistenthum," p. 22.

24. Wilfried Teicher, "Untersuchungen zur ärztlichen Spezialisierung im Spiegel des Reichsmedizinalkalenders am Beispiel Preußens im ersten Drittel des 20. Jahrhunderts" (PhD thesis, Johannes-Gutenberg-Universität, Mainz, 1992), p. 40; Claudia Huerkamp, *Der Aufstieg der Ärzte im 19. Jahrhundert: Vom gelehrten Stand zum professionellen Experten. Das Beispiel Preußens* (Göttingen: Vandenhoeck & Ruprecht, 1985), pp. 190–93; Hüllmann, "Das moderne Specialistenthum," p. 20.

25. "Verhandlungen des XX. Aerztetages: (Referent Dr. Stimmel)," p. 424; Körner, *Arbeitsteilung*, pp. 21–24.

26. "Verhandlungen des XX. Aerztetages: (Referent Dr. Stimmel)," p. 424.

27. J. Schwalbe, "Standesangelegenheiten," *DMW*, 28 (1902), 16.

28. E. Stimmel, "Die Einrichtung einer besonderen Prüfung für Specialärzte," *ÄVD*, 21 (1892), 124–27; and his remarks in "Verhandlungen des xx. Aerztetages: (Referent Dr. Stimmel)," pp. 420–24. The commission's original wording was, after vigorous discussion, reformulated in order to make clearer and harsher the conclusion that special examinations should be rejected. Ibid., pp. 434, 441.

29. "Verhandlungen des XX. Aerztetages: (Referent Dr. Stimmel)," p. 427.

30. "Verhandlungen des XX. Aerztetages: (Referent Dr. Stimmel)," pp. 421–25, 431; Stimmel, "Einrichtung einer besonderen Prüfung," pp. 125–26; Hüllmann, "Das moderne Specialistenthum," p. 23; Hartmann, "Medicinische Ausbildung," pp. 66–67. On these debates generally, see Riedl, "Auseinandersetzungen um die Spezialisierung," pp. 25–50.

31. Stimmel, "Einrichtung einer besonderen Prüfung," p. 127.

32. Dr. Goepel, "Zur Frage einer besondern Prüfung für Specialärzte," *ÄVD*, 21 (1892), 207–11.

33. Hüllmann, "Das moderne Specialistenthum," pp. 23–24; Körner, *Arbeitsteilung*, pp. 21–24.

34. "Verhandlungen des XX. Aerztetages: (Referent Dr Stimmel)," p. 426; Becher, in "Verhandlungen des XX. Aerztetages," *ÄVD*, 21 (1892), 438.

35. Becher, in "Verhandlungen des XX. Aerztetages," p. 441.

36. H. Löbker, "Referat," *ÄVD*, 37 (1908), 650.

37. J. Schwalbe, "Die Spezialistenfrage," *DMW*, 33 (1907), 1643–45.

38. Friedrich Prinzing, "Die Aerzte Deutschlands im Jahre 1907," *DMW*, 33 (1907), 2187–88.

39. Among many works on this subject, see Dr. Gutkind, "Der Spezialarzt für Kinderkrankheiten vom Standpunkte der Praxis aus betrachtet," *ÄVD*, 35 (1906), 497–99; H. Bartsch, "Zum Kapitel: Spezialarzt für Kinderheilkunde," *ÄVD*, 35 (1906), 543–45; F. Siegert, "Der 'Spezialarzt für Kinderkrankheiten,'" *ÄVD*, 35 (1906), 545–48; and Dr. Krecker, "Hausarzt und Spezialarzt," *ÄVD*, 36 (1907), 566–69.

40. Among the many articles on this subject are Dr. Mohr, "Freie Arztwahl und Honorierung der Spezialärzte," *ÄVD*, 32 (1903), 372–73, 556–57; Dr. Bewerunge, "Freie Arztwahl und Honorierung der Spezialärzte," *ÄVD*, 32 (1903), 421; Dr. Busch: "Die Honorierung der Spezialärzte in der Kassenpraxis," *ÄVD*, 33 (1904), 13–17, 44–49, and "Ueber die einheitliche Honorierung der praktischen Aerzte und Spezialärzte in der Kassenpraxis," *ÄVD*, 35 (1906), 247–53; Neumann, "Zur Frage der freien Arztwahl und der Honorierung der Aerzte," *ÄVD*, 33 (1904), 229–32; and Edouard Mueller, "Ueber eine einheitliche Honorierung der praktischen Aerzte und Spezialärzte in der Kassenpraxis," *ÄVD*, 35 (1906), 371–78.

41. Busch, "Ueber die einheitliche Honorierung," and "Entgegnung," *ÄVD* 35 (1906), 393–400; Dr. Beshoren, "Zur Spezialarztfrage," *ÄVD*, 35 (1906), 470–72.

42. Dr. Schroeder, "Situation der Spezialisten gegenüber den Krankenkassen- und praktischen Aerzten," *ÄVD*, 36 (1907), 696–702, and the response of the editor, ibid., pp. 702–4; Dr. Keil, "Zur Spezialarztfrage," *ÄVD*, 36 (1907), 798.

43. An anonymous article, "Welcher Arzt soll sich 'Spezialist' nennen dürfen?" *ÄVD*, 33 (1904), 308–9, cited the political press to this effect.

44. "The Specialist in Health Insurance Practice," *JAMA*, 66 (1916), 1984.

45. K. Jaffé, "Die Spezialarztfrage in der Hamburger Aerztekammer," *ÄVD*, 37 (1908), 4.

46. E. von Bergmann, "Die Wahrheit über das ärztliche Fortbildungswesen in Preußen," *ÄVD*, 34 (1905), 570–79. Also see "Kaiserin-Friedrich-Haus für das Aerztliche Fortbildungswesen," *ÄVD*, 35 (1906), 154–56.

47. Among many articles on this subject, see Landsberger, "Die erste 'Akademie für praktische Medizin,'" *ÄVD*, 33 (1904), 138–40; "Die Akademie für Praktische Medizin

in Cöln," *ÄVD*, 33 (1904), 575–78; F. Burkart, "Die Akademien für pracktische Medizin," *ÄVD*, 33 (1904), 604–9; "Die Eröffnung der Akademie für Praktische Medizin und der Allg. Ärztliche Verein zu Cöln," *ÄVD*, 33 (1904), 631–34; "Die Akademie für Praktische Medizin zu Cöln und der Allgemeine Ärztliche Verein," *ÄVD*, 34 (1905), 124–27.

48. Von Bergmann, "Wahrheit über das ärztliche Fortbildungswesen," p. 572.

49. "Zur Frage der Akademien für Praktische Medizin," *ÄVD*, 34 (1905), 330–32. Dr. H. Lobkers announced this decision to cheers in his presidential address to the Strasbourg *Ärztetag*, in "Verhandlung des XXXIII. deutschen Aerztetages," *ÄVD*, 34 (1905), 1–2.

50. Riedl, "Auseinandersetzungen um die Spezialisierung," pp. 52–56; "33. Deutsche Aerztetag," *DMW*, 31 (1905), 1136.

51. Hans-Heinz Eulner, "Das Spezialistentum in der ärztlichen Praxis," in *Der Arzt und der Kranke in der Gesellschaft des 19. Jahrhunderts*, ed. Walter Artelt und Walter Rüegg (Stuttgart: Ferdinand Enke Verlag, 1967), pp. 24–27; Huerkamp, *Aufstieg der Ärzte*, p.181.

52. *ÄVD*, 36 (1907), 865; Emmanuel Fink, "Die Spezialistenfrage in der Hamburger Aerztekammer," *ÄVD*, 36 (1907), 981–83.

53. "Standesordung für das Herzogthum Anhalt," *DMW*, 28 (1902), 475.

54. Teicher, "Untersuchungen zur ärztlichen Spezialisierung," p. 47.

55. Wilhelm Ebstein, "Das Spezialistentum in der ärztlichen Praxis," *DMW*, 30 (1904), 396.

56. Eulner, "Spezialistentum in der ärztlichen Praxis," p. 27; Riedl, "Auseinandersetzungen um die Spezialisierung," p. 74.

57. Dr. Mohr, "Freie Arztwahl und Honorierung der Spezialärzte," *ÄVD*, 32 (1903), 373; "Welcher Arzt soll sich 'Spezialist' nennen dürfen?" *ÄVD*, 33 (1904), 308–9; "Aus den Preußischen Aerztekammern," *ÄVD*, 34 (1905), 53–54; M. Sperling, "Spezialisten in der Aussenpraxis," *ÄVD*, 37 (1908), 238; Löbker, "Referat," pp. 653–54.

58. The best summary and discussion of all these various plans is Dr. Esch, "Spezialisten in der Aussenpraxis: Kritischer Literaturauszug," *ÄVD*, 36 (1907), 926–32, 946–50. Also see Heinrich Quincke, "Ueber ärztliche Spezialitäten und Spezialärzte," *MMW*, 53 (1906), 1213–17, 1260–64. For specific plans, see "Aus den Vereinen," *ÄVD*, 36 (1907), 410–15 (for the Verein Schleswig-Holsteinischer Aerzte); "Hamburgische Aerztekammer," *ÄVD*, 36 (1907), 859–61; and K. Jaffé, "Die Spezialarztfrage in der Hamburger Aerztekammer," *ÄVD*, 37 (1908), 4–6.

59. He chaired the annual *Ärztetage* from 1900 to 1909. See Robert Jütte, ed., *Geschichte der deutschen Ärzteschaft: Organisierte Berufs- und Gesundheitspolitik im 19. und 20. Jahrhundert* (Cologne: Deutscher Ärzte-Verlag, 1997), p. 290.

60. "Zur Behandlung der Spezialistenfrage in Preußen," *ÄVD*, 37 (1908), 603–5. Löbker's report ("Referat") and the final recommendations of the deputation are in *ÄVD*, 37 (1908), 644–60. This matter is discussed briefly in Huerkamp, *Aufstieg der Ärzte*, p. 182.

61. Löbker suggested that in Prussia, seven chambers responded positively and three negatively, and two did not respond (note in *ÄVD*, 39 [1910], 5). But subsequent reports suggested that even his own Westphalian chamber, which he listed as supporting the measure, rejected the proposal (*ÄVD*, 39 [1910], 93). For reports of widespread opposition among local medical societies in Dresden, see *ÄVD*, 39 (1910), 20–21.

62. For example, Dr. Loewenthal, "Zur Spezialarztfrage," *ÄVD*, 38 (1909), 232–34; "Der Württembergische ärztlicher Landesausschuß," *ÄVD*, 39 (1910), 35–39.

63. For instance, "Praktische Aerzte und Spezialärzte," *ÄVD*, 37 (1908), 564–65.

64. J. Schwalbe, "Die Spezialistenfrage," *DMW*, 22 (1907), 1691–93; Riedl, "Auseinandersetzungen um die Spezialisierung," p. 78.

65. Sperling, "Spezialisten in der Aussenpraxis " p. 238.

66. Quincke, "Ueber ärztliche Spezialitäten."

67. Löbker, "Referat," pp. 646–47; also Dr. Pentz, "Zur Spezialistenfrage," *ÄVD*, 37 (1908), 765–69.

68. The first definition is in Loewenthal, "Zur Spezialarztfrage"; the second, in Dr. W., "Zur Spezialarztfrage," *ÄVD*, 38 (1909), 444–47, 468–69.

69. Dr. W., "Zur Spezialarztfrage," pp. 447, 468–69.

70. Dr. W., "Zur Spezialarztfrage," pp. 444–47.

71. Dr. W., "Zur Spezialarztfrage," p. 447.

72. Dr. W., "Zur Spezialarztfrage," p. 447.

73. On professional conditions during this period, see Eberhard Wolff, "Mehr als nur materielle Interessen: Die organisierte Ärzteschaft in Ersten Weltkrieg und in der Weimarer Republik 1914–1933," in *Geschichte der deutschen Ärzteschaft*, ed. Robert Jütte (Cologne: Ärzte-Verlag, 1997), pp. 97–142; and Paul Weindling, "Bourgeois Values, Doctors and the State: The Professionalization of Medicine in Germany, 1848–1933," in *The German Bourgeoisie: Essays on the Social History of the German Middle Class from the Late Eighteenth to the Early Twentieth Century*, ed. David Blackbourn and Richard J. Evans (London and New York: Routledge, 1991), pp. 198–223.

74. Friedrich Prinzing, "Die Aerzte Deutschlands im Jahre 1925," *DMW*, 52 (1926), 499.

75. Carl Prausnitz, "Die ärztliche Ausbildung in Deutschland, Frankreich und Großbritannien im Lichte der Reformbestrebungen des medizinischen Studiums," *DMW*, 58 (1932), 1534.

76. John M. Efron, *Medicine and the German Jews: A History* (New Haven, Conn.: Yale University Press, 2001), pp. 234–64; Wilfried Teicher, "Der Anteil der jüdischen Arzte an der Spezialisierung im ersten Drittel dieses Jahrhunderts in Preußen," in *Medizinsche Wissenschaft und Judentum*, ed. Nora Goldenbogen et al. (Dresden: Verein für Regionale Politik und Geschichte Dresden, 1996), pp. 14–29.

77. For an international overview, see Christopher Lawrence and George Weisz, "Medical Holism—the Context," in *Greater Than the Parts: Holism in Biomedicine, 1920–1950*, ed. Christopher Lawrence and George Weisz (New York: Oxford University Press, 1998), pp. 3–24. Among many works about German holism, see Anne Harrington, "Kurt Goldstein's Neurology of Healing and Wholeness: A Weimar Story," and Cay-Rudiger Pruell, "Holism and German Pathology (1914–1933)," in *Greater Than the Parts*, pp. 25–45 and 46–67, respectively.

78. Michael Moran, *Governing the Health Care State: A Comparative Study of the United Kingdom, the United States and Germany* (Manchester: Manchester University Press, 1999), pp. 36–37.

79. The term *Facharzt* began to be used after the war in the *ÄVD*, the official publication of the national doctors' association, and then spread to other journals such as the *DMW*. This change occurred without comment.

80. See, for instance, W. Hoffmann, "Die Neuorganisation des Gesundheitswesens in der Stadtgemeinde Berlin," *DMW,* 47 (1921), 1268–70; and E. Galewsky, "Der neue Gesetzentwurf zur Bekämpfung der Geschlechtskrankheiten," *DMW* 48 (1922), 326–28.

81. Teicher, "Untersuchungen zur ärztlichen Spezialisierung," p. 73; Gustav Tugendreich, "Ist der Kinderarzt Facharzt? " *ÄVD* 48 (1919), 125–129.

82. Hans-Heinz Eulner, *Die Entwicklung der medizinischen Spezialfächer an den Universitäten des deutschen Sprachgebietes* (Stuttgart: Ferdinand Enke Verlag, 1970), pp. 233–34. Some of these effects are discussed in chapter 11 of this volume.

83. Efron, *Medicine and the German Jews,* pp. 251–53.

84. J. Schwalbe, "Der Stand der medizinischen Studienreform," *DMW,* 49 (1923), 1523.

85. Announcements appeared regularly in major journals.

86. The quote is from "An de Fachärzte Deutschlands!" *ÄVD,* 49 (1920), 139. The foundation of the Verein der Spezialärzte von Hamburg-Altona was announced in *ÄVD,* 49 (1920), 102–3.

87. O. Stuelp, "Zur Facharzte Frage," *ÄVD,* 51 (1922), 48–49.

88. Riedl, "Auseinandersetzungen um die Spezialisierung," p. 92.

89. R. Schaeffer, "Die 'Facharztfrage,'" *ÄVD,* 51 (1921), 12.

90. "Zur Facharztfrage," *ÄVD,* 51 (1922), 197–98. The initial text is printed in "Leitsätze zur Anerkennung und praktischen Tätigkeit von Fachärzten," *ÄVD,* 52 (1923), 117–20. The final draft is in *ÄVD,* 53 (1924), 85–88.

91. S. Alexander, "Dem 43. ordentlichen Deutschen Aerztetage," *DMW,* 50 (1924), 809.

92. Medicus Rusticus, "Gedanken zur Facharztfrage," *ÄVD,* 53 (1924), 159–61.

93. O. Schellong, "Die Facharztfrage vom Standpunkt des Allgemeinpraktikers," *DMW,* 50 (1924), 809–11.

94. Oscar Salomon, "Der 43. Deutsche Aerztetag am 20. und 21. VI in Bremen," *DMW,* 50 (1924) 963–64; "Die Facharztfrage," *MMW,* 71 (1924), 926–28.

95. "Die Facharztfrage," p. 927.

96. Salomon, "Der 43. Deutsche Aerztetag," p. 964.

97. The initial proposal stipulated thirteen categories ("Leitsätze zur Anerkennung," p. 118). These were internal medicine, gastroenterology, diseases of the lungs, pediatrics, surgery, gynecology and obstetrics, neurology and psychiatry, orthopedics, ophthalmology, ORL, dermatology and venereology, stomatology, and radiology and radium therapy. The one added was urology, which had initially been lumped together with dermatology/venereology.

98. Urology represented one of the few successful efforts to win approval. Alfred Rothschild, "Die Urologie und die Regelung der Facharztfragen," *ÄVD,* 52 (1923), 173–74. For less successful efforts, see Dr. Landt, "Der Facharzt für Kosmetik," *ÄVD,* 53 (1924), 338–39; W. Kühn, "Die elektrophysikalischen Heilmethoden und die Facharztfrage," *ÄVD,* 53 (1924), 339–40.

99. "Leitsätze der Berichterstatter Dr. Kustermann (München) und Professor Dr. Stuelp . . . ," *ÄVD,* 53 (1924), 85–88.

100. "Prague: Conditions of Medical Practice," *JAMA,* 84 (1925), 765.

101. "Vienna: Regulations Concerning Use of the Term Specialist," *JAMA*, 99 (1932), 1007–8; *JAMA*, 98 (1932), 749–50.

102. "The Title of Specialist in Hungary," *JAMA*, 84 (1925), 1587.

103. Friedrich Prinzing, "Die Aerzte in Deutschlands im Jahre 1926," *DMW*, 52 (1926), 1393.

104. Dr. Richter, "Richtlinien für ärztliche Anzeigen und Schilder," *ÄVD*, 27 (1928), 203–5; T. Brunner, "Zu den Richtlinien für ärztliche Anzeigen und Schilder," *ÄVD*, 27 (1928), 301–302; "Die Mißstände im Schilderwesen und die Wege zu ihrer Abhilfe," *ÄVD*, 27 (1928), 344–46.

105. "Umschau: Ist die Prüfung der Facharztausbildung durch die kassenärztliche Zulassungsstelle aufrechtzuerhalten?" *DÄ*, 61 (1932), 438–39; "Berlin: Qualification of Specialists," *JAMA*, 84 (1925), 764–65; "The Requirements for Recognition as a Specialist," *JAMA*, 84 (1925), 1143; "Berlin: The Regulation of Medical Specialties," *JAMA*, 99 (1932), 1007–8; Riedl, "Auseinandersetzungen um die Spezialisierung," pp. 97–98.

106. This very complex issue is discussed in Dr. Schläger, "Der Facharzt," *DMW*, 61 (1935), 386–87.

107. Kurt Möhring, "Die Berechtigung zur Führung der Facharztbezeichnung in Preußen," *ÄVD*, 56 (1927), 155–57; for a response, Vollman, ibid., 157–60.

108. Prausnitz, "Die ärztliche Ausbildung," p. 1729; "Gesetzliche Regelung des Facharztwesens in der Tschechoslowakei," *DÄ*, 61 (1932), 235–36, 307–8.

109. Dr. Th. B. "Die Bremer Leitsätze zur Facharztfrage " *ÄVD*, 55 (1926), 8–10.

110. Dr. Th. B., "Die Bremer Leitsätze," 9.

111. Prof. Dr. Stuelp, "Bisherige Erfahrungen mit den Bremer Leitsätzen zur Facharztfrage" *ÄVD*, 54 (1925) 427–28; Karl Jacobs, "Bisherige Erfahrungen mit den 'Bremer Leitsätzen zur Facharztfrage,'" *ÄVD*, 54 (1925), 507–10.

112. Prof. Dr. Stuelp, "Bisherige Erfahrungen mit den 'Bremer Leitsätzen zur Facharztfrage': II," *ÄVD*, 54 (1925), 489.

113. For the case of orthopedists, see Verein der Spezialärzte für Beinleiden, "Der Facharzt für Beinleiden: Ein Aufruf!" *ÄVD*, 56 (1927), 180–81; and "Kleine Mitteilungen," *ÄVD*, 56 (1927), 363.

114. "Auflösung des Verbandes der Fachärzte Deutschlands," *ÄVD* 57 (1928), 78; note in *MMW*, 75 (1928), 289.

115. "Leitsätze zu dem Referat 'Die Abgrenzung der Facharztgebiete der inneren Medizin und der Kinderkrankheiten' für den 47. Deutschen Ärztetag in Danzig," *ÄVD*, 57 (1928), 275–77. Discussions of this issue include Professor Strube, "Praktischer Arzt und Facharzt," *ÄVD*, 57 (1928), 327–32.

116. Dr. Mühlhausen, "Praktische Aerzte, Fachärzte und die Bremer Richtlinien," *ÄVD*, 57 (1928), 331–34.

117. Dr. Mühlhausen, "Praktische Aerzte . . . und die Bremer Richtlinien," pp. 331–34.

118. "47. Deutscher Ärztetag," *MMW*, 75 (1928), 1318–20.

119. For instance, the double titles "surgeon and gynecologist" and "surgeon and orthopedist" were allowed only in hospitals that were too small to have separate wards in each category. The combination of internal medicine and nervous diseases was disal-

lowed, as was the combination of internal medicine and roentgenology. "Auslegungen and Begutachtungen von Facharztfragen durch den Geschäftsausschuß und den ständigen Gutachterausschuß des Deutschen Aerztevereinsbundes," *ÄVD*, 58 (1929), 791–92.

120. "Auslegungen and Begutachtungen."

121. Hans J. Sewering, "Von der 'Bremer Richtlinien' zur Weiterbildungsordnung," *DÄ*, 84 (1987), B1597.

122. "Richtlinien zur Verhütung von Röntgenschäden," *DÄ*, 59 (1930), 337; "Aus der Sitzung des Vorstandes des Deutschen Ärztevereinsbundes am 21. November 1930 in Berlin," *DÄ*, 59 (1930), 433–34.

123. "Erlasse des Preußischen Ministers für Volkswohlfahrt," *DÄ*, 61 (1932), 302.

124. "Bericht über der Sitzung des Geschäftsausschußes des Deutschen Ärztevereinsbundes am 7. Februar 1932 in Berlin," *DÄ*, 61 (1932), 77. Further discussions are in Dr. Vrons, "Vorschläge zur Änderung der Facharztrichtlinien," *DÄ*, 62 (1933), 58–59.

125. Heinz Jaeger, "Die Eintragung in das Arztregister nach dem neuen Arztrecht," *DÄ*, 61 (1932), 164–66; "Aus der Sitzung des Vorstandes des Deutschen Ärztevereinsbundes am 20. Mai in Potsdam," *DÄ*, 61 (1932), 257; "Eintragung in das Arztregister für ein bestimmtes Fachgebiet?" *DÄ*, 61 (1932), 306; "Umschau: Ist die Prüfung der Facharztausbildung durch die kassenärztliche Zulassungstelle aufrechtzuerhalten?" *DÄ*, 61 (1932), 438–39.

126. In Westphalia, the answer to the first question was that an internist had to be called in unless the surgery had been on the lungs. The answer to the second was that the surgeon was responsible if any surgical procedure was required. Dr. Vusz, "Über die Abgrenzung fachärztlicher Arbeitsgebiete," *DÄ*, 62 (1933), 143.

127. The answer in Westphalia was that while gynecologists were normally limited to the genitalia and reproductive system, if in the course of normal surgery they came across other surgical problems, such as the need for an appendectomy or problems of the urinary tract, they were allowed, and in fact were obligated, to act. Vusz, "Über die Abgrenzung," p. 143.

128. It depended on the severity of the pain. Vusz, "Über die Abgrenzung," p. 143.

129. F. Schied, "Die Ziele des medizinischen Studiums und die Ausbildung in sozialer Medizin," *DÄ*, 60 (1931), 198–200, especially 199.

130. "Aus der Sitzung des Vorstandes und des Geschäftsausschußes des Deutschen Ärztevereinsbundes am 9. und 10. Mai 1930 in Berlin," *DÄ*, 60 (1931), 200–1. The pressure group in question was the Verband der Deutschen Berufsgenossenschaften.

131 "Bericht über der Sitzung des Geschäftsausschußes des Deutschen Ärztevereinsbundes am 7. Februar 1932 in Berlin," *DÄ*, 61(1932), 79; G. U. Weltz, "Zur Ausbildung der Teilröntgenologen," *DÄ*, 61 (1932), 272–74.

132. Dr. Th. Schreus, "Fortbildung des praktischen Arztes in Röntgenologie," *DÄ*, 65 (1935), 67–68.

133. See, for instance, Georg Bessau, "Von der Bedeutung und dem Wesen der Kinderheilkunde," *DMW*, 58 (1932), 1892–96.

134. Walter Löhlein, "Die Stellung der Augenheilkunde im Rahmen der gesamten Heilkunde," *DMW*, 61 (1935), 1125–29.

135. "Denkschrift der Deutschen Gesellschaft für Chirurgie," *DMW*, 59 (1933), 1136–38; H. Gocht, "Antwort der Deutschen Orthopädischen Gesellschaft auf die Denkschrift der Deutschen Gesellschaft für Chirurgie," *DMW*, 60 (1934), 449–51;

"Antwort der Deutschen Gesellschaft für Chirurgie auf die Erklärung der Deutschen Orthopädischen Gesellschaft," *DMW*, 60 (1934), 527–28. Also see J. Hadrich, "Die Fachärzte für Orthopädie," *DÄ*, 64 (1934), 801–3.

136. "Chirugie—Orthopädie," *DÄ*, 65 (1935), 367.

137. "Aus der Sitzung des Vorstandes und des Geschäftsauschußes des Deutschen Ärztevereinsbundes am 24. und 25. Januar 1931 in Berlin," *DÄ*, 60 (1931), 65–66.

138. "Aus der Sitzung . . . in Berlin," p. 66.

139. U. Schagen, "Die ärztliche Weiterbildung," in *Reform der Ärzteausbildung: Neue Wege in den Fakultäten*, ed. D. Halbeck, U. Schagen, and G. Wagner (Berlin: Blackwell Wissenschaft, 1993), 401–25, at 402. I return to this subject in my epilogue to this book.

140. "Revision der Facharztrichtlinien unter Berücksichtigung der Röntgentätigkeit," *DÄ*, 61 (1932), 428.

141. Teicher, "Untersuchungen zur ärztlichen Spezialisierung," p. 80.

142. R. Syller, "Zur Frage der Facharzt-Doppelbezeichnungen," *DÄ*, 65 (1935), 64.

143. For some examples, see Eduard Seidler, *Kinderärzte, 1933–1945: Entrechtet, geflohen, ermordet* (Bonn: Bouvier, 2000); Wolfgang Weyers, *Death of Medicine in Nazi Germany: Dermatology and Dermatopathology Under the Swastika*, ed. Bernard Ackerman (Philadelphia: Madison Books, 1998).

144. Löhlein, "Die Stellung der Augenheilkunde," p. 1127.

145. Löllke, "Grundsätze zur Facharztanerkennung in Berlin," p. 245.

146. Moran, *Governing the Health Care State*, p. 38; Deborah Stone, *The Limits of Professional Power: National Health Care in the Federal Republic of Germany* (Chicago: University of Chicago Press, 1980), pp. 39–40.

147. "Anordnung der Kassenärztlichen Vereinigung Deutschlands über die Standes- und Facharztordnung," *DÄ*, 65 (1935), 459–61; "Standes- und Facharztordnung," *DÄ*, 65 (1935), 633.

148. Löllke, "Grundsätze zur Facharztanerkennung," p. 244.

149. Löllke, "Grundsätze zur Facharztanerkennung, " p. 244

150. Kurt Blome, "Neue Richtlinien über ärztliche Fortbildung: Ärztliche Pflichtfortbildung," *DÄ*, 65 (1935), 773–77.

151. Kurt Blome, "Rückblick und Ausblick unserer ärztlichen Fortbildung und Schulung," *DÄ*, 67 (1937), 2–6, especially 4. Also see E. Sehrt, "Ein Facharzt über die ärztliche Pflichtfortbildung," *DÄ*, 67 (1937), 26–28; and Dr. Grote, "Die ärztliche Fortbildung in ihren Beziehungen zur Reichsärztekammer und Kassenärztlichen Vereinigung Deutschlands," *DÄ*, 67 (1937), 28–31.

152. Dr. Sonnenberg, "Die Stellung der Fachärzte in der Zulassungsordnung," *DÄ*, 66 (1936), 313–14.

153. Dr. Grote, "Die ärztliche Fortbildung"; Löllke, "Grundsätze zur Facharztanerkennung," p. 244.

154. The terms that specialists could use to describe themselves were severely restricted. Sewering, "Von der 'Bremer Richtlinien,'" B1597.

155. *JAMA*, 110 (1938), 221–23.

156. Sewering, "Von der 'Bremer Richtlinien,'" B1597.

157. Michael Kater, *Doctors Under Hitler* (Chapel Hill: University of North Carolina Press, 1989), pp. 29–30.

158. Kater, *Doctors Under Hitler*, p. 31.

1. Entrepreneurial writers offered GPs easy access to specialist knowledge in such books as J. D. Albright, *The General Practitioner as a Specialist: A Treatise Devoted the Consideration of Medical Specialties*, 3rd ed. (Philadelphia: n.p., 1904).

2. Lewis H. Taylor, "Work of the Section on Ophthalmology," *JAMA*, 46 (1906), 1897–98.

3. Among American medical graduates of 1915, between 66 and 75 percent eventually became or planned to become full-time or part-time specialists. H. G. Weiskotten, "Tendencies in Medical Practice," *JAMA*, 90 (1928), 1046, and "Tendencies in Medical Practice: A Study of 1925 Graduates," *Journal of the Association of American Medical Colleges*, 7 (1932), 72–73. For comparable figures, see Rosemary Stevens, *American Medicine and the Public Interest*, updated ed. (Berkeley: University of California Press, 1998), p. 116.

4. James G. Burrow, *Organized Medicine in the Progressive Era: The Move Toward Monopoly* (Baltimore: Johns Hopkins University Press, 1977).

5. George Rosen, *The Structure of American Medical Practice, 1875–1941*, ed. Charles E. Rosenberg (Philadelphia: University of Pennsylvania Press, 1983), pp. 88–90.

6. George E. Shambaugh, "The Specialist in Medicine," *JAMA*, 59 (1912), 1088–89.

7. Shambaugh, "The Specialist in Medicine," p. 1090.

8. Sydney A. Halpern, *American Pediatrics: The Social Dynamics of Professionalism* (Berkeley: University of California Press, 1988), pp. 50–54, 57–61, 65–69.

9. "Following in the wake of other specialties, pediatrics has gradually attained proper maturity and is second to no branch in energy, enthusiasm and progress, not only in the annual literary output, but in the teaching in the clinic and laboratory" (W. C. Hollopeter, "The Pediatric Outlook," *JAMA*, 47 [1906], 397). For a less optimistic view of the scientific output of the specialty that nevertheless viewed the field in equally academic terms, see David Edsall, "Presidential Address: American Pediatric Society," *JAMA*, 54 (1910), 1709–10.

10. Thomas S. Southworth, "The Role of Pediatrics in Preventive Medicine," *JAMA*, 55 (1910), 179. Also see Thomas Morgan Rotch, "The Opportunity of the Pediatrician," *JAMA*, 47 (1906), 729. Other examples can be found in Halpern, *American Pediatrics*, pp. 72–75.

11. Rosemary Stevens, "The Curious Career of Internal Medicine: Functional Ambivalence, Social Success," in *Grand Rounds: One Hundred Years of Internal Medicine*, ed. Russell C. Maulitz and Diana E. Long (Philadelphia: University of Pennsylvania Press, 1988), pp. 339–64.

12. William Graves, "Some Factors Tending Toward Adequate Instruction in Nervous and Mental Diseases," *JAMA*, 63 (1914), 1707–13.

13. Samuel H. Greenblatt, "Harvey Cushing's Paradigmatic Contribution to Nuerosurgery and the Evolution of His Thoughts About Specialization," *BHM*, 77 (2003), 810–19.

14. Franklin G. Ebaugh, "The Importance of Introducing Psychiatry into the General Internship," *JAMA*, 102 (1934), 982–85. On this issue more generally, see Jack D. Pressman, *Last Resort: Psychosurgery and the Limits of Medicine* (Cambridge: Cambridge

University Press, 1998), ch. 1, and "Human Understanding: Psychosomatic Medicine and the Mission of the Rockefeller Foundation," in *Greater Than the Parts: Holism in Biomedicine, 1920–1950*, ed. Christopher Lawrence and George Weisz (New York: Oxford University Press, 1998), pp. 189–208.

15. Lodilla Ambrose, "Instruction in Roentgenology," *JAMA*, 63 (1914), 651–53; Preston M. Hickey, "Education in Roentgenology," *JAMA*, 85 (1925), 557–58.

16. Fred M. Hodges, "The Section on Radiology," *JAMA*, 95 (1930), 833.

17. Ralph H. Waters et al., "The Relation of Anesthesiology to Medical Education," *JAMA*, 112 (1939), 1671.

18. J. Whitridge Williams, "Medical Education and the Midwife Problem in the United States," *JAMA*, 58 (1912), 1.

19. Charles Edward Ziegler, "The Elimination of the Midwife," *JAMA*, 60 (1913), 32–34.

20. Ziegler, "Elimination of the Midwife," p. 6 Edward P. Davis, "Obstetric Science and Art in the Service of the Nation," *JAMA*, 71 (1918), 1871.

21. S. MacCuen Smith, "Specialism in Its Relation to General Medicine," *JAMA*, 48 (1907), 2173.

22. Hugh Cabot, "Specialism in General and Genito-urinary Surgery in Particular," *The Lancet* (1912), 2, 398–99.

23. Barbara Bridgman Perkins, "Shaping Institution-Based Specialism: Early Twentieth-Century Economic Organization of Medicine," *SHM*, 10 (1997), 425–28.

24. Edward Jackson, "The Proper Provision for the Teaching of Ophthalmology in the Medical Schools," *JAMA*, 59 (1912), 1056.

25. George N. Jack, "The Established Specialist vs. the 'Developing Physician,'" *JAMA*, 49 (1907), 508.

26. Hugh Cabot, "Report of the Committe on Sections and Section Work," *JAMA*, 65 (1915), 115.

27. Greenfield Sluder, "The Specialists' Relation to the American Medical Association," *JAMA*, 71 (1918), 1785–86.

28. Thomas B. Cooly, "Relation of the Infant Welfare Movement to Pediatrics," *JAMA*, 59 (1912), 2218–19.

29. Halpern, *American Pediatrics*, ch. 5; figures are on p. 82.

30. On orthopedics, see Roger Cooter, *Surgery and Society in Peace and War: Orthopaedics and the Organization of Modern Medicine, 1880–1948* (London: Macmillan, 1993), pp. 142–51.

31. Joel Howell, "Hearts and Minds: The Invention and Transformation of American Cardiology," in *Grand Rounds: One Hundred Years of Internal Medicine*, ed. Russell C. Maulitz and Diana E. Long (Philadelphia: University of Pennsylvania Press, 1988), pp. 244–45, 248; W. Bruce Fye, *American Cardiology: The History of a Specialty and Its College* (Baltimore: Johns Hopkins University Press, 1996), chs. 1–3.

32. William G. Rothstein, *American Medical Schools and the Practice of Medicine: A History* (New York: Oxford University Press, 1987), pp. 299–300.

33. "American Roentgen Rau Society: Annual Meeting," *JAMA*, 59 (1912), 1209.

34. George M. MacKee and Erlin J. Stone, "Surgery in Dermatological Practice," *JAMA*, 95 (1930), 1315–17; Elmore B. Tauber, "Dermatology: Its Past, Its Present, Its Future," *JAMA*, 97 (1931), 3.

35. Bordon Veeder, "Discussion: The Teaching of Pediatrics," *JAMA*, 96 (1931), 702. For the case of gynecology, see note 38.

36. Walter G. Stern, "Orthopedics of Today," *JAMA*, 93 (1929), 1110.

37. Leonard W. Ely, "Orthopedic Surgery: Its Scope and Its Future," *JAMA*, 63 (1914), 2265.

38. George E. Shambaugh, "The Preparation of the Specialist: A Problem in Medical Education," *JAMA*, 49 (1907), 540–43.

39. The first figure applies to Harvard Medical School, and the second applies to Johns Hopkins. Association of American Medical Colleges, Commission on Medical Education, *Final Report of the Commission on Medical Education* (New York: Association of American Medical Colleges, 1932), p.115. See also Weiskotten, "Tendencies in Medical Practice: 1925 Graduates," p. 76.

40. Albert E. Bulson, "Some Comments and Suggestions Concerning the Welfare of the Section on Ophthalmology," *JAMA*, 57 (1911), 781.

41. J. Stitt Wishart, Charles Richardson, and S. MacCuen Smith, "Teaching of Otolaryngology," *JAMA*, 61 (1913), 535–37; J. M. T. Finney, "The Standardization of Surgery," *JAMA*, 63 (1914), 1433–37.

42. "Current Comment: Higher Degrees in Medicine," *JAMA*, 63 (1914), 1399. By 1917 a seventh was in place.

43. "Special Training for the Specialist," *JAMA*, 52 (1914), 1792.

44. E. P. Lyon, "Graduate Education in the Clinical Branches, and the Minnesota Experiment," *JAMA*, 69 (1917), 1310.

45. Lyon, "Graduate Eduation," pp. 1307–13.

46. Lyon, "Graduate Education," p. 1308.

47. "Annual Congress on Medical Education and Licensure: The Function of Special Boards of Examiners, by Sanford R. Gifford," *JAMA*, 100 (1933), 1111.

48. Perkins, "Shaping Institution-Based Specialism," p. 422; Rosen, *Structure of American Practice.*

49. Stevens, *American Medicine,* p. 79.

50. A superb and detailed account of the issues discussed below can be found in part II of Stevens, *American Medicine.* Rosen, *Structure of American Practice,* pp. 81–87, provides a summary version.

51. On the early standardization movement, see Rosemary Stevens, *In Sickness and in Wealth: American Hospitals in the Twentieth Century* (New York: Basic Books, 1989), pp. 52–79, 114–20.

52. Stevens, *American Medicine,* pp. 77–92.

53. Stevens, *American Medicine,* pp. 91–95. Also see Stevens, "Curious Career of Internal Medicine," pp. 345–47.

54. Stevens, *American Medicine,* pp. 98–114; Rosen, *Structure of American Practice,* pp. 83–84.

55. For example, "A Proposed Section on Genito-Urinary and Venereal Diseases," *JAMA*, 54 (1910), 1459–60.

56. "Archives of Pathology," *JAMA*, 85 (1925), 1400–1.

57. The request of industrial physicians for a section at the annual meeting and recognition in the *AMD* is discussed in "Report of Reference Committee on Sections and Section Work," *JAMA*, 70 (1918), 1942. The size of the associations making such re-

quests seems to have been an important factor in determining whether recognition was accorded or not. However, the number of existing sections and fears about overloading the program of annual meetings constituted a major impediment to the claims of new specialty groups.

58. Jonathan Engel, *Doctors and Reformers: Discussion and Debate over Health Policy, 1925–1950* (Columbia: University of South Carolina Press, 2002), p. 300, makes the point that by 1948 half the organization's members were general practitioners but 90 percent of the delegates were full-time specialists.

59. Stevens, *American Medicine*, pp. 115–27.

60. Arthur Dean Bevan, "Report of the Council on Medical Education and Hospitals," *JAMA*, 84 (1925), 1657.

61. Fye, *American Cardiology*, p. 44.

62. Arthur Dean Bevan, "The Organization of the Medical Profession for War," *JAMA*, 70 (1918), 1806.

63. Stevens, *American Medicine*, pp. 127–28.

64. "Fifteenth Annual Conference of the Council on Medical Education of the American Medical Association, Edward L. Munson, 'The Needs of Medical Education as Revealed by the War,'" *JAMA*, 72 (1919), 822–23

65. Robert W. Lovett, "A Plea for a More Fundamental Method in Medical Teaching," *JAMA*, 70 (1918), 1070–71.

66. Cooter, *Surgery and Society*, p. 130.

67. "Fifteenth Annual Conference of the Council on Medical Education of the American Medical Association, Comments by John M. Dobson," *JAMA*, 72 (1919), 821.

68. "The Navy Encourages Specialization," *JAMA*, 91 (1928), 1473.

69. Pressman, *Last Resort*, pp. 22–23.

70. Glen R Shepherd, *A History of the Council on Medical Education and Hospitals of the American Medical Association, 1904–1959* (Chicago: American Medical Association, 1960), p. 27.

71. Before World War I there were few residency programs available, and these were almost exclusively in major hospitals. They did not begin to develop in significant numbers until the 1920s. Rothstein, *American Medical Schools*, pp. 136–37.

72. Arthur Dean Bevan, "Report of the Council on Medical Education and Hospitals," *JAMA*, 84 (1925), 1657.

73. Terminology varied among schools and hospitals. But according to the list of graduate programs in *JAMA*, 85 (1925), 598–600, there were fourteen programs in laryngology and rhinology as well as fifteen in otolaryngology and another eighteen in ophthalmology and otology; there were also eighteen programs in general surgery, seventeen in neurology and psychiatry, sixteen in pediatrics with another four in infant feeding, and sixteen in public health and preventive medicine.

74. AMA Commission on Graduate Medical Education, *Graduate Medical Education: Report of the Commission on Graduate Medical Education* (Chicago: University of Chicago Press, 1940), p. 101.

75. Shepherd, *History of the Council on Medical Education*, p. 28.

76. Editorial, "Internships, Residencies and Fellowships," *JAMA*, 112 (1939), 997–98.

77. Editorial, "Internships, Residencies and Fellowships," p. 998.

78. Weiskotten, "Tendencies in Medical Practice: 1925 Graduates," p. 78.

79. Stevens, *American Medicine*, pp. 158–64.

80. Stevens, *American Medicine*, pp. 165–67.

81. Stevens, *American Medicine*, pp. 180–81.

82. Alphonse M. Schwitalla, "Basic Considerations in the Minority Report of the Committee on the Costs of Medical Care," *JAMA*, 100 (1933), 863.

83. Stevens, *American Medicine*, pp. 183–88. For a different perspective on the work of this committee, see Daniel M. Fox, *Health Policies, Health Politics: The British and American Experience, 1911–1965* (Princeton, N.J.: Princeton University Press, 1986), pp. 45–51. Also see Engel, *Doctors and Reformers*, ch. 2.

84. Engel, *Doctors and Reformers*, p. 38, suggests that the majority report's emphasis on the importance of specialization was largely introduced as a justification for the proposal to support group practice.

85. One of the leaders of CCMC, Ray Lyman Wilbur, played a significant role in the AMA's efforts to coordinate specialist training. But there is no evidence that he linked this effort with the CCMC's efforts to increase access to health care. His memoirs devote a chapter to this latter issue without once mentioning his work on AMA certification. Ray Lyman Wilbur, *The Memoirs of Ray Lyman Wilbur, 1875–1949*, ed. Edgar Eugene Robinson and Paul Carroll Edwards (Stanford, Calif.: Stanford University Press, 1960).

86. It is probably significant that only one year separated the creation of this board from that of the British Royal College of Obstetrics and Gynecology in 1929. Stevens, *American Medicine*, p. 200.

87. Stevens, *American Medicine*, p. 542, table A1.

88. Stevens, *In Sickness and in Wealth*, pp. 116, 139; David P. Adams, "Community and Professionalization: General Practitioners and Ear, Nose, and Throat Specialists in Cincinnati, 1945–1947," *BHM*, 68 (1994), 664–84.

89. Harry E. Mock, "The Council on Physical Therapy of the American Medical Association: Its Problems and Its Progress," *JAMA*, 100 (1933), 1433–43.

90. "Report of the Committee on the Present Status of Physical Therapy," *JAMA*, 107 (1936), 584–85.

91. "Report of of the Committee . . . Physical Therapy," pp. 584–85. On the relationship between physiotherapists and the medical profession more generally, see Beth Linker, "Strength and Science: Gender, Physiotherapy, and Medicine in the United States, 1918–35," *Journal of Women's History*, forthcoming.

92. Irving S. Cutter and John S. Coulter, "The Teaching of Physical Therapy to Undergraduate Medical Students" (Authorized by the Council on Physical Therapy), *JAMA*, 102 (1934), 1849. Also see Linker, "Strength and Science."

93. "Physicians Specializing in Pathology: Report by the Council on Medical Education and Hospitals," *JAMA*, 99 (1932), 1425–26.

94. Walter M. Simpson, "The Training of Technicians for the Clinical Laboratory," *JAMA*, 100 (1933), 1433.

95. "Radiologic Service in the United States: Report by the Council on Medical Education and Hospitals," *JAMA*, 100 (1933), 413–15. On the AMA's activities in pathology and radiology, see Stevens, *American Medicine*, pp. 207–8.

96. Ray Lyman Wilbur, "Report of the Chairman of the Council on Medical Education and Hospitals," *JAMA*, 100 (1933), 1040. This was in fact a direct quote from a resolution of 1931 by the AMA's House of Delegates: "Report of the Council on Medical Education and Hospitals," *JAMA*, 100 (1933), 1424.

97. Ray Lyman Wilbur, "The Relation of the Council on Medical Education and Hospitals of the American Medical Association to the Special Practice of Medicine," *JAMA*, 100 (1933), 1113. Also see "Report of the Council on Medical Education and Hospitals," *JAMA*, 100 (1933), 1424.

98. "Abstract of the Minutes of Council Business Meeting, June 9," *JAMA*, 108 (1935), 142; "Certification of Radiologists," *JAMA* 108 (1935), 630.

99. "Advisory Board on Medical Specialties," *JAMA*, 102 (1934), 702.

100. Council for Medical Education and Hospitals, "Certification of Specialists," *JAMA*, 102 (1934), 1085.

101. "Advisory Board for Boards Certifying Specialists,' *JAMA*, 102 (1934), 1326.

102. Ray Lyman Wilbur, "Report of the Council on Medical Education and Hospitals," *JAMA*, 102 (1934), 1065.

103. Stevens, *American Medicine*, pp. 212–17, 218, 542.

104. Stevens, *American Medicine*, pp. 244–48.

105. "Report of the Council on Medical Education and Hospitals, by Dr. Ray Lyman Wilbur," *JAMA*, 111 (1938), 62. For similar statements, see Wilbur, "Report of the Council on Medical Education and Hospitals," *JAMA*, 110 (1938), 1328.

106. "The Roentgenologist, the Pathologist and the Anesthetist Under Hospital Insurance Plans," *JAMA*, 111 (1938), 158–59; Council on Physical Therapy, "Physical Therapy Departments in Hospitals with Fifty or More Beds," *JAMA*, 110 (1938), 896–99.

107. Paul B. Beeson and Russell C. Maulitz, "The Inner History of Internal Medicine," in *Grand Rounds: One Hundred Years of Internal Medicine*, ed. Russell C. Maulitz and Diana E. Long (Philadelphia: University of Pennsylvania Press, 1988), pp. 28–29. More generally, see George F. Lull, "Fifty Thousand Doctors and Half a Million Personnel," in *Doctors at War*, ed. Morris Fishbein (New York: E. P. Dutton 1945), pp. 91–108.

108. Fox, *Health Policies, Health Politics*, p. 116; Rothstein, *American Medical Schools*, p. 187.

109. Stevens, *American Medicine*, pp. 213–15.

110. *JAMA*, 105 (1935), 723.

111. *Graduate Medical Education*, p. 117.

112. *Graduate Medical Education*, p. 110.

113. *Graduate Medical Education*, p.100.

114. Stevens, *American Medicine*, pp. 258–62.

115. Stevens, *American Medicine*, pp. 261–64.

116. H. G. Weiskotten et al., "Trends in Medical Practice: An Analysis of the Distribution and Characteristics of Medical College Graduates, 1915–1950," *Journal of Medical Education*, 35 (1960), 1071–1121.

117. W. B. Schwartz et al., "The Changing Geographic Distribution of Board-Certified Physicians," *New England Journal of Medicine*, 303 (1980), 1033.

118. Stevens, *American Medicine*, pp. 252–56.

119. Stevens, *American Medicine*, pp. 256–57, 277–80, 281–85.

120. Shepherd, *History of the Council on Medical Education*, pp. 29–30.

121. For an insider's view of certification examinations during this period, see Allan B. Weisse, "Certification and Recertification in Medicine: Self-Improvement, Self-Delusion, or Self-Strangulation?" *Perspectives in Biology and Medicine*, 41 (1998), 579–83.

122. Stevens, *American Medicine*, p. 216.

123. Rothstein, *American Medical Schools*, pp. 321–24.

124. Shepherd, *History of the Council on Medical Education*, pp. 29–30; Howell, "Hearts and Minds," p. 255.

125. Stevens, *American Medicine*, pp. 324–27.

126. The President's Commission on the Health Needs of the Nation, *Building America's Health: A Report to the President*, 5 vols. (Washington, D.C: Government Printing Office, 1952–53), vol. 3, pp. 160–65, gives a figure of 31 percent full-time specialists in 1949. Later statistics for this same year, cited by Stevens, *American Medicine*, p.181, give a figure of 36 percent.

127. *Graduate Medical Education*, pp. 106–7, 262–66.

128. Stevens, *American Medicine*, p. 257.

129. Fox, *Health Policies, Health Politics*, adds a useful antidote to discussions about American particularism by showing some of the parallels between policies in the United States and those of the United Kingdom.

130. Engel, *Doctors and Reformers*, p. 313.

Chapter 8

1. Christian Bonah, *Instruire, guérir, servir: Formation et pratique médicales en France et en Allemagne* (Strasbourg: Presses Universtaires de Strasbourg, 2000), pp. 116, 247.

2. This is the argument in Pierre Guillaume, *Le rôle social du médecin depuis deux siècles: 1800–1945* (Paris: Association pour l'Étude de l'Histoire de la Sécurité Sociale, 1996), pp. 209–10.

3. George Weisz, "The Development of Medical Specialization in Nineteenth-Century Paris," in *French Medical Culture in the Nineteenth Century, Clio Medica* 25, ed. Ann La Berge and Mordechai Feingold (Amsterdam and Atlanta: Rodopi, 1994), pp. 148–88.

4. Archives Nationales, Paris/Archives de l'Ordre des Médecins (hereafter ANP/ AOM), Circulaire no. 17, June 8, 1944, #3, "Lettre de Dr. Oberlin au ministre de la santé"; also see Dr. Menegaux, "Le certificat de chirurgien," *BOM*, 1947–48, 29–33. *BOM* appeared sporadically during the war, and postwar volumes were labeled unsystematically and without volume numbers. I identify volumes by the year(s) and, where it seems necessary (because monthly issues are paginated separately), the month.

5. On this prewar state of affairs, see George Weisz, *The Emergence of Modern Universities in France, 1863–1914* (Princeton, N.J.: Princeton University Press, 1983), pp. 341–68.

6. On elite careers in France, see George Weisz, *The Medical Mandarins: The French Academy of Medicine in the Nineteenth and Early Twentieth Centuries* (New York and Oxford: Oxford University Press, 1995).

7. These specialties were surgery, obstetrics, psychiatry, ophthalmology, otorhinolaryngology, electroradiology, and stomatology. The examinations were competitive ex-

aminations (*concours*) on the model of those that traditionally controlled access to hospital positions.

8. The leading medical directory of the period *Guide Rosenwald* of 1920, contains a list of Parisian hospital physicians, the vast majority of whom are described as specialists.

9. Weisz, "Development of Medical Specialization."

10. The decree is reprinted in *PMd*, 14 (1914), 719–25. On the wider context of this reform, see Paul Carnot, "Les nouveaux décrets relatifs à l'agrégation . . . ," *PMd*, 14 (1914), 731–32.

11. See, for instance, the many reports on the teaching of the different specialties in *Congrès des praticiens*, 2 vols. (Paris, 1907). Medical journals also sought to educate GPs in specialist knowledge. See the series of articles by Dr. Boudin throughout *CMd*, 32 (1910), titled "Le médecin de campagne et l'exercise de la spécialité." Also see J.-L. Faure, "L'enseignement de la chirurgie," *PrM*, 27 (1919), 401–3.

12. "Reportage médical," *CMd*, 31 (1909), 620.

13. A survey of such courses is in Paul Carnot, "Rapport sur l'organisation des enseignements de perfectionnement dans les facultés de médecine," *PMd*, 14 (1914), 146–47, 177–83, 249–53.

14. For example, H. Besnier, "A quoi sert le diplôme de médecine-légiste," *PrM*, 20 (1912), 1369–70. On these programs more generally, see Carnot, "Rapport sur l'organisation," pp. 180, 249–50. The situation was unchanged years later. "Association des diplômés de l'Institut d'hygiène de l'Université de Paris," *PMd*, 84 (1932), 615.

15. "Special Commission for Surveillance of Outcome of Nervous and Mental Disease in Soldiers," *JAMA*, 70 (1918), 1554.

16. Patrice Pinell, *Naissance d'un fléau: Histoire de la lutte contre le cancer en France* (Paris: Métaillié, 1992). This book has been published in English as *The Fight Against Cancer: France, 1890–1940*, trans. David Madell (London: Routledge, 2002).

17. The figure was 37 percent, compared with 35 percent fifteen years before. On the reasons for this stability, see George Weisz, "Mapping Medical Specialization in Paris in the Nineteenth and Twentieth Centuries," *SHM*, 7 (1994), 177–211.

18. The figure in the largest provincial cities was 46 percent in 1935, compared with 12 percent in 1905. On the growing number of specialists more generally, see Weisz, "Mapping Medical Specialization."

19. *Syndicats* were established for spa physicians in 1896; for oculists in 1905; for electroradiologists, ORL, and stomatologists in 1907; for urologists in 1913; for biologists (pathologists and bacteriologists) in 1924; for surgeons in 1925; for dermatologist-venereologists in 1929; for gynecologists in 1930; and for pneumologists (including TB) in 1931.

20. *Tout-Paris: Annuaire de la société parisienne, 1921* (Paris: A. Lafare, 1921), pp. 724–35.

21. G. Linossier, "Libres propos: Médecins spécialistes,' *PMd*, 42 (1921), 271–72.

22. Guillaume, *Rôle social*, p. 201.

23. Donna Evleth, "Vichy France and the Continuity of Medical Nationalism," *SHM*, 8 (1995), 95–116, and "'The Romanian Privilege' in French Medicine and Anti-Semitism," *SHM*, 11 (1998), 213–32.

24. Timothy B. Smith, "The Social Transformation of Hospitals and the Rise of Medical Insurance in France, 1914–1943," *The Historical Journal*, 41 (1998), 1055–87. In

1919 the Municipal Council of Paris discussed the creation of posts for ophthalmologists and stomatologists for the schools of Paris. Note in *PrM*, 27 (1919), 375.

25. See the series of articles "Applications du tarif des pensionés de guerre," in the issues of *Médecin syndicalist* of 1923 and 1924. For a retrospective view, see Dr. Caillaud, "Le C2 et les spécialistes," *CMd*, 70 (1948), 515–16.

26. A major dispute was provoked in the council of the Union des Syndicats Médicaux when the president published an article suggesting that specialists accept a reduction in their fees. "Tarifs des spécialistes," *MdS*, 8 (1926), 364–65. Also see F. Decourt, "Un omnipraticien ne serait-il qu'un 'demi-médecin': IV—Spécialisation n'est pas études 'supérieures' mais études 'fragmentaires,'" *CMd*, 66 (1944), 189–90.

27. See, for instance, "Question 53: Criterium du spécialiste," *MdS*, 5 (1923), 375; and the long quote from a judgment by the Commission Supérieure de Surveillance des Soins Gratuits aux Mutilés, reproduced in *MdFr*, 37 (1931), 915.

28. "Belgium: Diplomas for Specialists," *JAMA*, 99 (1933), 1706.

29. In 1928 there were specialist trade unions representing biologists, surgeons, electroradiologists, ophthalmologists, otorhinolaryngologists, spa physicians, stomatologists, and urologists. Together they had about 2,300 members (G. Renon, "Le statut des médecins spécialistes," *MdS*, 9 [1927], 274–80, especially 277–78; "Liste des syndicats médicaux," *MdS*, 10 [1928], 564). Two issues that proved especially thorny were whether members of national specialist *syndicats* also had to belong to (and pay dues to) local general *syndicats*, and what kind of voting rights, if any, specialist representatives had on the administrative councils.

30. This was the Groupement des Syndicats des Spécialistes ("Le statut des spécialistes," *MdS*, 9 [1927], 167–69). The best discussion of the intricacies of medical trade unionism during this period is Guillaume, *Rôle social*. Also see Bénédicte Vergez, *Le monde des médecins au XXe siècle* (Brussels: Éditions Complexe, 1996), pp. 236–46.

31. See the collection of reports and discussions grouped under the heading "Les médecins spécialisés et l'Union des Syndicats Médicaux," *MdS*, 9 (1927), 270–88.

32. "Les médecins spécialisés," p. 276.

33. "Les médecins spécialisés," p. 276.

34. "Les médecins specialisés," pp. 282–85.

35. "Notre revue," *Revue internationale de médecine professionnelle et sociale*, 1 (1928), 1–3.

36. In 1934, for instance, the annual meeting of the APIM voted unanimously that diagnosis and prescription for glasses should be under the control of doctors rather than opticians. "L'Association Professionnelle Internationale des Médecins," *PMd*, 94 (1934), 479.

37. Fernand Decourt, "Association Professionnelle Internationale des Médecins: La spécialisation en médecine et les spécialistes," *MdS*, 10 (1928), 518–57. The article was reprinted in *Revue internationale de médecine professionnelle et sociale*, 4 (1931), 10–44.

38. Dr. Vuilleumier, "Les médecins spécialistes," *Revue internationale de médecine professionnelle et sociale*, 1 (1928), 30–37, followed by discussion at 38–41. Also see Fernand Decourt, "Causeries professionnelles: De la multiplication dangereuse des catégories de 'spécialistes' en médecine," *Revue internationale de médecine professionnelle et sociale*, 11 (1938), 7–12.

39. See, for example, "Définition et qualification du médecin specialisé," *MdFr,* 37 (1931), 834–35. Foreign examples were not necessarily viewed positively. Decourt in 1938 used the result of a second survey he had prepared to warn the Confederation that unless appropriate steps were taken, France could easily end up with twenty to twenty-five specialties, as was the case in most of the countries in his survey. *MdFr,* 44 (1938), 714.

40. J. Couturat, "Les dermatologistes en face de l'exercise illégal ou commercial de la médecine," *PrM,* 43 (1935), 1309.

41. On the history of French dentistry, see François Vidal et al., *Histoire d'une diplôme, 1699–1892: De l'expert pour les dents au docteur en chirurgie dentaire* (Paris: n.p., 1993); Raymond Boissier, *L'évolution de l'art dentaire* (Paris: Omnès, 1927); and Charles Godin, *L'évolution de l'art dentaire: L'École dentaire, son histoire, son action, son avenir* (Paris: J.-B. Baillière, 1901).

42. This issue generated a huge polemical literature. See, for example, T. Raynal, *Rapport sur la réforme de l'enseignement et la refonte du statut professionnel de l'art dentaire en France* (Paris: A. Maloine, 1923). For a similar though less intense version of the same controversy in the United States, see Norman Gevitz, "Autonomous Profession or Medical Specialty: The Stomatological Movement and American Dentistry," *BHM,* 62 (1988), 407–28. For a comparative analysis of these conflicts in the four nations under discussion, see chapter 11 in this volume.

43. Syndicat Général des Médecins Stomatologistes Français, "Lettre ouverte au corps médical," *PMd,* 62 (1926), 18.

44. P. Boudin, "Mouvement syndical de l'année," *CMd,* 50 (1928), 3198–99. A good summary of the various attempts at reform is M. Mordagne, "La qualification des spécialistes," *PrM,* 46 (1938), 1517–18.

45. "Une note de M. le professeur Balthazard à l'Académie de Médecine," *MdFr,* 36 (1930), 155–57.

46. "Candidature du syndicats des gynécologues," *MdFr,* 38 (1932), 205, 280.

47. *PrM,* 41 (1933), 509, 967.

48. See Mordagne, "La qualification des spécialistes," p. 1517, for explicit links between this holism and opposition to specialization. On holism in France more generally, see George Weisz, "A Moment of Synthesis: Holism in Interwar France," in *Greater Than the Parts: Holism in Biomedicine, 1920–1950,* ed. Christopher Lawrence and George Weisz (New York and Oxford: Oxford University Press, 1998), pp. 68–93.

49. "Commission de droit syndical," *MdFr,* 38 (1932), 202–5.

50. G. Roussy, "Réforme des études médicales," *PrM,* 40 (1932), 1807–9; *PrM,* 41 (1933), 571–74.

51. "Commission de l'enseignement," *MdFr,* 39 (1933), 271–73; debate and conclusions, *MdFr,* 39 (1933), 357–78.

52. "Certificat de spécialités" *MdFr,* 39 (1933), 644–48.

53. *PMd,* 90 (1933), 403, with discussion in "Études et certificats de spécialités," *MdFr,* 39 (1933), 966–72; "Brevet de chirugien " *MdFr,* 40 (1934), 186–95.

54. "Enseignement des spécialités," *MdFr,* 40 (1934), 27–29; "Assemblée générale de la Confédération des Syndicats Médicaux Français. 15–17 dec. 1933," *MdFr,* 40 (1934), 165–85.

55. G. Roussy, "La réforme des concours d'agrégation des facultés de médecine," *PrM*, 42 (1934), 1545–49.

56. Secretary-general's comments, *MdFr*, 43 (1937), 148; Dr. Béliard, untitled report, *MdFr*, 43 (1937), 149–54.

57. Béliard, untitled report, p. 152; *MdFr*, 45 (1939), 414.

58. "Qualification des spécialistes," *MdFr*, 44 (1938), 161–69; "Proposition de loi," *MdFr*, 44 (1938), 288–93.

59. "La qualification du spécialiste," *MdFr*, 44 (1938), 586–89.

60. Discussions are in "Certificats de spécialités," *MdFr*, 44 (1938), 706–25.

61. The possibility of obtaining a specialist certificate before obtaining the MD was mainly directed at hospital interns, who normally did not graduate until after the completion of the internship. "Qualification du spécialiste," *MdFr*, 45 (1939), 268.

62. In this version, the Confederation recognized only seven specialties: surgery, ophthalmology, otorhinolaryngology, stomatology, electroradiology, neuropsychiatry, and laboratory biology.

63. Mordagne, "La qualification des spécialistes," pp. 1517–18.

64. "La qualification du spécialiste," *MdFr*, 44 (1938), 931–37, at 932. The article is unsigned but was certainly written by Paul Cibrie, secretary-general of the Confederation.

65. "Accord interconfédéral sur l'intégration de l'art dentaire dans le doctorat en médécine," *MdFr*, 44 (1938), 937–39; "Il n'y aura pas de docteurs-dentistes," *MdFr*, 45 (1939), 225–26. Developments during the postwar period are discussed in chapter 11 of this volume.

66. "Statut général des specialités," *BOM*, June 1941, 95–98 ; see also p. 42.

67. There were twenty-two specialist categories of this sort, and no doctor was allowed to practice more than two.

68. I summarize very superficially many pages of rather inconclusive discussions from the minutes of the Conseil Supérieur de l'Ordre des Médecins from mid-March to mid-December 1941 in the Archives de l'Ordre des Médecins (AOM). Donna Evelth has prepared a detailed (so far unpublished) study of the various projects discussed by this council and the diverse ideological tendencies represented within it.

69. Brief notes on the Ordre in *PrM*, 52 (1943), 174, 239.

70. "École de chirurgie," *BOM*, August 1942, 142–43; ANP/AOM, Circulaire no. 17, June 8, 1944, "Projet d'enseignement de la chirurgie."

71. These were surgery, phtisiology, dermato-venerology, ORL, and ophthalmology. ANP/AOM, Circulaire no. 17, July 1942.

72. ANP/AOM, Circulaire no. 7, April 19, 1944.

73. Fernand Decourt, "Un omnipraticien ne serait-il qu'un demi-médecin," *CMd*, 66 (1944), 274–75. The Council did in fact intervene on several occasions when an administrative body decided that some specialties did not merit the high fees specialists usually received. For a case involving the Veterans' Administration, see ANP/AOM, Circulaire no. 3, January 3, 1944. On the composition of the Ordre at this time, see Bénédicte Vergez, "Internes et anciens internes des hôpitaux de Paris" (PhD thesis, Institut des Études Politiques, 1995), p. 373.

74. ANP/AOM, Circulaire no. 7, April 19, 1944.

75. ANP/AOM, Circulaire no. 20, June 12, 1944.

76. "De la qualification des spécialistes: Rapport de Dr. Carlotti," *BOM*, 1946–47, 77–87, at 77. Also see the brief editorial note, "Qualifications des spécialistes," *MdFr*, 52 (1946), 593.

77. While surgery, radiology, biology, stomatology, ophthalmology, ORL, and gyne-cology-obstetrics could be practiced only as exclusive specialties, dermato-venereology, neurology, urology, and phtisiology could be exclusive specialties or competencies combined with general practice. (Obstetrics, by itself, could also be a competence.) Up to two competencies could be combined with general medicine.

78. "De la qualification des spécialistes . . . Carlotti," pp. 77–87.

79. "Définition du médecin spécialiste: Rapport du Dr. Carlotti," *BOM*, 1947, 231–33, at 231.

80. "Définition du médecin spécialiste . . . Carlotti, " p. 233.

81. Menegaux, "Le certificat de chirurgien," p. 30.

82. "Arrête du 23 août 1947," *MdFr*, 53 (1947), 1225–27; "Lettre du ministère de la santé publique," *MdFr*, 53 (1947), 1228–30; *BOM*, 1947, 10.

83. Carlotti, in discussion, "De la qualification des specialistes," *BOM*, 1946–47, 74; "Définition du médicin spécialiste . . . Carlotti," 86. These decisions did not put an end to vigorous debate and campaigning around these issues. See Dr. Demarque, "L'homéopathie est-elle une spécialité?" *CMd*, 70 (1948), 358–59.

84. "De la qualification des specialistes . . . Carlotti," p 79.

85. Carlotti in discussion, "Qualification du spécialiste," BOM 1946–47, 209.

86. "Conseil national," *BOM*, 1947–48, 241–42.

87. Ophthalmology and ORL, however, could be combined into a single practice.

88. Although combining competencies with general practice was permitted, the specialist trade unions still considered exclusive practice as the norm for specialists. The Groupement des Syndicats Nationaux des Médecins Spécialisés excluded as member groups the *syndicats* of neurologists and gastroenterologists, which admitted members who combined their specialty with general practice. Dr. Courtois, "Quelques problèmes qui se posent au spécialités," *MdFr*, 60 (1954), 7901–5, at 7902. Eventually physicians practicing a competency exclusively came to be considered a special category. To complicate matters still further, it turned out that it was possible to combine competencies (psychiatry and neurology, ORL and ophthalmology) and a specialty (such as surgery) with a competency (such as urology or gynecology).

89. These were published throughout *BOM*, 1947–48.

90. Dr. Hude, "L'avenir de la radiologie," *CMd*, 71 (1949), 1025–26.

91. "Qualification des spécialistes: État des travaux," *BOM*, 1948–49, 9–10. By 1949, the figure had reached 7,000. R. Garaud, "Toujours à propos des spécialisations," *CMd*, 71 (1949), 449–50.

92. C. Blondel, "Qualification des spécialistes," *BOM*, 1955, 6–9. It was not until 1958 that certificates formally became the fundamental prerequisite for specialization, and even then important exceptions remained.

93. Courtois, "Quelque problèmes qui se posent au spécialités," p. 7901.

94. J. R. Debray, "Étude de la répartition des médecins en France en 1953," *BOM*, 1954, 36–44.

95. Dr. Durand, "La spécialisation," *CMd*, 80 (1958), 3095–3106, at 3105.

96. An initial decision to this effect was taken by the Ordre in 1950 ("Séance du 9 juillet [après-midi]," *MdFr*, 56 [1950], 3673–75). It took some years for this decision to come into effect. "Information et documentation: Pédiatrie," *MdFr*, 64 (1958), 1954–56.

97. Durand, "La spécialisation," pp. 3095–3106. For protests about this situation, see Dr. Kreis, "Bruits de pot fêlé dans la symphonie des spécialisations," *CMd*, 72 (1950), 1537–44.

98. J. Mignon, "Organisation professionnelle: Les praticiens devant le problème de la spécialisation," *CMd*, 70 (1948), 2053–54.

99. "Qualification des spécialistes," *MdFr*, 55 (1949), 2872–73.

100. P. Douriez, "Tout ne va pas pour le mieux en matière de la qualification des spécialistes," *CMd*, 79 (1957), 57–60, at 58.

101. P. Douriez, "Comment se trouvent rétablie la dualité des qualifications des spécialistes," *CMd*, 71 (1949), 2541–45; "Circulaire N. 63 SS du 4 avril 1950," *MdFr*, 56 (1950), 3529–30. A decree of July 29, 1957, tried to realign the social insurance regulations to follow those of the Ordre. *BOM*, 1957, 251–52.

102. P. Douriez, "Actualité professionnelle: Pour l'intégrité du diplôme," *CMd*, 73 (1951), 1409–11; "Le certificat d'études spéciales n'est plus exigé des radiologistes hospitaliers," *CMd*, 80 (1958), 2043.

103. Discussion in *BOM*, 1955, 150–51.

104. The three administrative modifications of the regulatory basis of specialization that had been introduced in 1947 and 1948 were promulgated in 1952, 1955, and 1957. For legal difficulties provoked by the system, see H. Meillet, "La procédure de la qualification des spécialistes devra-t-elle être modifiée?" *CMd*, 74 (1952), 2817–19; J. Mignon, "Qualifications des spécialistes ou qualifications des consultants," *CMd*, 77 (1955), 1351–53; and P. Douriez, "Tout ne va pas pour le mieux," pp. 57–59, and "Le quatrième régime de qualification des spécialistes a vu le jour," *CMd*, 79 (1957), 403–4.

105. A few examples are R. Jodin, "Pour une spécialité de médecine interne," *CMd*, 70 (1948), 17–19; Dr. Kreiss, "À propos de la spécialisation surveillée," *CMd*, 71 (1949), 145–47; Robert Durand, "Défense du praticien," *CMd*, 71 (1949), 1665–66; R. Salins and F. Michaud, "Pour un dialogue constructif entre omnipraticiens et spécialistes," *CMd*, 80 (1958), 3223–27.

106. Dr. Caillaud "Le C2 et les spécialistes," pp. 515–16.

107. The first was bemoaned by Kreiss, "À propos," p. 445. The second was mentioned by several speakers in the account of "Colloque tenu à l'abbeye de Royaument, 22 oct. 1960," *PrM*, 69 (1961), 264–66. On earlier opposition of Paris interns to specialty diplomas that did not distinguish interns from noninterns, see Comité des Internes en Exercice des Hôpitaux de Paris, "L'internat des hôpitaux de Paris et la création de nouveaux diplômes de spécialité," *Journal des praticiens*, 63 (1949), 189. The complexity of this issue is underlined by the fact that the latter statement is followed immediately by another (Syndicat National des Médecins des Hôpitaux Libre, "À propos de la qualification des chirurgiens et spécialistes," pp. 189–90), complaining that many of those who interned outside of the official Paris hospitals (especially those in the suburbs) were being denied qualifications as surgeons.

108. Mignon, "Organisation professionnelle," pp. 1852–53; Courtois, "Quelques problèmes," p. 7902.

109. "Les internes et la qualification des spécialités," *CMd*, 77 (1955), 2789–90.

110. Kreiss, "À propos de la qualification," pp. 446–47.

111. Pequignot's comments are in "Colloque tenu à l'abbeye de Royaument," p. 264.

112. J.-P. Carlotti and H. Lafitte, "De la qualification des médecins spécialistes," in Ordre National des Médecins, *Premier Congrès International de Morale Medicale: Paris, octobre 1955*, vol. 1, *Rapports* (Paris: Masson, 1955), pp. 35–40. On this congress, see George Weisz, "The Origins of Medical Ethics in France: The International Congress of *Morale Médicale* of 1955," in *Social Science Perspectives on Medical Ethics*, ed. George Weisz (Dordecht: Kluwer, 1990), pp. 145–62.

Chapter 9

1. Originally published in the *Atlantic Monthly* and cited in "The English Side of Medical Education," *JAMA*, 56 (1915), 1391–92.

2. "Special Hospitals for Officers: Lord Knutford's Appeal," *The Lancet* (1915), 2, 1155. Similarly, demands for rationality led to new emphasis in the military on full and standardized clinical records. "Special Hospitals for Officers," p. 1157.

3. Joel D. Howell, "'Soldier's Heart': The Redefinition of Heart Disease and Specialty Formation in Early Twentieth-Century Great Britain," in *The Emergence of Modern Cardiology*, ed. W. F. Bynum, C. Lawrence, and V. Nutton, *Medical History*, supp. no. 5 (London: Wellcome Institute for the History of Medicine, 1985), pp. 34–52; Christopher Lawrence, "Moderns and Ancients: The 'New Cardiology' in Britain, 1880–1930," in *Emergence of Modern Cardiology*, pp. 1–33

4. "Letter from London," *JAMA*, 66 (1916), 1716.

5. Roger Cooter, *Surgery and Society in Peace and War: Orthopaedics and the Organization of Modern Medicine, 1880–1948* (London: Macmillan, 1993), pp. 105–36.

6. Howell, "'Soldier's Heart,'" pp. 44–47; Lawrence, "Moderns and Ancients," pp. 31–32.

7. Royal College of Surgeons (RCS), Correspondence, 1921 B no. 779, letter from the War Office to the chancellor—recruiting for general hospitals of Reconstructed Territorial Force.

8. RCS, Correspondence, 1918 B no. 859, letter from George Cronshaw to George Makins, May 16, 1918.

9. RCS, Correspondence, 1918 B no. 858; and Minutes of Council, 1917–19, pp. 159, 170.

10. On this conflict more generally see Cooter, *Surgery and Society*, pp. 130–36.

11. For example, Lauristen E. Shaw, "Medicine and the State," *The Lancet* (1918), 2, 87–90, especially 90; "The Need for Special Hospitals," *The Lancet* (1926), 1, 188 (summary of speech by Dr. I. Harris).

12. "An Institute for Otology," *JAMA*, 85 (1925), 688. "The Ferens Institute of Otology," *JAMA*, 88 (1927), 1091.

13. Henry Cohen, "Specialization—Its Value and Abuse," *BMJ* (1949), 1, 587.

14. Michael Worboys, "The Emergence of Tropical Medicine: A Study in the Establishment of a Scientific Specialty," in *Perspectives on the Emergence of Scientific Disciplines*, ed. G. Lemaine et al. (The Hague and Paris: Mouton, 1976), pp. 75–97; Douglas M.

Haynes, *Imperial Medicine: Patrick Manson and the Conquest of Tropical Disease* (Philadelphia: University of Pennsylvania Press, 2001).

15. Anne Digby, *The Evolution of British General Practice, 1850–1948* (Oxford: Oxford University Press, 1999), p. 61.

16. Sir Norman Walker, "Medical Education in Great Britain and Ireland," *JAMA*, 90 (1928), 1187; Digby, *Evolution of British General Practice*, p. 62.

17. Rosemary Stevens, *Medical Practice in Modern England and the Impact of Specialization and State Medicine* (New Haven, Conn.: Yale University Press, 1966), p. 42.

18. Frank Honigsbaum, *The Division in British Medicine: A History of the Separation of General Practice from Hospital Care* (London: Kogan Page, 1979), pp. 12, 14.

19. Honigsbaum, *Division in British Medicine*, pp. 163, 316. An influx of medical refugees from Germany and Austria artificially increased the number of GP-specialists in the country. But they were in no position to effectively defend their professional interests. Honigsbaum, *Division in British Medicine*, pp. 301, 311–12.

20. "Specialism in Germany," *BMJ* (1908), 2, 764–65.

21. "Berlin: Proposed New Regulations for Specialists," *BMJ* (1908), 2, 771–72.

22. Honigsbaum, *Division in British Medicine*, p. 117.

23. For a foreign account of the poor quality of specialty teaching in Britain, see Carl Prausnitz, "Die ärztliche Ausbildung in Deutschland, Frankreich und Großbritannien im Lichte der Reformbestrebungen des medizinischen Studiums," *DMW*, 58 (1932), 1689.

24. "Education in Ophthalmology," *The Lancet* (1919), 1, 578–79.

25. Holger Mygind, "The Education of the Specialist on the Continent," *BMJ* (1912), 2, 413–15.

26. Watson-Williams, "Education of the Specialist," pp. 415–19.

27. Watson-Williams, "Education of the Specialist," pp. 419–21.

28. St. Clair Thomson, "Education of the Specialist," p. 420.

29. Herbert Tilley, "Education of the Specialist," p. 420.

30. Mr. Wagget "Education of the Specialist," 420.

31. D. B. McGrigor, "Training in Radiology," *BMJ* (1936), 1, 476.

32. CMAC (Contemporary Medical Archives Centre, Wellcome Institute), SA/BMA/B70, meeting of the Physical Medicine Group, Apr. 6, 1932.

33. CMAC, SA/BMA/B71, memorandum by Frank Howitt, meeting of the Group Committee, May 24, 1934.

34. For an account of many such programs, see Stevens, *Medical Practice in Modern England*, pp. 48–50.

35. Archives of the BMA (ABMA), James Galloway, "Report on Special Diplomas and Certificates of Proficiency," Minutes of Council 1919–21, p. 73 (Jan. 6, 1920).

36. ABMA, Minutes of Council 1919–21, p. 257. The matter is briefly discussed in file 93, 1944–47, "Inception of FRCS (Ophth.)."

37. Frank Wellman and Paul Palmer, *The London Specialist Postgraduate Hospitals: A Review and Commentary on Their Future* (London: King Edward's Hospital Fund, 1975), p. 22.

38. Wellman and Palmer, *London Specialist Postgraduate Hospitals*, p. 23.

39. Wellman and Palmer, *London Specialist Postgraduate Hospitals*, p. 23.

40. "Discussion on the Treatment of Fractures: With Special Reference to Its Organisation and Teaching," *BMJ* (1925), 2, 317–31. On this issue more generally, see Cooter, *Surgery and Society*, pp. 180–98.

41. George Newman, *Recent Advances in Medical Education in England* (London: His Majesty's Stationery Office, 1923), and "The Formation of the Medical and Surgical Professorial Units in the London Teaching Hospitals," *Annals of Science*, 26 (1970), 1–22; Geoffrey Rivett, *The Development of the London Hospital System, 1823–1982* (London: King Edward's Hospital Fund for London, 1986), pp. 189–91.

42. Charles Webster, ed., *Caring for Health: History and Diversity*, 2nd ed. (Buckingham, U.K., and Philadelphia: Open University Press, 1993). p. 137.

43. On these matters, see Charles Webster, *The Health Services Since the War*, vol. 1, *Problems of Health Care: The National Health Service Before 1957* (London: Her Majesty's Stationery Office, 1988), pp. 6–10, 17.

44. "Hospitals Under the New Regime," *The Lancet* (1929), 1, 508; Stevens, *Medical Practice in Modern England*, pp. 58–61; Rivett, *Development of London Hospital System*, pp. 184–227.

45. Rivett, *Development of London Hospital System*, pp. 133–83.

46. E. Graham Little, "An Address on the Present Position of the Voluntary Hospitals," *The Lancet* (1927), 2, 1275–79.

47. "Hospitals Under the New Regime," p. 508; also 612, 682–83.

48. "Hospital Readjustment in London," *The Lancet* (1931), 1, 477.

49. Rivett, *Development of London Hospital System*, p. 202.

50. Stevens, *Medical Practice in Modern England*, p. 61.

51. Cooter, *Surgery and Society*, pp. 166–68.

52. Stevens, *Medical Practice in Modern England*, pp. 62–63.

53. Steve Sturdy and Roger Cooter, "Science, Scientific Management, and the Transformation of Medicine in Britain c. 1870–1950," *History of Science*, 36 (1998), 421–66, especially 432. For a discussion of the difference between Dawson's brand of professionally oriented rationalization and the more public health variant espoused by George Newman, see Cooter, *Surgery and Society*, pp. 166–68.

54. "The Optical Practitioners Bill," *The Lancet* (1928) 1, 89–90; *JAMA*, 85 (1926), 837.

55. A version of this list marked "Private and Confidential" is in CMAC, SA/BMA/B11; also see "British Medical Association Annual Meeting," *The Lancet* (1931), 2, 242.

56. "The Consultants List," *BMJ* (1933), 2, supp., 30C–2.

57. Letters in *BMJ* (1933), 2, supp., 310–11.

58. British Medical Association, *Consultant and Specialist Services* (London: BMA, Jan. 1938), in CMAC, SA/BMA/B11.

59. Of those on the medical list, 99 out of 147 indicated a specialty interest. Among surgeons the figure was 49 out of 127. BMA, *Consultant and Specialist Services*, pp. 4–19.

60. BMA, *Consultant and Specialist Services*, pp. 4–19.

61. The vast majority of initial applications were accepted. But by 1936 a considerable number were being rejected or postponed. ABMA, B/153/1/1.

62. All these cases occurred at the meeting of Sept. 27, 1932. ABMA, B/153/1/1.

63. ABMA, B/153/1/2.

64. Clinical reports publicized the fact that large numbers of patients who consulted the Service for errors of refraction also had other defects that would not have been picked up by opticians. N. Bishop Harman, "The Findings of Eye Examinations," *BMJ* (1936), 1, supp., 69–70.

65. The *BMJ* included many discussions of this issue at the end of 1935 and throughout 1936.

66. "The Place of the Physician in Ophthalmology," *The Lancet* (1919), 2, 1093–94; H. R Kenwood, "Abstract of the Milroy Lectures on the Teaching and Training in Hygiene," *The Lancet* (1918), 1, 695–99.

67. Digby, *Evolution of British General Practice*, pp. 289–92, notes that the two terms were interchangeable by the interwar years.

68. "The Profession of Medicine," *BMJ* (1937), 2, 444.

69. BMA, *Consultant and Specialist Services*.

70. "Hospital Reorganization in Manchester," *BMJ* (1935), 2, 353.

71. Stevens, *Medical Practice in Modern England*, pp. 48–52.

72. Stevens, *Medical Practice in Modern England*, p. 48.

73. Ministry of Health, *Report of the Inter-departmental Committee on Medical Schools* (Goodenough Report) (London: His Majesty's Stationery Office, 1944), pp. 231–32.

74. Ornella Moscucci, *The Science of Woman: Gynaecology and Gender in England, 1800–1929* (Cambridge: Cambridge University Press, 1990), pp. 165–206.

75. Stevens, *Medical Practice in Modern England*, pp. 43–45.

76. "Proceedings of the Council," *BMJ* (1935), 2, supp., 234–35.

77. Stevens, *Medical Practice in Modern England*, pp. 46–47.

78. "Consultants and the Association," *BMJ* (1934), 1, supp., 73; "Proceedings of the Council," *BMJ* (1934), 1, supp., 146–47. Minutes of meetings leading up to it are in CMAC, SA/BMA/B6.

79. "Meeting, Nov. 23," *BMJ* (1934), 2, supp., 295.

80. "Meeting, Dec. 17," *BMJ* (1937), 2, supp., 7.

81. "Proceedings of the Council," *BMJ* (1935), 1, supp., 35–36; "Report of Eligibility Subcommittee, 11 January 1935," CMAC, SA/BMA/B6; letters of 1943 in CMAC, SA/BMA/B11.

82. See the manuscript "Private and Confidential: Memorandum on the Provision of Consultant and Specialist and Pathologist Services for Insured Persons," by the Joint Committee (n.d., but probably written in 1937–38), CMAC, SA/BMA/B6.

83. Consultants and Specialists Group meetings of May 22, 1936, and Jan. 15, 1937, CMAC, SA/BMA/B6.

84. Stevens, *Medical Practice in Modern England*, pp. 67–73.

85. CMAC, SA/BMA/A30, 1947.

86. Amended rules, Apr. 1947, CMAC, SA/BMA/A30.

87. "Annual Representative Meeting," *BMJ* (1937), 2, supp., 51–53.

88. "Proceedings of the Council," *BMJ* (1937), 2, supp., 123.

89. *BMJ* (1937), 2, supp., 311. Also "Organization Committee, Dec. 28, 1937," CMAC, SA/BMA/A30.

90. "The following proposals are based on the assumption that the field of specialist and consultant practice will soon be completely 'covered' by groups." "Memorandum on the Constitution of Groups, Dec. 28, 1937," CMAC, SA/BMA/A30.

91. Annual report of the BMA Council, CMAC, SA/BMA/B108.

92. "Annual Report of the Council," *BMJ* (1946), 1, supp., 91.

93. "Annual Report of the Council." The BMA, however, did evenutally set up a part-time specialist roll for service at reduced fees.

94. Webster, *Health Services*, vol. 1, pp. 22–23.

95. Ministry of Health, *On the State of Public Health During Six Years of War: Report of the Chief Medical Officer of the Ministry of Health, 1939–45* (London: His Majesty's Stationery Office, 1946), p. 8.

96. Ministry of Health, *State of Public Health*, pp. 8, 135.

97. Ministry of Health, *Report of the Inter-departmental Committee on Medical Schools* (London: His Majesty's Stationery Office, 1944).

98. Ministry of Health, *Report of Inter-departmental Committee*, pp. 148–52.

99. Ministry of Health, *Report of Inter-departmental Committee*, pp. 32–33.

100. Ministry of Health, *Report of Inter-departmental Committee*, p. 32.

101. The report does not take a clear stand on this point but does mention that most witnesses appearing before it suggested that one of the higher degrees of the royal colleges should be an essential qualification. Ministry of Health, *Report of Inter-departmental Committee*, p. 212.

102. "Note A: Interim Planning Report of the Medical Planning Commission, 1944," CMAC, SA/BMA/B108; "Note C [no title]," CMAC, SA/BMA/B108. For a more elaborate proposal by Professor Henry Cohen of Liverpool, see "Note B [no title]," CMAC, SA/BMA/B108.

103. Special Practice Committee, Feb. 4, 1944, note 4. CMAC, SA/BMA/B108.

104. Consultant Services Committee, *A Consultant Service for the Nation, Feb. 1 1946*, p. 17, CMAC, SA/BMA/B.1.

105. The standard account is Webster, *Health Services*, vol. 1, ch. 4. But the relevant chapters of Stevens, *Medical Practice in Modern England*, remain essential.

106. Stevens, *Medical Practice in Modern England*, pp. 80–94. Charles Webster gives an interesting twist to this conventional interpretation in "Note on 'Stuffing Their Mouths with Gold,'" in *Aneurin Bevan on the National Health Service*, ed. Charles Webster (Oxford: University of Oxford-Wellcome Unit for the History of Medicine, 1991), pp. 219–22. Also see Charles Webster, *The National Health Service: A Political History* (Oxford: Oxford University Press, 1998), pp. 25–34.

107. Consultant Services Committee, *A Consultant Service for the Nation*, p. 11. Also see Webster, *Health Services*, vol. 1, ch. 4; and Cooter, *Surgery and Society*, pp. 233, 237.

108. According to the *BMJ* reporting on the work of a Commons committee in 1946: " . . . if the ministry was going to pay, as it probably would have to pay, a higher sum for consultants . . . it was necessary to have some objective definition of what was a consultant; whether the word used was specialist or consultant did not seem to matter." "Health Services Bill in Committee," *BMJ* (1946), 1, 819.

109. "Consultants and Specialists Committee," *BMJ* (1947), 1, supp., 49.

110. Stevens, *Medical Practice in Modern England*, p. 96.

111. "Representation of Consultants and Specialists," *BMJ* (1948), 2, 343, 1070.

112. Letter from N. Ross Smith, "Organization of Consultants and Specialists," *BMJ* (1948), 2, 438; P. H. Wilson, "Remuneration of Specialists," *BMJ* (1948), 2, 48.

113. "Consultants and Specialists Committee " *BMJ* (1947), 1, supp., 112.

114. Ministry of Health, *National Health Service: The Development of Consultant Services* (London: His Majesty's Stationery Office, 1950), p. 25.

115. Ministry of Health, *National Health Service: Development of Consultant Services*, p. 2.

116. Ministry of Health, *National Health Service: Development of Consultant Services*, p. 6.

117. Ministry of Health, *National Health Service: Development of Consultant Services*, pp. 11–13.

118. Stevens, *Medical Practice in Modern England*, pp. 85–86.

119. Ministry of Health, *National Health Service: Development of Consultant Services*, pp. 14, 21.

120. Ministry of Health, *National Health Service: Development of Consultant Services*, pp. 31–32.

121. Ministry of Health, *National Health Service: Development of Consultant Services*, p. 33.

122. Charles Webster, *The Health Services Since the War*, vol. 2, *Government and Health Care: The National Health Service 1958–1979* (London: The Stationery Office, 1996), p. 17.

123. Stevens, *Medical Practice in Modern England*, pp. 86, 98.

124. General Medical Council, report of the Special Committee on the Registration of Specialists, May 25, 1944, ABMA, B/263/1/2.

125. Radiological Group, Oct. 19, 1944, ABMA B/297/1/7.

126. Letter from Lord Moran, May 10, 1945, CMAC, SA/BMA/B11. Also see Consultant Services Committee, *A Consultant Service for the Nation*, Feb. 1, 1946, p. 17.

127. Letter of Mar. 21, 1944, from the standing committee of the three royal colleges, CMAC, SA/BMA/B9; minutes of the BMA Consultant and Specialist Committee, Apr. 12, 1945, CMAC, SA/BMA/B9.

128. "Consultants and Specialists Committee," *BMJ* (1947), 1, supp., 49.

129. Medico-Psychological Association, Jan. 1949, ABMA, B/61/49/20. Also see the letter from Lord Moran on behalf of the RCP, May 26, 1943, CMAC, SA/BMA/B9.

130. Consultant Services Committee, *A Consultant Service for the Nation*, p. 18.

131. Ministry of Health, "Memorandum: Review of Hospital Medical and Dental Staff," Jan. 1949, ABMA B/61/11. For parliamentary unhappiness with this refusal, see "Health Services Bill in Committee," *BMJ* (1946), 1, 819.

132. Consultant Services Committee, *A Consultant Service for the Nation*, p.19.

133. Wellman and Palmer, *London Specialist Postgraduate Hospitals*, p. 24.

134. Consultant and Specialist Group, Mar. 20, 1947, CMAC, SA/BMA/B18.

135. Orthpaedics Group, Nov. 7, 1950, ABMA B/263/1/3, p. 4.

136. "The Grading of Specialists," *BMJ* (1948), 2, 220–21.

137. "Committee of the RCP on Training of General Physicians," *BMJ* (1946), 1, 363; Consultant Services Committee, *A Consultant Service for the Nation*, p. 19.

138. "Special Representative Meeting," *BMJ* (1946), 1, supp., 133; "Annual Representative Meeting," *BMJ* (1947), 2, supp., 34–35.

139. Stevens, *Medical Practice in Modern England*, p. 98.

140. Some notes by the secretary of the Central Consultants and Specialists Commission, meeting of the Psychological Medicine Group Commission, Apr. 11, 1949,

ABMA B/287/1/4; meeting of the BMA organization Committee, Mar. 2, 1948, AMBA B/287/1/4.

141. Stevens, *Medical Practice in Modern England*, p. 98.

142. Thus the RCP's Committee on Neurology was opposed to a special diploma and preferred the MRCP in general medicine. Stevens, *Medical Practice in Modern England*, p. 116.

143. Stevens, *Medical Practice in Modern England*, pp. 110–19.

144. Stevens, *Medical Practice in Modern England*, p. 114 For the case of orthopedics, see Cooter, *Surgery and Society*, p. 242.

145. Stevens, *Medical Practice in Modern England*, pp. 107–8; Wellman and Palmer, *London Specialist Postgraduate Hospitals*, p. 23.

146. Stevens, *Medical Practice in Modern England*, p. 108.

147. This is discussed in the Epilogue of this volume.

148. Stevens, *Medical Practice in Modern England*, p. 357.

149. "The Spens Prizes for Specialists," *BMJ* (1948), 2, 31–32.

150. Stevens, *Medical Practice in Modern England*, pp. 218–20.

151. Charles Webster, "Note on 'Stuffing Their Mouths with Gold,'" p. 222.

Chapter 10

1. George Weisz, "Mapping Medical Specialization in Paris in the Nineteenth and Twentieth Centuries," *SHM*, 7 (1994), 177–211, especially 202.

2. Anne Digby, *The Evolution of British General Practice, 1850–1948* (Oxford: Oxford University Press, 1999), p. 162.

3. In 1968, the French figure was 13.7 percent; in the United Kingdom, the figure in 1958 was 16 percent; in West Germany in 1965, it was 17.2 percent. The sources for these figures are, respectively: Annick Vilain, "La féminisation du corps médical," *Solidarité santé* 1 (1995), 23; Charles Webster, *The Health Services Since the War*, vol. 2 (London: The Stationer's Office, 1996), p.18; Udo Schagen, "Frauen im ärztlichen Studium und Beruf : Quantitative Entwicklung und politische Vorgaben in DDR und BRD," in *Geschlechterverhältnisse in Medizin, Naturwissenschaft und Technik*, ed. Christoph Meinel and Monika Renneberg (Bassum: Verlag für Geschichte der Naturwissenschafter und der Technik, 1996), p. 328.

4. Women made up 6.8 percent of the medical workforce in 1960 and 7.6 percent in 1970. Ellen S. More, *Restoring the Balance: Women Physicians and the Profession of Medicine, 1850–1995* (Cambridge, Mass.: Harvard University Press, 1999), p. 225.

5. By 1935 women made up 7 percent of the Parisian specialist population. Among practitioners without specialty designations, 5 percent were women. The tendency for French women doctors to be specialists continued; in 1977, women constituted over 15 percent of all specialists, and only 9 percent of generalists. Caisse Nationale de l'Assurance Maladie des Travailleurs Salariés, *Le secteur libéral des professions de santé en 1982*, vol. 1, *Démographie* (Paris: 1983), p. 31.

6. The figure would be a little higher if one counted nonrecognized specialties, such as hydrotherapy, that were occasionally mentioned in words rather than pictograms. Also see Johanna Bleker and Sabine Schleiermacher, *Ärztinnen aus dem Kaiserreich: Lebensläufe einer Generation* (Weinheim: Deutscher Studien Verlag, 2000), p. 214.

7. In 1940, only 6.5 percent of hospital residency programs were open to women. More, *Restoring the Balance*, pp. 108–11.

8. More, *Restoring the Balance*, pp. 108–11.

9. National figures are based on as Bleker and Schleiermacher, *Ärztinnen aus dem Kaiserreich*, p. 214. These are largely confirmed in Friedrich Prinzing, "Die Aerzte in Deutschlands im Jahre 1926," *DMW*, 52 (1926), 1395; and Michael Kater, *Doctors Under Hitler* (Chapel Hill: University of North Carolina Press, 1989), p. 91. The figures for Berlin, based on my own analysis of a small sample of women specialists listed in the Reichs-Medizinal-Kalender (*RMK*), are very similar.

10. Bleker and Schleiermacher, *Ärztinnen aus dem Kaiserreich*, p. 214; Kater, *Doctors Under Hitler*, p. 91.

11. Wilfried Teicher, "Der Anteil der jüdischen Ärzte an der Spezialisierung im ersten Drittel dieses Jahrhunderts in Preußen," in *Medizinsche Wissenschaft und Judentum*, ed. Nora Goldenbogen et al. (Dresden: Verein für Regionale Politik und Geschichte Dresden, 1996), pp. 14–29.

12. More, *Restoring the Balance*, p. 293, n. 66.

13. More, *Restoring the Balance*, p. 293, n. 66.

14. According to one report, in 1900 about one-quarter of 133 institutions dealing with the insane employed women doctors. Regina Morantz-Sanchez, *Conduct Unbecoming a Woman: Medicine on Trial in Turn-of-the-Century Brooklyn* (New York: Oxford University Press, 1999), pp. 154–55, based on Constance M. McGovern, *Masters of Madness: Social Origins of the American Psychiatric Profession* (Hanover, N.H.: University Press of New England, 1981).

15. Mary Ann Elston, "'Run by Women, (Mainly) for Women': Medical Women's Hospitals in Britain, 1866–1948," in *Women and Modern Medicine*, ed. Anne Hardy and Lawrence Conrad (Amsterdam and New York: Rodopi, 2001), pp. 73–108.

16. Wendy Alexander, *First Ladies of Medicine* (Glasgow: Wellcome Unit for the History of Medicine, 1987), p. 49.

17. Alexander, *First Ladies of Medicine*, p. 50.

18. M. H. Kettle, "The Fate of a Population of Women Medical Students," *The Lancet*, 230 (1936), 1370–74.

19. Ulrich Tröhler, "Surgery (Modern)," in *Companion Encyclopedia of the History of Medicine*, ed. W. F. Bynum and Roy Porter, 2 vols. (London: Routledge, 1993), vol. 2, pp. 984–1028, especially p. 995.

20. George Weisz, "The Development of Medical Specialization in Nineteenth-Century Paris," in *French Medical Culture in the Nineteenth Century, Clio Medica 25*, ed. Ann La Berge and Mordechai Feingold (Amsterdam and Atlanta: Rodopi, 1994), p. 179.

21. On surgical teaching staffs at German universities, see Johannes Müller, *Statistische Untersuchungen über Vorlesungen und Dozenten der medizinischen Fakultäten der deutschen Universitäten in den Jahren 1927 bis 1931–32* (Berlin: Struppe & Winckler, 1933).

22. Weisz, "Mapping Medical Specialization," p. 202, table 3.

23. Wilfried Teicher, "Untersuchungen zur ärztlichen Spezialisierung im Spiegel des Reichsmedizinalkalenders am Beispiel Preußens im ersten Drittel des 20. Jahrhunderts" (MD thesis, Johannes-Gutenberg-Universität Mainz, 1992), pp. 68–69.

24. The percentage of surgeons rose from 10 percent in 1935 to over 16 percent in 1940. Teicher, "Untersuchungen zur ärztlichen Spezialisierung," p. 68; Kater, *Doctors Under Hitler*, p. 29.

25. Teicher, "Untersuchungen zur ärztlichen Spezialisierung," p. 69; Weisz, "Mapping Medical Specialization," pp. 202–3.

26. On this point see Christopher Lawrence and Tom Treasure, "Surgeons," in *Medicine in the Twentieth Century*, ed. Roger Cooter and John Pickstone (Amsterdam: Harwood, 2000), pp. 653–70.

27. On surgical incomes in the early nineteenth century, see George Weisz, *The Medical Mandarins: The French Academy of Medicine in the Nineteenth and Early Twentieth Centuries* (New York and Oxford: Oxford University Press, 1995), pp. 273–74.

28. Weisz, *Medical Mandarins*, p. 274.

29. Bradford Hill, "The Evidence Committee on Remuneration of Consultants and Specialists," interim report submitted Oct. 7, 1947, p. 20, in ABMA/163. According to his figures, 18.6 percent of surgeons earned over £5,000 annually, as did 17.8 percent of gynecologists. The next largest group was orthopedists, at 8 percent.

30. R. G. Leland, "Income from Medical Practice," *JAMA*, 96 (1931), 1683–91. The data on specialties are on pp. 1686–87 and are from 1928.

31. Kater, *Doctors Under Hitler*, p. 31.

32. R. Syller, "Zur Frage der Facharzt-Doppelbezeichnungen," *DÄ*, 65 (1935), 64.

33. For some examples, see Rosemary Stevens, *American Medicine and the Public Interest*, updated ed. (Berkeley: University of California Press, 1998), p. 234.

34. "Denkschrift der Deutschen Gesellschaft für Chirurgie," *DMW*, 59 (1933), 1136–37; H. Gocht, "Antwort der Deutschen Orthopädischen Gesellschaft auf die Denkschrift der Deutschen Gesellschaft für Chirurgie, *DMW*, 60 (1934), 449–51; "Antwort der Deutschen Gesellschaft für Chirurgie auf die Erklärung Deutschen Orthopädischen Gesellschaft," *DMW*, 60 (1934), 527–28. Others, however, were willing to limit themselves to care for chronic problems resulting from fractures (information communicated by Thomas Schlich).

35. "Discussion on the Treatment of Fractures: With Special Reference to Its Organization and Teaching," *BMJ* (1925), 2, 317–31. On the NHS, see chapter 9 of this volume.

36. Rosemary Stevens, "The Curious Career of Internal Medicine: Functional Ambivalence, Social Success," in *Grand Rounds: One Hundred Years of Internal Medicine*, ed. Russell C. Maulitz and Diana E. Long (Philadelphia: University of Pennsylvania Press, 1988), p. 339.

37. Russell C. Maulitz, "Introduction: Historical Perspectives," in *Grand Rounds: One Hundred Years of Internal Medicine*, ed. Russell C. Maulitz and Diana E. Long (Philadelphia: University of Pennsylvania Press, 1988), p. 4.

38. See, for instance, H. E. Bock, "Die Einheit der inneren Medezin—eine langjärige Kontroverse? Historische Entwicklung und Status Quo," in *Internisten und innere Medizin im 20. Jahrhundert*, ed. Meinhard Classen (Munich and Vienna: Urban & Schwarzenberg, 1994), pp. 186–11, especially pp. 190–91.

39. Wilhelm His, "50 jährigen Bestehen des Vereins für innere Medizin in Berlin," *DMW*, 57 (1931), 641.

40. Hans-Heinz Eulner, *Die Entwicklung der medizinischen Spezialfächer an den Universitäten des deutschen Sprachgebietes* (Stuttgart: Ferdinand Enke Verlag, 1970), p. 183; K.-H. Usadel and E. Wetzels, "Das Berufsbild des Internisten im Wandel der Zeit," in *Internisten und innere Medizin im 20. Jahrhundert,* ed. Meinhard Classen (Munich and Vienna: Urban & Schwarzenberg, 1994), p. 472.

41. Eulner, *Entwicklung der medizinischen Spezialfächer,* pp.180–83.

42. These figures are from Teicher, "Untersuchungen zur ärztlichen Spezialisierung," p. 64.

43. Müller, *Statistische Untersuchungen,* pp. 56–60.

44. Teicher, "Untersuchungen zur ärztlichen Spezialisierung," p. 71.

45. Stevens, "Curious Career," p. 342.

46. Arnd Schulte-Bockholt and Axel Bauer, "Innere Medizin in den deutschsprachigen Ländern und in den USA," *Gesnerus,* 52 (1995), 94–115.

47. Department of Health, *2001 Medical and Dental Workforce Census,* table 1, "Hospital Medical Staff by Specialty and Grade; England at 30 September 2001." Data for 2002 were kindly sent to me by Claire Thompson: "Hospital, Public Health Medicine and Community Health Services, England as of 31 March 2002," available at http://www.doh.gov.uk/ AH1890.xls.

48. Ordre National des Médecins, *La démographie médicale française: Situation au 1er janvier 1991* (Paris: Ordre National des Médecins, 1992), pp. 29–30.

49. Direction de la Recherche des Études et de l'Évaluation Statistique, *Données sur la situation sanitaire en France en 2001* (Paris: La Documentation Française, 2001), p. 148.

50. Bock, "Einheit der inneren Medizin," pp. 186–211.

51. Johannes Pantel, "Neurologie, Psychiatrie und innere Medizin: Verlauf und Dynamik eines historischen Streites," *Würzburger medizinhistorische Mitteilungen,* 11 (1993), 77–94.

52. See chapter 9 in this volume.

53. This emerges very clearly in the essays collected in Meinhard Classen, ed., *Internisten und innere Medizin im 20. Jahrhundert* (Munich and Vienna: Urban & Schwarzenberg, 1994).

54. See especially Usadel and Wetzels, "Berufsbild des Internisten," pp. 478–81.

55. Recent statistics on numbers of specialists are easily available on the official Web site of the Kassenärztliche Bundesvereinigung, http://www.kbv.de/home/home.htm.

56. The process is described in Stevenson, "Curious Career"; and W. Bruce Fye, *American Cardiology: The History of a Specialty and Its College* (Baltimore: Johns Hopkins University Press, 1996), pp. 88–92.

57. Stevens, "Curious Career," p. 339.

58. On these matters, see Fye, *American Cardiology,* pp. 295–334.

59. B. Stimmel et al., "The Practice of General Internal Medicine by Subspecialists," *Journal of Urban Health,* 75 (1998), 184–90.

60. R. C. Bates, "My Specialty Is Doomed," *Medical Economics,* 60 (1983), 101–11.

61. A. M. Fogelman, "Strategies for Training Generalists and Subspecialists," *Annals of Internal Medicine,* 120 (1994), 579–83.

62. Alex Robinson, "Forging a New Subspecialty: General Internal Medicine," *Canadian Medical Association Journal,* 150 (1994), 1995–98.

63. E. B. Larson, "General Internal Medicine at the Crossroads of Prosperity and Despair: Caring for Patients with Chronic Diseases in an Aging Society," *Annals of Internal Medicine*, 134 (2001), 997–1000.

64. Teicher, "Untersuchungen zur ärztlichen Spezialisierung," p. 35.

65. Teicher, "Untersuchungen zur ärztlichen Spezialisierung," pp. 31–32.

66. "Report of the Inaugural Meeting of the Obstetrical Society of London, 1858," *Transactions of the Obstetrical Society of London*, 1 (1859), vi.

67. Charlotte G. Borst, *Catching Babies: The Professionalization of Childbirth, 1870–1920* (Cambridge, Mass.: Harvard University Press, 1995).

68. On this development in the United States, see Judith Walzer Leavitt, *Brought to Bed: Childbearing in America, 1750 to 1950* (New York: Oxford University Press, 1986). Also see William Ray Arney, *Power and the Profession of Obstetrics* (Chicago: University of Chicago Press, 1982).

69. Ministry of Health, *National Health Service: The Development of Consultant Services* (London: His Majesty's Stationery Office, 1950), p. 13.

70. "Report of the Inaugural Meeting of the Obstetrical Society of London," p. v.

71. The situation in France is discussed in Weisz, "Mapping Medical Specialization," pp. 186–90. Data on Germany and the United States can be found in chapters 3 and 4 of this volume.

72. Howard A. Kelly, "History of Gynecology in America," in Howard Atwood Kelly, *Cyclopedia of American Medical Biography* (Philadelphia and London: W.B. Saunders, 1912), p. xl. The best introduction to gynecology in the late nineteenth-century United States is Morantz-Sanchez, *Conduct Unbecoming a Woman*, pp. 88–137. Also see Frederick N. Dyer, *Champion of Women and the Unborn: Horatio Robinson Storer, M.D.* (Canton, Mass.: Science History Publications, 1999).

73. Archives of the BMA, minutes of the Council and subcommittees, 1885–87; see meetings of Apr. 8, 1885, p. 971.

74. This argument is made explicitly in Müller, *Statistische Untersuchungen*, p. 107.

75. J. Whitridge Williams, "Has the American Gynecological Society Done Its Part in the Advancement of Obstetrical Knowledge?" *JAMA*, 52 (1914), 1771.

76. Ornella Moscucci, *The Science of Woman: Gynaecology and Gender in England, 1800–1929* (Cambridge: Cambridge University Press, 1990).

77. Dyer, *Champion of Women*, p. 166, discusses the identification of gynecology and quackery in the United States. In chapter 6 of this volume, I provide examples of such criticism in Germany; in the case of France, see below.

78. For a French example, see Weisz, "Mapping Medical Specialization," pp. 191–200.

79. In the words of one professor who taught both subjects at the University of Michigan: "Gynecology separated from obstetrics, will tend to become more and more a surgical specialty. . . . Inevitably the chairs of gynecology will disappear. . . . United with obstetrics, gynecology will survive; separated, it will gradually cease to exist." Harold Speert, *Obstetrics and Gynecology in America: A History* (Chicago: American College of Obstetricians and Gynecologists, 1980), pp 86–87.

80. Such arguments by the French obstetrician Bar are discussed below. Similar arguments by an American, J. Whitridge Williams, are discussed in Speert, *Obstetrics and Gynecology*, p. 87.

81. Teicher, "Untersuchungen zur ärztlichen Spezialisierung," p. 31.

82. F. Winkel, "The Necessity of the Union of Obstetrics and Gynecology as Branches of Medical Instruction," *American Journal of Obstetrics*, 27 (1893), 781–95, cited in Speert, *Obstetrics and Gynecology*, pp. 86–87.

83. Dr. Hansberg, "Die praktische Ausbildung in der Gerburthilfe—IV," *ÄVD*, 52 (1923), 113–14.

84. David Innes Williams, "RSM 1907: The Acceptance of Specialization," *Journal of the Royal Society of Medicine*, 93 (2000), 645.

85. Moscucci, *Science of Woman*.

86. Ministry of Health, *National Health Service*, p.13.

87. Royal College of Obstetricians and Gynaecologists, *Overall Statistics for England and Wales as at 14 May 2001*, available at http://www.rcog.org.uk/resources/public/England%20and%20Wales.doc.

88. Speert, *Obstetrics and Gynecology*, pp. 86–87.

89. Curiously, in its first specialist list of 1909, only gynecology was mentioned. Neither obstetrics alone nor gynecology combined with obstetrics made an appearance until the volume of 1911.

90. Speert, *Obstetrics and Gynecology*, pp. 86–87.

91. Speert, *Obstetrics and Gynecology*, p. 88. On similar tendencies in Canada, see Wendy Mitchinson, "The Sometimes Uncertain World of Canadian Obstetrics, 1900–1950," *Canadian Bulletin of Medical History*, 17 (2000), 193–208.

92. Speert, *Obstetrics and Gynecology*, p. 88.

93. The argument about gynecology in France is made in greater detail in Weisz, "Mapping Medical Specialization," pp. 194–96, 199–200.

94. This is discussed in chapter 7 of this volume.

95. Paul Bar, "Évolution de l'obstétrique en France," *L'obstétrique*, 16 (1911), 1–23.

Chapter 11

1. Helen Corlett, "'No Small Uncertainty': Eye Treatments in Eighteenth-Century England and France," *MH*, 42 (1998), 221.

2. Corlett, "'No Small Uncertainty,'" p. 231.

3. Corlett, "'No Small Uncertainty,'" pp. 217, 219.

4. For American examples, see chapter 4 of this volume.

5. Wilfried Teicher, "Untersuchungen zur ärztlichen Spezialisierung im Spiegel des Reichsmedizinalkalenders am Beispiel Preußens im ersten Drittel des 20. Jahrhunderts" (MD thesis, Johannes-Gutenberg-Universität Mainz, 1992), p. 31.

6. Jan E. Goldstein, *Console and Classify: The French Psychiatric Profession in the Nineteenth Century* (New York: Cambridge University Press, 1987), pp. 60–62.

7. Teicher, "Untersuchungen zur ärztlichen Spezialisierung," p. 64.

8. Adolf Reche, "Die Lage des Spezialistentums," *ÄVD*, 35 (1906), 173–77.

9. This is discussed in detail in George Weisz, "Medical Directories and Medical Specialization in France, Britain, and the United States," *BHM*, 71 (1997), 65–66.

10. George Weisz, "The Development of Medical Specialization in Nineteenth-Century Paris," in *French Medical Culture in the Nineteenth Century, Cleo Medica 25*, ed. Ann La Berge and Mordechai Feingold (Amsterdam and Atlanta: Rodopi, 1994), p. 173.

11. However, appendix 1 suggests that the practice was gradually disappearing in large cities such as New York and Boston.

12. In 1877 one of the hospitals for the throat in London was renamed the Hospital for Diseases of the Throat and Chest. Donald Harrison, *Felix Semon 1849–1921: A Victorian Laryngologist* (London: Royal Society of Medicine Press, 2000), p. 23. Also see George Weisz, "Mapping Medical Specialization in Paris in the Nineteenth and Twentieth Centuries," *SHM*, 7 (1994), 193, fig. 2.

13. Harrison, *Felix Semon*, p. 29.

14. Otto Körner, *Die Arbeitsteilung in der Heilkunde* (Wiesbaden: Verlag von J.F. Bergmann, 1909), pp.15–18 and, for bibliography, p. 26.

15. Teicher, "Untersuchungen zur ärztlichen Spezialisierung," pp. 17–18.

16. Archives of the British Medical Association (ABMA), minutes of the Council and subcommittees, no. 3, 1885–87, p. 1048.

17. ABMA, minutes of the Council, p. 1438.

18. See the comments in his autobiography, Felix Semon, *The Autobiography of Sir Felix Semon*, ed. Henry C. Semon and Thomas A. McIntyre (London: Jarrolds, 1926), p. 84.

19. Penelope Hunting, *The History of the Royal Society of Medicine* (London: Royal Society of Medicine Press, 2001), pp. 272, 275.

20. British Medical Association, *Consultant and Specialist Services* (London: BMA, 1938); Consultant Services Committee, *A Consultant Service for the Nation*, Feb. 1 1946, app. 3, (CMAC), SA/BMA/B; Ministry of Health, *National Health Service: The Development of Consultant Services* (London: His Majesty's Stationery Office, 1950), pp. 24–25.

21. Teicher, "Untersuchungen zur ärztlichen Spezialisierung," p. 64.

22. Weisz, "Mapping Medical Specialization," p. 185.

23. Andrew Aisenberg, "Syphilis and Prostitution: A Regulatory Couplet in Nineteenth-Century France," in *Sex, Sin and Suffering: Venereal Disease and European Society Since 1870*, ed. Roger Davidson and Lesley A. Hall (London and New York: Routledge, 2001), pp. 15–28. Also see Claude Quétel, *History of Syphilis*, trans. Judith Braddock and Brian Pike (Cambridge: Polity Press, 1990), pp. 288–98.

24. Lutz Sauerteig, *Krankheit, Sexualität, Gesellschaft: Geschlechtskrankheiten und Gesundheitspolitik in Deutschland im 19. und frühen 20. Jahrhundert* (Stuttgart: Franz Steiner Verlag, 1999), p. 38; Hans-Heinz Eulner, *Die Entwicklung der medizinischen Spezialfächer an den Universitäten des deutschen Sprachgebietes* (Stuttgart: Ferdinand Enke Verlag, 1970), pp. 222–56.

25. Sauerteig, *Krankheit, Sexualität, Gesellschaft*, pp. 38–40; Teicher, "Untersuchungen zur ärztlichen Spezialisierung," pp. 18–19.

26. Lutz D. H. Sauerteig, "'The Fatherland Is in Danger, Save the Fatherland!': Venereal Disease, Sexuality and Gender in Imperial and Weimar Germany," in *Sex, Sin and Suffering: Venereal Disease and European Society Since 1870*, ed. Roger Davidson and Lesley A. Hall (London and New York: Routledge, 2001), pp. 76–92, especially pp. 79–80.

27. Teicher, "Untersuchungen zur ärztlichen Spezialisierung," p. 32.

28. Sauerteig, "'The Fatherland Is in Danger,'" pp. 85–86.

29. Sauerteig, *Krankheit, Sexualität, Gesellschaft*, pp. 40–41; Albrecht Scholz, *Geschichte der Dermatologie in Deutschland* (Berlin: Springer, 1999), pp. 86–88; Johannes Müller, *Statistische Untersuchungen über Vorlesungen und Dozenten der medizinischen*

Fakultäten der deutschen Universitäten in den Jahren 1927 bis 1931– 32 (Berlin: Struppe & Winckler, 1933), p. 84.

30. Teicher, "Untersuchungen zur ärztlichen Spezialisierung," p. 77.

31. Friedrich Prinzing, "Die Aerzte Deutschlands in Jahre 1928," *DMW,* 55 (1929), 280.

32. Nearly 18 percent of Jewish physicians still in Germany in 1937 were listed as specialists in this field in the *RMK;* among non-Jews the figure was slightly over 10 percent. Wilfried Teicher,"Der Anteil der jüdischen Ärzte an der Spezialisierung im ersten Drittel dieses Jahrhunderts in Preußen," in *Medizinische Wissenschaften und Judentum,* ed. Nora Goldenbogen et al. (Dresden: Einverlag des Vereins für Regionale Politik und Geschichte Dresden, 1996).

33. Teicher, "Untersuchungen zur ärztlichen Spezialisierung," p. 79.

34. That the autonomous existence of venereology was something of an issue is suggested by the fact that an American Medical Association section founded in 1886 had the following sequence of titles: Dermatology and Venereal Diseases; Dermatology and Syphilography; Cutaneous Medicine and Surgery; Dermatology; Dermatology and Syphilis; Dermatology and Syphilology.

35. Allan M. Brandt, *No Magic Bullet: A Social History of Venereal Disease in the United States Since 1880,* enl. ed. (New York and Oxford: Oxford University Press, 1987), pp. 132– 33.

36. J. E. Lane, "The Dermatologist-Syphilologist in the United States," *JAMA,* 84 (1925), 1616– 19.

37. "A Proposed Section on Genito-Urinary and Venereal Diseases," *JAMA,* 54 (1910), 1459– 50.

38. H. H. Hazen, "Duties of the Dermatologist," *JAMA,* 70 (1918), 1990.

39. Lane, "The Dermatologist-Syphilologist," p. 1617.

40. Brandt, *No Magic Bullet,* pp. 143– 44.

41. Rosemary Stevens, *American Medicine and the Public Interest,* updated ed. (Berkeley: University of California Press, 1998), p. 162.

42. Calculated from Stevens, *American Medicine,* p. 162.

43. W. P. W. Phillimore, ed., *The Dictionary of Medical Specialists: Being a Classified List of London Practitioners Who Chiefly Attend to Special Departments of Medicine and Surgery* (London: Chas. J. Clark, 1889).

44. C. Bracebridge Allen, *London Medical Specialists* (London: Ward and Lock, 1890).

45. David Evans, "Tackling the Hideous Scourge: The Creation of the Venereal Disease Treatment Centres in Early Twentieth-Century Britain," *SHM,* 5 (1992), 413– 33.

46. Lesley A. Hall, "Venereal Diseases and Society in Britain, from the Contagious Diseases Acts to the National Health Service," in *Sex, Sin and Suffering: Venereal Disease and European Society Since 1870,* ed. Roger Davidson and Lesley A. Hall (London and New York: Routledge, 2001), pp.120– 36, especially pp. 125– 27.

47. Hall, "Venereal Diseases and Society," p. 128.

48. *The Medical Who's Who, 1925* (London: Grafton, 1925).

49. Hunting, *History of the Royal Society of Medicine,* pp. 259– 60.

50. David Evans, "Sexually Transmitted Disease Policy in the English National Health Service, 1948– 2000: Continuity and Social Change," in *Sex, Sin and Suffering:*

Venereal Disease and European Society Since 1870, ed. Roger Davidson and Lesley A. Hall (London and New York: Routledge, 2001), p. 239.

51. "Annual Meeting of the Council," *BMJ* (1947), 1, supp., 70.

52. Ministry of Health, *National Health Service: The Development of Consultant Services* (London: His Majesty's Stationery Office, 1950). According to the cover, this was first circulated as a memorandum in 1948.

53. Evans, "Sexually Transmitted Disease Policy," p. 241.

54. Central Consultants and Specialists Commission, meeting of Nov. 4, 1948, p. 8, ABMA, B61.

55. Evans, "Sexually Transmitted Disease Policy," p. 242.

56. Roger Davidson, *Dangerous Liaisons: A Social History of Venereal Disease in Twentieth-Century Scotland*, Clio Medica 57 (Amsterdam: Rodopi, 2000), especially pp. 91–97, 259–65.

57. Evans, "Sexually Transmitted Disease Policy," p. 243.

58. Evans, "Sexually Transmitted Disease Policy," pp. 247–48.

59. Roger King, *The Making of the Dentiste, c. 1650–1760* (Aldershot, U.K.: Ashgate, 1998), pp. 34–48.

60. M. D. K. Bremner, *The Story of Dentistry from the Dawn of Civilization to the Present*, 2nd ed. (Brooklyn, N.Y.: Dental Items of Interest, 1947); L. Laszlo Schwartz, "The Historical Relations of American Dentistry and Medicine," *BHM*, 28 (1954), 542–49.

61. Harry P. Carlton, "The Dentistry of Tomorrow," *JAMA*, 45 (1905), 1055–57; Frank L. Platt, "A Common Ground for Medicine and Dentistry," *JAMA*, 45 (1905), 512–13; Calvin William Knowles, "The Physician as Dentist," *JAMA*, 45 (1905), 514; William C. Fisher, "The Section on Stomatology: Its Needs, Its Duties and Its Opportunities," *JAMA*, 63 (1914), 2104–6.

62. The organization's policy was to keep the number of specialty sections stable. "Report of the Council on Scientific Assembly," *JAMA*, 84 (1925), 1660–61.

63. Norman Gevitz, "Autonomous Profession or Medical Specialty: The Stomatological Movement and American Dentistry," *BHM*, 62 (1988), 407–28.

64. Erna Lesky, *The Vienna Medical School of the Nineteenth Century*, trans. L. Williams and I. S. Levij (Baltimore: Johns Hopkins University Press, 1976), pp. 204–9, 450–56.

65. Lesky, *Vienna Medical School*, p. 209.

66. Prof. Walkhoff, "Gedanken zur Reform des zahnärztlichen Studiums," *DMW*, 52 (1926), 970–71.

67. Dominik Groß, *Die schwierige Professionalisierung der deutschen Zahnärzteschaft (1867–1919)* (Frankfurt and Berlin: Peter Lang, 1994), pp. 40–43.

68. Groß, *Die schwierige Professionalisierung*, pp. 50–51.

69. Ilona Marz, "Das Studium der Beflissenen der Zahnheilkunde, Chirurgie und Pharmazie und Direktorium für Nichtimmatrikulierte," in *Die Medizin an der Berliner Universität an der Charité zwischen 1810 und 1850*, ed. Peter Schneck and Hans-Uwe Lammel (Husum: Matthiesen Verlag, 1995), p. 192.

70. Heinrich Riedl, "Die Auseinandersetzungen um die Spezialisierung in der Medizin von 1862 bis 1925" (MD thesis, Fakultät für Medizin der Technischen Universität München, 1981), p. 7.

71. Groß, *Die schwierige Professionalisierung*, p. 112.

72. Groß, *Die schwierige Professionalisierung*, pp. 224–25.

73. Groß, *Die schwierige Professionalisierung*, pp. 219–24; S. Davidsohn, "Die Stellung der Zahnärzte zur Gewerbeordnung," *DMW*, 23 (1897), 45.

74. This specialty is so tiny that it is ignored in most histories of German specialization. Teicher, "Untersuchungen zur ärztlichen Spezialisierung," does not include statistics on it.

75. This represented less than 1 percent of all specialists. Dr. Hadrich, "Die Zahl der Ärzte Deutschlands und ihre Gliederung im Jahre 1935," *DÄ*, 65 (1935), 696–98. Also see Karl Keller, "Dozenten der Medizin und Zahnheilkunde an den deutschen Hochschulen," *DÄ*, 65 (1935), 695–96.

76. "Auslegungen and Begutachtungen von Facharztfragen durch den Geschäftsausschuß und den ständigen Gutachterausschuß des Deutschen Ärztevereinsbundes," *ÄVD*, 58 (1929), 792; "Sitzung des engeren Geschäftsausschußes des Deutschen Ärztevereinbundes, am 2 März 1930 in Berlin," *DÄ*, 59 (1930), 92. Also see "Aus der Sitzung des Vorstandes des Deutschen Ärztevereinsbundes am 21. November 1930 in Berlin," *DÄ*, 59 (1930), 434, for conflicts about the right of dentists to utilize purportedly medical substances such as narcotics and X-rays.

77. Only orthodontics and dental surgery were recognized as dental specialties. In the latter case, practitioners were prohibited from using the term "Facharzt für Chirurgie" and had to use the title "Fach*zahn*arzt für zahnärztliche Chirurgie." "Abkommen zwischen dem Deutschen Ärztevereinsbund und dem Reichsverband der Zahnärzte Deutschlands," *DÄ*, 60 (1931), 462–63.

78. For instance, Prof. Adloff, "Wer darf Kieferkrankheiten behandeln?" *DMW*, 57 (1931), 1335–36; Dr. Fabien, "Entgegnung auf den Aufsatz Dr. Baden: I," and Dr. Henn, "Entgegnung auf den Aufsatz Dr. Baden: II," *ÄVD*, 55 (1926), 54–57.

79. For an interesting debate on this point by two professors of dentistry, see Christian Bruhn, "Gedanken über Sinn und Notwendigkeit der stomatologischen Spezialisierung," *DMW*, 58 (1932), 668–70; and O. Loos, "Stomatologische Spezialisierung der Zahnärzte?" *DMW*, 58 (1932), 1811. When in 1930 the Association of Teachers in Dentistry proposed that the MD diploma no longer be a requirement for the right (*Habilitation*) to teach dentistry in medical schools, the only serious opposition I have come across is an article written by a stomatologist living in Amsterdam: L.de Ruyter-Mayer, "Die Habilitation für das Fach Zahnheilkunde," *MMW*, 77 (1930), 719–20.

80. Prof. Deick, "Zur Frage des 'Einheitsstandes' der Zahnärzte und Zahntechniker," *DMW*, 52 (1926), 293–94, estimated that the nation required about 15,000 dental practitioners.

81. Dieck, "Zur Frage des 'Einheitsstandes,'" pp. 293–94. As the number of dentists increased dramatically in the postwar period, they complained increasingly about this policy. Walter Lustig, "Die Gefährdung der zahnärztlichen Approbation in ihrer Bedeutung für den gesamten Aerztestand," *DMW*, 50 (1924), 1661; Groß, *Die schwierige Professionalisierung*, pp. 28, 220, 235–36; Eulner, *Entwicklung der medizinischen Spezialfächer*, p. 419.

82. L. Lührse, "Zahnheilkunde und Gesamtmedizin," *DMW*, 44 (1918), 245–46, 270–271; Dr. Richter, "Zahnheilkunde und Gesamtmedizin: Eine Erwiderung," *DMW*, 44 (1918), 662–63.

83. Groß, *Die schwierige Professionalisierung*, pp. 28, 220, 235–36; Eulner, *Entwicklung der medizinischen Spezialfächer*, p. 419.

84. Eulner, *Entwicklung der medizinischen Spezialfächer*, p. 419.

85. This development has been much discussed. For a short summary, see E. G. Forbes, "The Professionalization of Dentistry in the United Kingdom," *MH*, 29 (1985), 169–81.

86. Ernest G. Smith and Beryl D. Cottell, *A History of the Royal Dental Hospital of London and School of Dental Surgery, 1858–1985* (London: Athlone Press, 1997); Forbes, "Professionalization of Dentistry," p. 171.

87. Forbes, "Professionalization of Dentistry," p. 172.

88. Smith and Cottell, *History of the Royal Dental Hospital of London*, p. 39; Forbes, "Professionalization of Dentistry," p. 173. A letter from the RCS secretary dated Mar. 14, 1910, clearly explained this situation in response to a query from the Royal College of Surgeons of Ireland, RCS Archives, 1120. Claire Jackson, at the time archivist of the RCS, kindly made this letter available to me.

89. Smith and Cottell, *History of the Royal Dental Hospital of London*, p. 85.

90. Forbes, "Professionalization of Dentistry," p. 178.

91. Zachary Cope, "The Making of the Dental Profession in Britain," *Proceedings of the Royal Society of Medicine*, 57 (1964), 919–26.

92. "Stomatology in England," *JAMA*, 85 (1925), 630.

93. Wilfred Fish, "A Profession in the Making," *British Dental Journal*, 107 (1959), 19–30.

94. Joint Planning Committee of Dental Students, *An Investigation and Recommendation Concerning the Future of Dentistry*, part 1, *Dental Education*, Oct. 1942. Also see General Medical Council and Dental Board of the United Kingdom, *Memorandum of Evidence on Matters of Fact Submitted on Behalf of the Council and of the Board to the Interdepartmental Committee on Dentistry*, 1944.

95. British Medical Association, Consultant and Specialist Services (London, January 1938), CMAC, SA/BMA/B11.

96. Smith and Cottell, *History of the Royal Dental Hospital of London*, pp. 87, 102–4. Also see W. A. Bulleid, "The Separation of Dentisry from Medicine," *British Dental Journal*, 62 (1937), 113–21.

97. Forbes, "Professionalization of Dentistry," pp. 180–81.

98. Cope, "Making of the Dental Profession," p. 925.

99. Frank Wellman and Paul Palmer, *The London Specialist Postgraduate Hospitals: A Review and Commentary on Their Future* (London: King Edward's Hospital Fund, 1975), p. 23.

100. My account relies largely on François Vidal et al., *Histoire d'un diplôme, 1699–1892: De l'expert pour les dents au docteur en chirurgie dentaire* (Paris: n.p., 1993); Dr. Robert Weill, "Un siècle à réussir," in *Ordre National des Chirurgiens Dentistes, 1892–1992: Centenaire du diplôme du chirurgien dentiste* (Paris: Bulletin Officiel du Conseil National, 1992), pp. 12–30.

101. Like the French and British directories, the *Annuaire médical belge* of the 1930s included a stomatology section with a substantial number of practitioners. When, in 1925, Hungary regulated specialties, dentistry was among the fields recognized. "Foreign Letters. Budapest (from Our Regular Correspondent)," *JAMA*, 84 (1925), 1587.

102. "Stomatologistes des hôpitaux de Paris," *PMd*, 50 (1923), 21–22.

103. Dr. Hennion, "Syndicat National des Médecins Stomotologistes Qualifiés: Historique," *MdFr*, 104 (1954), 7923–25.

104. Weill, "Un siècle à réussir," pp. 19–21.

105. Michel Dechaume, "Sur la loi relative à l'exercise illégal de l'art dentaire," *BAM*, 150 (1966), 431.

106. Vidal et al., *Histoire d'un diplôme*, p. 235; Jean Jardine, "La capacité professionnelle: Un long combat," in *Ordre National des Chirurgiens Dentistes, 1892–1992: Centenaire du diplôme du chirurgien dentiste* (Paris: Bulletin Officiel du Conseil National, 1992), p. 32.

107. Weill, "Un siècle à réussir," p. 28.

108. Weill, "Un siècle à réussir," p. 14.

109. DREES, *Données sur la situation sanitaire et sociale en France en 2000* (Paris: La Documentation Française, 2001), p. 148, table 5.3. In 1986, there were 1,542 stomatologists; by 1989 there were almost 1,700. Patrick Guého, "Les professions de santé: Des évolutions contrastées selon le mode d'exercice," *Solidarité santé: études statistiques* (1995), no. 1, 9–22, at 20, annexe 1.

110. Jacqueline Gottely and Annick Vilain, "Les perspectives démographiques des professions médicales," *Dossiers Solidarité et santé: Les médecins, démographie et revenus* (1999), no. 1, 7–22, at 10, table 01.

111. B. Raphael, "Editorial: Indissociables, par définition et au travers de leur histoire, chirurgie maxillo-faciale et stomatologie doivent de bâtir en commun un projet d'avenir," *Revue de stomatologie et chirurgie maxillo-faciale*, 100 (1999), 266–67.

Epilogue

1. John Horder, "Developments in Other Countries," in *General Practice Under the National Health Service, 1948–1997*, ed. Irvine Loudon, John Horder, and Charles Webster (London: Clarendon Press, 1998), pp. 247–77, especially p. 276; Barbara Starfield, "Is Primary Care Essential?" *The Lancet*, 344 (1994), 1129–33.

2. Department of Health, Medical and Workforce Census; the figures for 1975 are on the Web site of the Department of Health, http://www.dh.gov.uk, while those for 2002 were kindly provided by Ms. Claire Thompson of the Department of Health.

3. In 1970, the proportion of GNP spent on health care was 6 percent in Germany, 5.9 percent in France, and 4.6 percent in the United Kingdom. By the year 2000 figures for the three countries respectively were 10.6 percent, 9.5 percent, and 7.3 percent. In 2000, per capita expenditure on health in the three countries (in US$) were Germany, 2,748; France, 2,349; and United Kingdom, 1,763. The figures for 2000 are from OECD, *Health Data 2002* (www.oecd.org), and those for 1970 are from Patrick Hassenteufel, *Les médecins face à l'état: Une comparaison européenne* (Paris: Presses de la Fondation Nationale des Sciences Politiques, 1997), p. 349.

4. Charles Webster, *The Health Services Since the War*, vol. 2, *Government and Health Care: The National Health Service, 1958–1979* (London: The Stationery Office, 1996), p. 311.

5. Brian Salter, *The Politics of Change in the Health Service* (London: Macmillan, 1998), p. 18.

6. A look under the term "Reorganization" in the index to Webster, *The Health Services*, vol. 2, pp. 984–85, shows how ubiquitous this notion was.

7. James Parkhouse and Robin A. Darton, "Specialist Medical Training in Britain: A Survey of the Hospital Specialties in 1975," Working Paper no. 16, Health Services Management Unit, Department of Social Administration, University of Manchester, 1976, p. 9.

8. John Lister, *Postgraduate Medical Education* (London: The Nuffield Provincial Hospitals Trust, 1993), pp. 40, 43.

9. Parkhouse and Darton, "Specialist Medical Training, 1975," p. 6.

10. Although one assumes that the majority of consultants received such training, it is striking that among the plethora of statistics that the Ministry of Health has produced, there are no data about the kind of training that consultants have received.

11. Lister, *Postgraduate Medical Education*, pp. 51–53.

12. Lister, *Postgraduate Medical Education*, pp. 51–53; Salter, *Politics of Change*, p.105.

13. Salter, *Politics of Change*; Lister, *Postgraduate Medical Education*; Christopher Ham, Judith Smith, and John Temple, *Hubs, Spokes and Policy Cycles: An Analysis of the Policy Implications for the NHS of Changes to Medical Staffing* (Birmingham: University of Birmingham Press, 1993); Alan Maynard and Arthur Walker, *The Physician Workforce in the United Kingdom: Issues, Prospects and Policies* (London: Nuffield Trust, 1997), especially pp. 38–43.

14. Audit Commission, *The Doctors' Tale: The Work of Hospital Doctors in England and Wales* (London: Her Majesty's Stationery Office, 1995), especially pp. 12–13.

15. Salter, *Politics of Change*, p. 117.

16. Audit Commission, "Medical Staffing Review: Acute Hospital Portfolio," at http://www.audit-commission.gov.uk/reports, pp. 3–4, 13–14 of the "accessible version"; the statistics are in "All NHS Doctors at a Glance," at http://www.doh.gov.uk/stats/doctors/htm; Royal College of Physicians, "Non-consultant Career Grade Doctors: Recommendations for an Improved Career Structure, June 2000," on RCP Web site: http://www.rcplondon.ac.uk. About three-quarters of these positions are "staff grade," which means they are at about the same level as registrars training to become specialists, but without possibility of advancement. The remaining quarter is made up of associate specialists who are closer to the consultant level.

17. Audit Commission, *Doctors' Tale*, p. 14.

18. Audit Commission, *Doctors' Tale*, pp. 35–48.

19. Audit Commission, "Medical Staffing Review," p. 9.

20. See, for instance, British Medical Association, "Memorandum of Evidence to the Doctors' and Dentists' Review Body, 2000: Career Grade Hospital Doctors," especially pp. 4–5, on the BMA Web site, www.bma.org.uk.

21. Royal College of Physicians, Medical Workforce Unit, "Summary of Information: Consultant Workforce in Medical Specialties in England, Wales and Ireland—1999," pp. 2–3 (typescript).

22. OCDE (Organisation de cooperation et de développement économique), *Panorama de la santé: Les indicateurs de l'OCDE 2003* (Paris: OCDE, 2003), p. 37. This gap was considerably less narrow than in previous years.

23. British Medical Association, "Workforce Planning Briefing Note for the ARM," pp. 1–3, on the BMA Web site, http://www.bma.org.uk.

24. British Medical Association, "Workforce Planning Briefing Note," p. 6.

25. BMA, "Memorandum of Evidence, 2000," p. 15.

26. Royal College of Physicians, "Training in Academic Medicine: Recommendations from the Academic Medicine Committee of the RCP," on RCP Web site, http://www.rcplondon.ac.uk.

27. Parkhouse and Darton, "Specialist Medical Training, 1975," p. 7.

28. Salter, *Politics of Change*, pp. 75, 88.

29. BMA, "Workforce Planning Briefing Note," pp. 1–5.

30. Department of Health, "The NHS Plan: A Progress Report. The NHS Modernisation Board's Annual Report," pp. 26–27, at www.doh.gov.uk/modernizationboard-report.

31. According to the summary statistics of the Department of Health, the proportion of GPs among all medical staff of the NHS (including trainees and dentists) declined from 37 to 31 percent between 1975 and 2001; that of consultants rose from 18 to 25 percent (18.5 to 31 percent if "other career grades" are lumped together with consultants). If only GPs and specialists (consultants and "others") are taken into account, the division is now about 50–50.

32. Trevor W. Lambert, Michael J. Goldacre, and Gill Turner, "Career Choices of United Kingdom Medical Graduates of 1999 and 2000: Questionnaire Surveys," *BMJ*, 326 (2003), 194–95; Trevor W. Lambert and Michael J. Goldacre, "Career Destinations and Views in 1998 of the Doctors Who Qualified in the United Kingdom in 1993," *Medical Education*, 36 (2002), 192–98; Royal College of General Practitioners (RCGP), "College Viewpoint, the Primary Care Workforce: An Update for the New Millennium" (2nd ed., 2000), on the College's Web site, www.rcgp.org.uk.

33. Ninety-four percent of men and 61 percent of women were working full-time in the late 1990s. RCGP, "College Viewpoint, the Primary Care Workforce."

34. RCGP, "College Viewpoint, the Primary Care Workforce."

35. "BMA Response to Consultation on the General Medical Practice and Specialist Medical Education, Training and Qualifications Order 2003," BMA Web site, www.bma.org.uk/.

36. Michael Ashley-Miller, "Health Workforce Policy Lessons from Britain," in *The U.S. Health Workforce: Power, Politics, and Policy*, ed. Marian Osterweis et al. (Washington, D.C.: Association of Academic Health Centers, 1996), pp. 57–61.

37. Derek Wanless, letter to the chancellor of the exchequer, in "Securing Our Future Health: Taking a Long-Term View, Final Report April 2002," at www.hmtreasury.gov.uk/consultations_and_legislation/wanless/consult_wanless_final.cfm.

38. At the beginning of the twenty-first century there were slightly less than 150 insurance funds in France and over 564 in German. This latter figure (which continues to fall) represented a huge drop from the pre-1990 period, when there were about 1,100 funds in existence. Françoise Bas-Theron, "Le système de santé et d'assurance maladie en Allemagne: Actions concernant la qualité des soins et la régulation des dépenses en ambulatoire," Inspection Générale des Affaires Sociales, Rapport no. 2002 052 (May 2002), p. 15 (www.ladocfrançaise.gouv.fr.brp/notices/024000448.shtml), Richard Freeman, *The Politics of Health in Europe* (Manchester: Manchester University Press, 2000), pp. 55, 66.

39. Horder, "Developments in Other Countries," p. 266.

40. Freeman, *Politics of Health*, p. 107.

41. For instance, Denis Durand de Bousingen: "French, German and Belgian Doctors Unite," *The Lancet*, 349 (1997), 483; and "French and German Doctors United in Fight," *The Lancet*, 353 (1999), 9146.

42. Freeman, *Politics of Health*, p. 98.

43. Cillian Twomey, "Credentialing of Specialists Throughout the World: The European Perspective," in *Credentialing Physician Specialists: A World Perspective, June 8–10 2000, Chicago, Proceedings*, ed. Philip G. Bashook et al. (Royal College of Physicians and Surgeons of Canada and American Board of Medical Specialties), pp. 33–35, at www.abms.org. National variation is also discussed in Peter Glogner, "Weiterbildung: Europa wächst zusammen," *DÄ*, 98 (2001), A2095–96.

44. "Mission sur la démographie des professions de la santé (Rapport Berland), November 2002," p. 62, at http://orthoptie.net/pro/rapport/berland.htm.

45. Twomey, "Credentialing Specialists," pp. 33–35.

46. Alain Letourmy, "Les politiques de santé en Europe Une vue d'ensemble," *Sociologie du travail*, 42 (2000), 13–30, at 17.

47. The Committee for Practice Guidelines and Policy Conferences (CPGPC) was established by the board of the European Society of Cardiology. European cooperation for clinical practice guidelines in cancer is currently being set up. More generally, the AGREE collaboration has been producing guidelines on preparing practice guidelines.

48. The best accounts of these issues are Anne-Chantal Dubernet: "Faire (quelle?) médecine: À propos de la loi de 1982 sur la réforme du troisième cycle des études médicales," in *Professions et institutions de santé face à l'organisation du travail: Aspects sociologiques*, ed. Geneviève Cresson and François-Xavier Schweyer (Paris: Ed. de l'Ecole Nationale de la Santé Publique (ENSP), 2000), pp. 87–96; and "L'internat de médecine ou la formation par la concurrence," in *Coopérations, conflits et concurrences dans le système de santé*, ed. Geneviève Cresson, Marcel Drulhe, and François-Xavier Schweyer (Paris: ENSP, 2003), pp. 75–87.

49. *Le secteur libéral des professions de santé (au 31.12.1982)*, vol. 1, *Démographie*, Caisse Nationale de l'Assurance Maladie des Travailleurs, pp. 3, 12, 13.

50. This led to yet another diploma, the DESC.

51. France is awash in divergent medical manpower statistics. I use the statistics produced by DREES (Direction de la Recherche des Études de l'Évaluation et des Statistiques), which are published annually and quoted widely. See especially DREES, *Données sur la situation sanitaire et sociale en France en 2001* (Paris: La Documentation Française, 2001), p. 145.

52. Jean de Kervasdoué, "Symptômes et origines 'objectives' de la crise," in *La crise des professions de santé*, ed. Jean de Kervasdoué (Paris: Dunod, 2003), pp. 5–23, at p. 19.

53. Dubernet: "Faire (quelle?) médecine," pp. 92–95; and "Cooperations, conflits et concurrences," pp. 76–77.

54. Dubernet, "Cooperations, conflits et concurrences," p. 81.

55. Among older women doctors (forty-five and over), a majority are specialists; among those under the age of forty-four, general practitioners are the majority (*Mission Démographie des professions de la santé [Rapport Berland]*, p.15); also see Dubernet, "Cooperations, conflits et concurrences," p. 85.

56. On general practice in France, see Martine Bungener and Isabelle Baszanger, "Médecine générale, le temps des redéfinitions," in *Quelle médecine voulons-nous?* ed. Is-

abelle Baszanger, Martine Bungener, and Anne Paillet (Paris: La Dispute, 2002), pp. 19–34; Michel Arliaud and Magali Robelet, "Réformes du système de santé et devenir du 'corps médicale,'" *Sociologie du Travail*, 42 (2000), 91–112; Magali Robelet, "La grande désillusion des médecins libéraux: Entre la tentation de la division et l'espoir de l'unité retrouvée," in *La crise des professions de santé*, ed. Jean de Kervasdoué (Paris: Dunod, 2003), p. 225.

57. Arliaud and Robelet, "Réformes du système de santé," p. 104.

58. Robelet, "La grande désillusion," p. 225.

59. *Mission Démographie (Rapport Berland)*, p. 81.

60. In 1998, the net annual income for specialists was 78,259€, and for GPs, 51, 007€ (Philippe Ulmann, "La crise des professions santé a-t-elle une origine économique?" in *La crise des professions de santé*, ed. Jean de Kervasdoué [Paris: Dunod, 2003], p. 42). In 2002, the gross annual income of specialists was 203,700€, and for generalists, 115, 000€; this followed a major increase in generalists' fees in 2002 that raised their average annual income nearly 7 percent. Cyrille Dupuis, "Honoraires 2002," *Quotidien du médecin*, Oct. 17, 2003.

61. Robelet, "La grande désillusion," p. 224.

62. Ulmann, "La crise des professions," p. 48. According to figures dating from 2000, psychiatrists are the lowest-paid private practitioners in France, followed by pediatricians and then GPs. Also see Robelet, "La grande désillusion," pp. 208–10.

63. Paul C. Sorum, "Two Tiers of Physicians in France: General Pediatrics Declines, General Practice Rises," *JAMA*, 280 (1998), 1099–1101.

64. The development of these specialties is discussed in chapter 10 of this volume.

65. "Arrête du 8–4–2003, Diplômes d'études spécialisées de médecine", at http://www.education.gouv.fr.bo/2003/19/MENA0300781A.htm. For the number of places for each specialty, see CNCI, (Centre National des Concours d'Internat), "Actualité des concours d'internat," http://www.sante.gouv.fr/htm/actu/concours/dh/internat/medecine/places_2003.pdf.

66. *Mission Démographie (Rapport Berland)*; "Spécialités en crise: Quelles solutions pour l'avenir ?" 10e jeudi de l'Ordre des Médecins, Jan. 18, 2001, at www.conseil-national.medecin.fr/CNOM/Actu.nsf/.

67. *Mission Démographie (Rapport Berland)*, p. 26.

68. François-Xavier Schweyer, "Crises et mutations de la médecine hospitalière," in *La crise des professions de santé*, ed. Jean de Kervasdoué (Paris: Dunod, 2003), pp. 256–57.

69. For an interesting American take on this situation, see Paul G. Sorum, "Striking Against Managed Care: The Last Gasp of La Médecine Libérale," *JAMA*, 280 (1998), 659–64.

70. Patrick Hassenteufel and Frédéric Pierru, "De la crise de la représentation à la crise de la régulation de l'assurance maladie?" in *La crise des professions de santé*, ed. Jean de Kervasdoué (Paris: Dunod, 2003), pp. 77–120; Robelet, "La grande désillusion," pp. 213–17; Arliaud and Robelet, "Réformes du système," pp. 91–112.

71. Kervasdoué, "Symptômes et origines," pp. 5–23; Hassenteufel and Pierru, "De la crise," p. 102.

72. A brief description of this system is in Thomas Schlich, *Surgery, Science, and Industry: A Revolution in Fracture Care, 1950s–1990s* (Houndmills, U.K., and New York:

Palgrave Macmillan, 2002), pp. 169–70. The most detailed recent study is Anne-Sabine Ernst, *"Die beste Prophylaxe ist der Sozialismus": Ärzte und medizinische Hochschullehrer in der SBZ/DDR, 1945–1961* (Münster: Waxman, 1997).

73. Michael Moran, *Governing the Health Care State: A Comparative Study of the United Kingdom, the United States and Germany* (Manchester: Manchester University Press, 1999), p. 34.

74. On these developments, see Eberhard Wolff, "Mehr als nur materielle Interessen: Die organisierte Ärzteschaft im Ersten Weltkrieg und in der Weimarer Republik 1914–1933," in *Geschichte der deutschen Ärzteschaft*, ed. Robert Jütte (Cologne: Ärzte-Verlag, 1997), pp. 131–34; Martin Rüther, "Ärztliches Standeswesen im Nationalsozialismus," ibid, pp. 174–75; Thomas Gerst, "Neuaufbau und Konsolidierung: Ärztliche Selbstverwaltung und Interessenvertretung in den drei Westzonen und der Bundesrepublik Deutschland, 1945–1995," ibid, pp. 230–32; Moran, *Governing the Health Care State*, pp. 38–41. Also see chapter 6 in this volume.

75. Hans J. Sewering, "Von der 'Bremer Richtlinie' zur Weiterbildungsordnung," *DÄ*, 84 (1987), B1595–1602, at B1595; Moran, *Governing the Health Care State*, p. 39.

76. Moran, *Governing the Health Care State*, pp. 111–13.

77. On the consequences of the separation between ambulatory and hospital care, see Frédéric Rupprecht, Bruno Tissot, and Frédéric Chatel, "German Healthcare System: Promoting Greater Responsibility Among All System Players," *INSEE Studies*, 42 (2000), 1–23; Arnold J. Heidenheimer, "Organized Medicine and Physician Specialization in Scandinavia and West Germany," *West European Politics*, 3 (1980), 376; and Hassenteufel, *Médecins face à l'état*, p. 123.

78. Sewering, "Von der 'Bremer Richtlinie,'" p. B1597. On the earlier decisions leading to this reform, see K.-H. Usadel and E. Wetzels, "Das Berufsbild des Internisten im Wandel der Zeit," in *Internisten und innere Medizin im 20. Jahrhundert*, ed. Meinhard Classen (Munich and Vienna: Urban & Schwarzenberg, 1994), pp. 471–75.

79. Sewering, "Von der 'Bremer Richtlinie,'" p. B1598; Marion Döhler, "Comparing National Patterns of Medical Specialization: A Contribution to the Theory of Professions," *Social Science Information*, 32 (1993), 203; Hans J. Sewering, "Die Weiterbildungsordnung," *DÄ*, 65 (1968), 1445–77.

80. U. Schagen, "Die ärztliche Weiterbildung," in *Reform der Ärzteausbildung: Neue Wege in den Fakultäten*, ed. D. Halbeck, U. Schagen, and G. Wagner (Berlin: Blackwell Wissenschaft, 1993), p. 402.

81. Döhler, "Comparing National Patterns," p. 203.

82. Sewering, "Von der 'Bremer Richtlinie,'" pp. B1598–99; Döhler, "Comparing National Patterns," pp. 198, 203; Heidenheimer, "Organized Medicine," pp. 378–79.

83. Heidenheimer, "Organized Medicine," p. 379.

84. Y. Bourgueil, U. Durr, G. de Pouvourville, and S. Rocamora-Houzard, "La régulation des professions de santé—études monographiques: Allemagne, Royaume-Uni, Québec, Belgique, États-Unis," Études DREES, Document de Travail no. 22 (2002), pp. 13–14, 28–29, available at http://www.sante gouv.fr/htm/publication/.

85. The Federal Chamber of Physicians is opposed to this requirement, but the Union of Insurance Physicians supports it. Bourgueil et al., "La régulation des professions de santé," pp. 29–30.

86. Bourgueil et al., "La regulation des professions de santé," p. 8.

87. Döhler, "Comparing National Patterns," pp. 211–12; I owe the insight about the role of the *Habilitation* to Cornelius Borck.

88. Three new specialties were introduced in 1949, 1953, and 1956 respectively. Sewering, "Von der 'Bremer Richtlinie,'" p. B1597. The logic of recognition of new specialties is discussed in Döhler, "Comparing National Patterns," pp. 215–16.

89. Heidenheimer, "Organized Medicine," p. 379, counted twenty-six in West Germany in 1980, as opposed to forty-four in Sweden and thirty-two in Denmark. According to Döhler, "Comparing National Patterns," p. 224, Germany in 1987 had thirty specialties and sixteen subspecialties, with another eighteen added qualifications ranging from homeopathy to medical genetics. The United Kingdom had fifty-three specialties (with no subspecialties), while the United States in 1990 had twenty-eight specialties and forty-five subspecialties, along with a handful of added qualifications. The latest figures are from Döhler, "Comparing National Patterns," p. 203.

90. Bourgueil et al., "Régulation des professions," pp. 13, 24–26. The role of court decisions has been explained to me by Cornelius Borck.

91. While France in 1998 had 5.1 medical students per 10,000 population, Germany had 10.2. Germany in 1997 had 464 doctors per 100,000 population. Bourgueil et al., "Régulation des professions," pp. 15–16.

92. Bas-Theron, "Le système de santé," p. 21.

93. OECD figures for 1996 are 9.4 beds per 1,000 inhabitants in Germany, as opposed to 4.5 per 1,000 in the United Kingdom and 4.1 per 1,000 in the United States. Germany also had the longest hospital stays, 14.3 days on average, as opposed to 9.8 and 7.8, respectively (Bas-Theron, "Le système de santé," p. 21). The figures remained high in 2000. OCDE, *Panorama de la santé,* p. 51.

94. Moran, *Governing the Health Care State,* p. 73. By 2002 the figure was 14.5 percent.

95. Freeman, *Politics of Health,* pp. 95–96.

96. Bourgueil et al., "Régulation des professions," pp. 40, 14.

97. "Entschliessungen zum Tagesordnungspunkt II: Ausbeutung junger Ärztinnen und Ärzte," *DÄ,* 98 (2001), A1466; Bourgueil et al., "Régulation des professions," p. 19. These measures have slowed the rate of growth of doctors contracting with the insurance system, from over 3 percent annually before the measures were passed to 1.2 percent in recent years. Bourgueil et al., "Régulation des professions," p. 43.

98. Heidenheimer, "Organized Medicine," pp. 380–81.

99. The figures are from "Statistik der BÄK 2001," section 1, table 7. This source is on the Web at http://www.kbv.de/publikationen/grunddaten.htm. I am grateful to Udo Schagen for calling it to my attention.

100. Bourgueil et al., "Régulation des professions," p. 31.

101. Bourgueil et al., "Régulation des profesions," p. 32.

102. Sandra Goldbeck-Wood: "General Practice Reforms Agreed in Germany," *BMJ* (1996), 2, 1560; and "Germany to Reform GP Training," *BMJ,* 314 (1997), 1709.

103. Several specialties, notably gynecology, will remain freely accessible.

104. Bourgueil et al., "Régulation des professions," pp. 13–14, 33; Bas-Theron, "Le système de santé," p. 29.

105. "Statement des GFB-Präsidenten Rüggeberg zur aktuellen Gesundheitspolitik," available at www.Facharztverband.de/content/articles.

106. Bourgueil et al., "Régulation des professions," pp. 33–34.

107. The number of appellations of all kinds dropped from 160 to 100. "Neue Weiterbildung soll zügig umgesetzt warden," *Ärzte Zeitung*, Sept. 12, 2003.

108. "DGIM Kämpft gegen Beschluss des Ärztetags," *Ärzte Zeitung*, Nov. 23, 2003; Wolfgang van den Bergh, "Noch Fragen zur Weiterbildung," *Ärzte Zeitung*, May 23, 2003.

109. There is serious resistance even in certain local chambers. "Ärztekammer Thüringen bremst bei Weiterbildungsordnung," *Ärzte Zeitung*, Oct. 25, 2003.

110. On this reform, which has been discussed at length in the medical press for the past few years, see especially Heike Korzilius: "Top II: Novellierung der (Muster-) Weiterbildungsordnung. Operation gelungen," *DÄ*, 100 (2003), A1478–82; and "Schmerzlicher Kompromis," *DÄ*, 99 (2002), A1568–71. The entire text of this reform is available at various locations online, including http://www.bundesaerztekammer.de/30/Weiterbildung/22MWBO2003.pdf and http://www.aerzteblatt.de/v4/plus/down.asp?typ=PDF&id=1110.

111. Hassenteufel and Pierru, "Crise de la représentaticn," pp. 97–98.

112. Germany has recently ranked last in Europe in terms of life expectancy. Rupprecht, Tissot, and Chatel, "German Healthcare System," pp. 1–23.

113. Françoise Bas-Theron, Carine Chevier-Fatome, and Gilles Duhamel, "L'encadrement et le contrôle de la médicine ambulatoire. Étude d'administration comparée: Allemagne, Angleterre, États-Unis, Pays Bas," Inspection Générale des Affaires Sociales, Rapport no. 2002 081 (May 2002).

114. Bas-Theron, "Le système de santé" emphasizes this point throughout.

115. Moran, *Governing the Health Care State*, p. 117.

116. Samir Rabbata, "Gesundheitsreform: Durchbruch erzielt," *DÄ*, 100 (2003), A1969; Walter Kannengießer, "Finanzpolitik: Steuern runter—Schulden rauf," *DÄ*, 100 (2003), A1981; Jane Burgermeister, "Germany Reaches Controversial Deal on Healthcare Reform," *BMJ*, 327 (2003), 250.

117. Moran, *Governing the Health Care State*.

118. Deborah A. Stone, *The Limits of Professional Power: National Health Care in the Federal Republic of Germany* (Chicago: University of Chicago Press, 1980), p. 63.

119. On its Web page dealing with maintenance of certification (http://www.abms.org/MOC.asp), the ABMS claims that over 85 percent of American physicians are certified by ABMS-approved boards. It is not clear, however, how many are practicing only the specialties for which they have been certified.

120. This point has been made by many commentators, including Stone, *Limits of Professional Power*, p. 65; and Döhler, "Comparing National Patterns," p. 193.

121. Fred G. Domini-Lenhoff and Hannah Hedrick, "Growth of Specialization in Graduate Medical Education," *JAMA*, 284 (2000), 1284–89, at 1288.

122. Döhler, "Comparing National Patterns," p. 217; Domini-Lenhoff and Hedrick, "Growth of Specialization," pp. 1287–88.

123. Daniel M. Fox, "The Political History of Health Workforce Policy," in *The U.S. Health Workforce: Power, Politics, and Policy*, ed. Marian Osterweis et al. (Washington, D.C.: Association of Academic Health Centers, 1996), pp. 31–46, at pp. 34–35.

124. Döhler, "Comparing National Patterns," p. 208; Rosemary Stevens, *American Medicine and the Public Interest*, updated ed. (Berkeley: University of California Press, 1998), p. 348.

125. Döhler, "Comparing National Patterns," p. 209.

126. American Medical Association, *Physician Characteristics and Distribution in the U.S., 2002–2003 Edition* (Chicago: AMA Press, 2002), p. 9.

127. The best expression of the mood during this period is Donald G. Langsley and James H. Darragh, eds., *Trends in Specialization: Tomorrow's Medicine* (Evanston, Ill.: American Board of Medical Specialties, 1985). The volume includes an annotated bibliography that gives some idea of how ubiquitous the issue was.

128. In January 2000, the ACGME accredited nearly 770 residency programs in 103 specialties and subspecialties. The ABMS in that year recognized twenty-four specialty boards offering thirty-seven general certificates and eighty-seven subspecialty certificates. Domini-Lenhoff and Hedrick, "Growth of Specialization," pp. 1286–87.

129. This section is based on Stevens, *American Medicine*, pp. 293–317; Eliana Riska and Nancy Buffenbarger, "Primary Care Delivery: Is Family Medicine the Solution," *Research in Sociology and Health Care* 2 (1982), 285–303; and D. P. Adams, *American Board of Family Practice: A History* (Lexington, Ky.: American Board of Family Practice, 1999).

130. Riska and Buffenbarger, "Primary Care Delivery," pp. 291–92.

131. Moran, *Governing the Health Care State*, p. 46.

132. David A. Kindig and Harmoz Movassaghi, "Will the Supply and Distribution of Physicians Be Appropriate for the National Needs in the Year 2000?" in *Beyond Flexner: Medical Education in the Twentieth Century*, ed. Barbara Barzansky and Norman Gevitz (New York and Westport, Conn.: Greenwood Press, 1992), pp. 158–59. Also see Daniel M. Fox, "The Political History of Health Workforce Policy," in *The U.S. Health Workforce: Power, Politics, and Policy*, ed. Marian Osterweis et al. (Washington, D.C.: Association of Academic Health Centers, 1996), pp. 31–46.

133. William G. Rothstein, *American Medical Schools and the Practice of Medicine: A History* (New York and Oxford: Oxford University Press, 1987), pp. 326–27.

134. Rothstein, *American Medical Schools*, pp. 328–29.

135. James F. Cawley, "The Evolution of New Health Professions: A History of Physician Assistants," in *The U.S. Health Workforce: Power, Politics, and Policy*, ed. Marian Osterweis et al. (Washington, D.C.: Association of Academic Health Centers, 1996), pp. 189–207; Bourgueil et al., "Régulation des professions," p. 209.

136. One of the three reports produced in 1966 (the Millis Report) suggested that the new general specialist being proposed should be called a "primary physician." It was the term proposed by the Willard Report, "family physician," that became accepted. Riska and Buffenbarger, "Primary Care Delivery," pp. 291–92, discuss the different terms that were employed.

137. Stevens, *American Medicine* (first published in 1971), also does not include the term "primary care" in its index, although one sporadically finds both the term and the idea in the text. In 1987, the ABMS issued a formal definition of "primary care."

138. For just a few of the many papers trying to define the scope of primary medicine and the fields eligible for government subsidies, see R. G. Petersdorf, "Internal Medicine and Family Practice: Controversies, Conflict and Compromise," *New England Journal of Medicine*, 293 (1975), 326–32; and U.S. Department of Health and Human Services, *Third Report to the President and Congress on the Status of Health Professions Personnel in the United States* (Washington, D.C.: Division of Health Profession Analysis, January 1982), pp. IV-2–IV-5.

139. J. M. Colwill, "Where Have All the Primary Care Applicants Gone?" *New England Journal of Medicine,* 326 (1991), 387–93.

140. Jack M. Colwill and James Cultice, "Increasing Numbers of Family Physicians— Implication for Rural America," in COGME, Update 2000, pp. 31–32, available at the COGME Web page, http://www.cogme.gov/rptmain.htm.

141. Riska and Buffenbarger, "Primary Care Delivery," p. 291.

142. Table 202, Number of Active Physicians, available at http://bhpr.hrsa.gov/ healthworkforce/reports/factbook02/GB102.htm.

143. AMA, *Physician Characteristics and Distribution, 2002–2003,* p. 288.

144. Deborah Gesensway, "PR Campaign for Internal Medicine: ACP Will Explain Why the Public Should Choose Internists," ACP Observer *(January 1997), available at* http://www.acponline.org/journals/news/jan97/printmed.htm.

145. On training, see Rothstein, *American Medical Schools,* pp. 325, 327, 329. On the urban-rural divide, see Colwell and Cultice, "Increasing Numbers of Family Physicians," p. 30.

146. The best recent discussion of the current state of family medicine is Rosemary A. Stevens, "The Americanization of Family Medicine: Contradictions, Challenges and Change, 1969–2000," *Family Medicine,* 33 (2001), 232–43. Also see David Pingitore, "Family Medicine: American Culture in American Medicine," *Science as Culture,* 4 (1993), 169–211.

147. This is the Future of Family Medicine Project, completed by the American Academy of Family Physicians in the spring of 2004. James C. Martin et al., "The Future of Family Medicine: A Collaborative Project of the Family Medicine Community," *Annals of Family Medicine,* 2 (2004), 3–32.

148. In Colwill and Cultice, "Increasing Numbers of Family Physicians," pp. 4–5. Recent reports confirm that declines have continued in the following years. Deborah S. McPherson et al., "Entry of U.S. Medical School Graduates into Family Practice Residencies: 2002–2003 and 3-Year Summary," *Family Medicine Journal,* 35 (2003), 555–63.

149. Colwill and Cultice, "Increasing Numbers of Family Physicians," pp. 30, 32–33.

150. Council on Graduate Medical Education (COGME), "2002 Summary Report" (June 2002), p. 18, available at http://www.cogme.gov/rptmain.htm, indicates that projections suggest there will be 125,000 practicing nurse practitioners and 69,000 physician assistants by 2010. On the easing of restrictions, see COGME, "2002 Summary Report," p. 19. Also see Colwill and Cultice, "Increasing Numbers of Family Physicians," p. 36.

151. John J. Frey III, "GP to FP to GP?" *Family Medicine* 35 (2003), 671–72.

152. For a review of COGME's activities and goals, see Council on Graduate Medical Education, "2002 Summary Report."

153. COGME, "2002 Summary Report," p. 5; Kenneth M. Ludmerer, *Time to Heal: American Medical Education from the Turn of the Century to the Era of Managed Care* (Oxford: Oxford University Press, 1999), p. 314.

154. The Balanced Budget Act of 1997 capped the number of residencies funded by Medicare. It also privileged primary care residencies COGME, "2002 Summary Report," p. 12.

155. Bourgueil et al., "Régulation des professions," pp. 219–20; Ludmerer, *Time to Heal,* p. 314.

156. Several cases of this sort are described in Marian Osterweis et al., eds., *The U.S. Health Workforce: Power, Politics, and Policy* (Washington, D.C.: Association of Academic Health Centers, 1996).

157. COGME, "2002 Summary Report," p. 4.

158. Council on Graduate Medical Education, Resource Paper Compendium, *Update on the Physician Workforce,* (Washington, D.C.: U.S. Department of Health and Human Services, August, 2000); COGME, "Fourteenth Report: Recent Developments and Remaining Challenges in Meeting National Goals" (March 1999), available at http://www.cogme.gov/rptmain.htm.

159. Philip G. Bashook et al., eds., "Credentialing Physician Specialists: A World Perspective, June 8–10 2000, Chicago, Proceedings" (The Royal College of Physicians and Surgeons of Canada and The American Board of Medical Specialties), available at www.abms.org.

160. For instance, "Repositioning for the Future of Continuing Medical Education," *position paper from Council of Medical Specialty Societies (Mar. 23, 2002),* available at http://www.cmss.org/.

161. The information about time-limited certificates has been provided by Rosemary Stevens.

162. "History of the ABMS," available at http://www.abms.org/history.asp.

163. This is based on a section of the AMBS Web site, http://www.abms.org/MOC.asp.

164. For instance, Allen B. Weisse, "Certification and Recertification in Medicine: Self-improvement, Self-delusion, or Self-strangulation," *Perspectives in Biology and Medicine,* 41 (1998), 580–90.

165. See, for instance, John Roberts, "Specialists in the United States: What Lessons?" *BMJ,* 310 (1995), 724–227 (followed by several other articles in the same vein); and Peter Schieper, "Die USA—eine Perspective für deutsche Ärzte," *DÄ,* 93 (1996), A241–42.

Index

Abbott, Andrew, xiv, xvii
ABMS. *See* American Board of Medical
Specialties
academic specialization, 59, 88, 128
accoucheurs, 4, 6, 64
Ackerknecht, Erwin, xix, 9, 10
Addison, Thomas, 27
advertising, 77, 79, 83, 91–92, 96, 97,
98, 109
Agnew, David Hays, 69
Albrecht, Heinrich, 220
Alibert, J.L.M., 18
Allgemeine Krankenhaus, 16, 47, 48,
49, 214
Almanach général de médecine, 93
Almanach royal, 92
almanacs, 92, 94, 99
Alsace and Lorraine, 56
Althoff, Friedrich, 112–13, 114
AMA. *See* American Medical Association
AMD. See American Medical Directory
American Academy of General Practice,
250
American Board of Dermatology and
Syphilology, 216
American Board of Family Medicine, 251
American Board of Internal Medicine, 251
American Board of Medical Specialties
(ABMS), 250, 254, 255
American Board of Pediatrics, 251
American College of Physicians, 135

American College of Surgeons, 135, 143
American Medical Association (AMA),
xxvi
and American College of Surgeons, 135
American Medical Directory, 95, 97,
101, 102, 128, 136, 141, 215, 216
and Association of Medical Superintendents, 67
directory of physicians, 93–94, 95
founding of, 72
General Practice Section, 250
majority report on specialties, 34, 35
and medical education, 75–76
position on advertising, 77, 79
position on obstetrics and gynecology,
207–8
position on specialization, 78, 80,
82–83, 98
*Principles Regarding Graduate Medical
Education*, 138
proclivity for self-regulation, 63
reorganization (1901), 128
scientific role, 80
and specialist certification, 127, 136
specialty journals, 136
specialty sections, 128, 131–32, 136
status of full section within, 42, 43
strictures against specialties in directories, 70
and struggle for regulatory dominance,
139–45, 146

American Medical Association (AMA)
(*continued*)
  system of sections, 80–81, 82
  treatment of midwifery, 66
  during World War I, 137
American Medical Directory, The (AMD),
  95, 97, 101, 102, 103, 128, 136,
  141, 192, 200, 207, 213, 215, 216
American Ophthalmological Society, 80
anatomy, 4, 5
anesthesiology, 130, 192, 211
Annals of Medicine, 135
Annuaire des familles, 99
*Annuaire des spécialités médicales et
  pharmaceutiques*, 100
Annuaire Roubaud, 93, 100
anti-Semitism, 116
antisepsis, 211
Ärztliches Vereinsblatt für Deutschland, 95
Askew, Henry, 78
Association Générale des Médecins, 150
Association of American Physicians, 81,
  200
Association of Medical Superintendents,
  67
Association of Superintendents of
  Asylums, 80
Association Professionnelle Internationale
  des Médecins, 152–53
associations, xxvi, 59, 80, 90, 229
  See also specific associations
Athlone Report, 172
Atkinson, William, 65–66, 68, 79
Austria, 119, 219
  See also Vienna (Austria)
Austro-Hungarian Empire, 53

bacteriology, 53, 123, 258
Baer, Karl Ernest von, 47
Barez, S., 46
Bartham, John, 64
Beer, Georg Joseph, 48
Belgium, 161, 223
Ben-David, Joseph, 13, 58
Berlin (Ger.), 45, 46, 48, 53, 55–56, 60,
  87, 88, 99, 106, 116
Berlin Academy of Sciences, 47
Billings, John Shaw, 72, 74, 76, 80
Billroth, Theodor, 55
biographies, 64, 79

biomedicine, xi, xii, 231
birthing. *See* midwifery; obstetrics
Blake, Clarence, 73–74
Bleker, Johanna, 46
blindness, 210–11
Blustein, Bonnie, 71
BMA. *See* British Medical Association
BMJ. See British Medical Journal
Boer, H.X., 47
Boër, J., 47
Börner, Paul, 60, 95, 96, 98
Borst, Charlotte, 89, 204
Boston (Mass.), 68, 88, 201, 208,
  257–58
Boston City Hospital, 68
Boston Eye and Ear Infirmary, 74
Bouland, P., 100
Bourdet, Étienne, 5
Bowditch, Henry, 34, 73, 77
Bremen Guidelines, 117–24, 194, 199,
  200, 207, 212, 214, 221, 243
Breteuil, Louis-August de, 16
Brigham, Amariah, 65
Bright, Richard, 27
Britain. *See* Great Britain
British Association of Dermatology and
  Syphilology, 217
British College of Obstetricians, 177
British Dental Association, 222
British Dental Journal, 223
British Gynaecological Society, 205, 207
*British Journal of Dermatology and
  Syphilis*, 217
British Journal of Venereology, 217
British Medical Association (BMA),
  xxv–xxvi, 36, 41, 42, 43, 97, 102,
  103, 164, 169, 170, 173–79, 181,
  183, 184, 205, 212, 217, 236
British Medical Directory, 43
British Medical Journal (BMJ), 33, 38, 39,
  40, 42, 60, 99, 168, 176, 183
British Postgraduate Medical Federation,
  185
British Postgraduate Medical School, 185
Broc, Pierre-Paul, 9
Brodie, Benjamin, 33
Broussais, F., 7, 14
bureaucratic rationality, xxvii–xxviii
Burkner, Kurt, 56
Butler, Samuel, 94

Cabot, Hugh, 131
Calman, Kenneth, 234
Calman reforms, 235
Cambridge University, 41
Canada, 203
Caraballi, Georg, 47
cardiology, 132, 165, 193, 202
cataracts, 4, 67, 210
CCMC. *See* Committee on the Costs of
    Medical Care
certification, xxvi–xxvii
    Bremen Guidelines, 117–24
    in dentistry, 149, 153–54, 157
    in family medicine, 251
    in France, xxvii, 147–63, 238
    in Germany, xxvi–xxvii, xxviii,
        105–26, 153, 168, 169, 244
    in Great Britain, 164–87, 234–35
    "maintenance," 255
    in ophthalmology, 136
    in radiology, 122
    in surgery, 160
    in U.S., xxvi–xxvii, 127–46, 248, 251,
        255
Channing, Walter, 65
Charenton Asylum, 18
charitable giving. *See* philanthropy
Charité Hospital (Berlin), 46, 55, 214
charlatanism, xix, 6, 91
Cheneau, Dr., 19
Chéreau, A., 24
Cheyne, John, 6
childbirth. *See* midwifery; obstetrics
children. *See* pediatrics
chirurgien dentiste, 5
Churchill, John, 93
cities, xiii, 71
Civil War, 71
Clément, Julien, 4
clinical guidelines, 232
clinical pathology, 258
clinical trials, xi
clinics, 51, 54, 55, 56, 57, 174
COGME. *See* Council on Graduate Medical
    Education
Cohen, Henry, 166
Collège de France, 14, 15
College of Obstetricians (Great Britain),
    207
College of Physicians of Philadelphia, 70

Cologne Academy, 112–13
Committee on the Costs of Medical Care
    (CCMC), 139, 146
Company of Surgeons (Great Britain), 29
competition, 133, 134
Confederation of Medical Trade Unions.
    See General Confederation of Medical
    Trade Unions (France)
Congress of American Physicians and
    Surgeons, 81, 82
Corlett, Helen, 211
Council on Graduate Medical Education
    (COGME), 253, 254
Cullerier, François, 6
Cushing, Harvey, 129
Czechoslovakia, 119, 120, 153

Daston, Lorraine, xx, 15
DÄV. *See* Deutsche Ärztevereinsbund
Daviel, Jacques, 4
Dawson Report, 174
Dechambre, Dr., 19
Decourt, Fernand, 153
Denmark, 105
dentistry, 218–25
    in France, 4–5, 6, 8, 149, 153–54,
        157, 223–25
    in Germany, 220–22
    in Great Britain, 41, 220, 222–23
    in U.S., 219
dermatology
    combined with venereology, 193,
        213–18
    in France, 24, 153, 213–14
    in German-speaking world, 53, 116,
        214–15
    in Great Britain, 216–18
    Neisser on, 108
    rapid spread of field, 106
    specialists in U.S., France, and Germany,
        257
    in U.S., 75, 215–16
    women practitioners, 195
Deutsche Ärztevereinsbund (DÄV), 61,
    95, 96, 107, 119, 120, 121, 122,
    123, 146, 202, 221
Deutsche medizinische Wochenschrift, 95,
    110, 221
Dewees, William Potts, 64
dictionaries, 7–8

Dictionnaire de médecine, 8, 19
Die medizinische Reform, 51
directories, xxv–xxvi, 83
    American Medical Association,
        93–94, 95
    cost of, 96, 97
    in France, 88, 93, 97, 98, 100, 102
    in Germany, 60, 95, 96, 97, 98, 101,
        104
    in Great Britain, 30, 38, 39–40,
        92–93, 96, 98, 99–100, 102–3
    as identifiers of specialists, 97–103
    natural history of, 92–97
    in Philadelphia, 70
    pictograms in, 101
    regulation of specialists in national,
        87–104
    specialist self-identification in, 89
    trade and business, 93
    in U.S., 93–95, 96, 97, 98, 101, 104
    without specialty listings, 79
    See also specific directories
Directory of Medical Specialists, 142
diseases, 33
division of labor, xiii, xx, 31, 33, 52, 108,
    168
doctors. See general practitioners; physi-
    cians; specialization
Drake, Daniel, 65
Dugès, Antoine, 8
Duhring, Louis, 70
Durkheim, Emile, xiii
Düsseldorf Academy, 112–13
Duval, Vincent, 7

economics, 228
Edinburgh Dental Hospital, 222
Edinburgh Medical Journal, 35
education. See medical education
Ehrlich, Paul, 216
electrical medicine, 192, 258
elite status, 72, 73, 74, 193
Elizabeth Children's Hospital, 46
encyclopedias, 7–8
Enfants Malades (Paris), 46
England. See Great Britain; London
Esquirol, J.E.D., 6, 18
ethics, 77, 79
Eulner, Hans, xiv, 50, 57
Europe, 153, 232, 237–48

European Union, 229, 232
European Union of Medical Specialists,
    238
evidence-based medicine, 232
examinations, for specialization, 109,
    110, 112, 114, 127, 234
expertise, 229
experts, 3–4, 5, 6
eye. See ophthalmology

family practice, 245–46, 251, 253
Fauchard, Pierre, 5
fees, 111, 162, 168, 198, 240
Fellowship of Medicine and Postgraduate
    Medical Association, 172
Feuchtersleben, Ernst von, 49
fistula surgery, 66
Flexner, Abraham, 165
Flint, Austin, 81
Foucault, Michel, xv
Fournier, Alfred, 23, 24
Fox, Daniel, 249
France
    certification in, xxvii, 147–63, 238
    decentralized insurance and health-
        care politics, 237, 238–42
    dentistry in, 4–5, 6, 8, 149, 153–54,
        157, 223–25
    directories in, 88, 93, 97, 98, 100,
        102
    early opposition to specialization, xxii
    experts, 3–4, 5, 6
    general practitioners in, 150, 156, 162,
        240
    hospitals in, 14, 16–19, 23, 149, 158,
        162
    internal medicine in, 201–2
    medical education in, 56, 147, 156,
        158, 239, 241
    medical trade union movement, 152,
        156
    obstetrics and gynecology in, 5, 6–7,
        8, 9, 204, 208–9
    ophthalmology in, 5, 7, 22, 211
    oversupply of doctors in, 151
    regulation of specialists in, 147–63,
        238
    scientific work in, xx, 13
    specialists compared with those in U.S.
        and Germany, 257–58

surgeons and surgery in, 4, 149, 156, 160, 197
venereology and dermatology in, 23, 24, 153, 213–14
Vichy regime, 158
women doctors in, 194
See also Paris (France)
Frank, Johann Peter, 49
Freidson, Elliot, xiv
Frick, Charles, 65
Frick, George, 67
Fried, Johann Jakob, 45
Furnari, S., 7

Galès, J.C., 18
gastroenterology, 193, 202
Gelfand, Toby, 4, 12
General Confederation of Medical Trade Unions (France), 154–57, 159, 161, 162, 208
general practitioners (GPs)
American Medical Association majority report on, 35
in France, 150, 156, 162, 240
in Germany, 110, 114, 120–24, 200, 244
in Great Britain, 37, 39–42, 166–69, 172, 174, 175, 177, 178, 180, 181, 186, 236, 237–38, 255
in obstetrics, 175, 177, 204, 207
in U.S., 74, 79, 81, 132, 249, 250, 251
German Society for Internal Medicine, 202
Germany
Bremen Guidelines, 117–24, 194, 199, 200, 207, 212, 214, 221, 243
certification in, xxvi–xxvii, xxviii, 244
decentralized insurance and health-care politics, 237, 238, 242–48
dentistry in, 220–22
directories in, 60, 95, 96, 97, 98, 101, 104
emergence of specialization in, 51, 63, 87
general practitioners in, 110, 114, 120–24, 200, 244
internal medicine in, 199–201, 202
laboratory sciences in, 54
medical directories in, 60
medical education in, 105–6

Nazi regime, 96, 124–26, 198, 243
obstetrics and gynecology in, 46, 48, 207
orthopedics in, 199
regulation of specialists in, 105–26, 153, 168, 169, 244
resources to support specialties in, 56
scientific institutes, 54
specialists compared with those in U.S. and France, 257–58
surgeons and surgery in, 196, 197, 198
universities as centers of specialization, xxiii, 55, 57
venereology and dermatology in, 214–15
Weimar Republic, 115–16, 117, 243
women doctors in, 194, 195
See also Prussia
Gilibert, Jean-Emmanuel, 5, 12, 14
Girtanner, Christoph, 6
Glasgow (Scotland), 195
Glasgow Dental School, 223
Goodenough Commission, 185
Goodenough Report, 179–80
Göttingen (Ger.), 46, 48
government, xi, 88, 112, 227–28
GPs. *See* general practitioners
Graefe, Albrecht von, 55, 59
Graefe, Johann Jüngken von, 55
Grafton (publisher), 102, 103
Great Britain
certification in, xxvii, xxviii, 234–35
dentistry in, 41, 220, 222–23
directories in, 30, 38, 39–40, 88, 92–93, 96, 98, 99–100, 102–3
early specialization in, xxi, 26–43
emergence of specialists and rising backlash, 28–34
general practitioners in, 37, 39–42, 166–69, 172, 174, 175, 177, 178, 180, 181, 186, 236, 237–38, 255
hospitals in, 27, 29–37, 39, 41–42, 165, 173–74, 181
internal medicine in, 201
laborious advance of specialization, 34–39
medical directories in, 38, 39–40
national health insurance, 167
National Health Service, 180–86, 199, 204, 211, 212, 217, 223, 233–37

Great Britain (*continued*)
   obstetrics and gynecology in, 29, 40,
      176–77, 204, 206, 207
   ophthalmology in, 30, 178, 211–12
   orthopedics in, 199
   otology and laryngology in, 212
   overworked doctors in, 236
   philanthrophic activity in, xx
   regulation of specialists in, 164–87
   resistance to specialization in, xxii, 196
   Royal College of Physicians, 29, 30,
      36, 41, 176, 236
   Royal College of Surgeons, 29, 30, 36,
      41, 166, 171, 172, 176, 197, 199,
      222, 223
   specialists during inter-war years, 259
   surgeons and surgery in, 40, 182, 196,
      197, 198, 199
   venereology and dermatology in,
      216–18
   women doctors in, 194, 195, 196
   See also London (England)
Great Transition, xix, 27
Greenwood Committee, 172
Gross, Samuel David, 65, 68, 71, 94
Guide médical, 99
Guide Rosenwald, 93, 97, 100, 101, 151,
   197, 213
Gulz, Ignaz, 49
Guy's Hospital (London), 27, 32, 34, 39
gynecology
   combined with obstetrics, 193, 206,
      207
   in France, 161, 194, 208–9, 241–42
   in Germany, 207
   in Great Britain, 176, 206, 207
   specialists in U.S., France, and Ger-
      many, 257
   in U.S., 66, 75, 207–8
   See also obstetrics

Halpern, Sidney, xv, 129, 132
Hamburg (Ger.), 60, 113, 117
Hammersmith Hospital (Great Britain),
   173
Handbook of Physical Therapy, 140
Hannover (Ger.), 48
Harris, Andrew, 64
Harvard Medical School, 70, 76, 134
Hays, Isaac, 67

health-care costs, 232
health-care politics, 237–48
health-care reform, 247
health-care systems, 228, 231, 248–55
health insurance. *See* insurance
Hebra, Ferdinand, 49, 214
Heider, Moritz, 49, 59, 219, 220
Henri IV, 16
hernia, 5, 6
Hess, Volker, 46
Hill, Bradford, 198
Himly, Carl, 46
Hodgkin, Thomas, 27
holistic movement, 155
Homberger, Julius, 77, 78
homeopathy, 81, 178
home visits, 120, 121
Hooker, Worthington, 77
Hospice de Vénériens, 16
Hospital for Diseases of the Eye and Ear
   (Phila.), 67
Hospital of the Protestant Episcopal
   Church, 68
hospitals
   in France, 14, 16–19, 23, 149, 158, 162
   in German-speaking world, 46, 53, 55,
      243
   in Great Britain, 27, 29–37, 39,
      41–42, 165, 173–74, 181
   lying-in, 45, 66, 203
   residency programs, 138, 143–44
   in U.S., 66, 68–69, 71, 74
   in Vienna, 48
Howard, E. Lloyd, 78
Howard Hospital and Infirmary for
   Incurables, 69
Hughes, Everett, xiv
Hungary, 119, 153, 223
Hunter, William, 29

infant mortality, 203, 208
Infant Welfare Movement, 132
infectious diseases, 106
insanity, 10, 64, 67
insurance, xi, 228
   in continental Europe, 237–48
   for dentistry, 221
   in German-speaking world, 62, 107,
      111, 112, 116, 124–25, 214, 221,
      243, 245

in Great Britain, 164, 167, 174
medicine, 106
in U.S., 145, 248
for venereal disease, 214
internal medicine, 53, 129, 192, 195, 196, 199–203, 252–53, 258
internationalism, 229
International Medical Congress (Phila.), 81
Itard, J.M.G., 18

Jackson, James, 65
Jackson, James Sr., 64
Jacobi, Abraham, 76, 129
JAMA. See Journal of the American Medical Association
James, Thomas, 64, 65
Jefferson Medical College, 69
Jews, xxviii, 116–17, 124, 195, 198
Johns Hopkins Medical School, 208
Johnston, Christopher, 78
Jones, Robert, 166
Joseph's Academy (Vienna), 46, 48
Journal of the American Medical Association (JAMA), 81, 82, 96, 132, 136, 165
journals, 7, 21–22, 38, 57
See also specific journals
Juppé reforms, 240, 241

Kaiser-Wilhelms-Universität (Strasbourg), 56
Kater, Michael, 126
Kennedy, James, 77
King, Roger, 5
Kurierfreiheit, 61, 107
Kurpfuscherei, 61

laboratory sciences, 54, 173
Laehr, Heinrich, 56
Lancet, The, 31, 33, 34, 35, 36, 38, 41, 96
Larsen, Magali, xiv
laryngology, 212
laryngoscope, 212
larynx, 212
legal medicine, 258
Leipziger Verband, 62
Lenoir, Timothy, 47, 52
L'esculape: Journal des spécialités médico-chirurgicales, 7, 10

Lesky, Erna, 50
Lesuer, Octave, 9
literature, xii–xv, 72
Liverpool University, 176
Lives of Eminent Physicians and Surgeons (Gross), 65
Löbker, H., 114
Lock Hospital (London), 216
London (England)
British Medical Association list of specialists in, 175
directories, 100, 102
expansion of specialists in, 88
hospitals in, 27, 35, 174
late acceptance of specialization, xxii
medical research in, 27–28
specialists during inter-war years, 259
specialization and its opponents in, 26–43
London and Provincial Medical Directory, The, 30, 96, 98
London Dermatological Society, 38
London Doctors and Dental Surgeons, 102
London Medical Specialists, 99
London Obstetrical Society, 32, 204, 207
London Postgraduate Association, 172
London University, 177
Louis XIV, 4
lying-in hospitals, 45, 66, 203

male midwifery, 4
Malgaigne, J.-F., 17
Maria Theresa, Empress, 48
Marjolin, J.N., 8
Massachusetts General Hospital, 68
mass media, xxiv
maternal mortality, 203, 208
Mauthier, Ludwig Wilhelm, 49
Mauthner, Ludwig, 49
McClellan, George, 67
McGregor, Deborah Kuhn, 66
médecins-accoucheurs, 7
Medicaid, 248, 251
Medical and Surgical Register of the United States, The, 94, 96, 98
medical associations. *See* associations
medical biographies. *See* biographies
medical directories. *See* directories
Medical Directory, The (Great Britain), 92, 93, 96, 97, 102, 103–4

medical education, 227
    foreign training of Americans, 72–74
    in France, 56, 147, 156, 158, 239,
        241
    in German-speaking world, 44,
        45–46, 52–55, 105–6
    graduate university training, 134, 138
    in Great Britain, 37, 40, 173, 236
    reform of, 72, 76, 106, 128, 129, 156,
        173
    specialist training, 232, 234
    specialty chairs, 22–23, 53–57, 147,
        150
    in U.S., 69, 72, 75–76, 250, 251, 254
    in Vienna, 46, 49, 55
medical ethics. *See* ethics
Medical Faculty of Montpellier, 4
medical literature, 72
*Medical Register and Directory of the
    United States, The,* 94
medical research, xi, 227
    in France, 15
    in German-speaking world, 51–52,
        173
    in Great Britain, 27–28, 173
    in U.S., 71, 75, 173
medical societies. *See* societies
Medical Society of New York State. *See*
    New York State Medical Society
medical specialization. *See* specialization
Medical Who's Who, The, 103
medical writing, 72
Medicare, 248, 251
Medicus, 102
mental illness, 34, 132
Meyer, Adolf, 137
Middlesex Hospital Medical School (Great
    Britain), 166
midwifery, 4, 6, 28–29, 45, 66, 130, 176,
    203, 204
Mikschik, Eduard, 49
military medicine, 137, 165–66
Milwaukee (Wis.), 89, 204
"Minority Report" (Bowditch), 34
Mitchell, Silas Weir, 69
Moorfields Hospital, 37
Moran, Lord, 180, 181, 183, 185
Moran, Michael, 248, 251
Morgan, John, 65
Morton, Thomas, 68–69

Moscucci, Ornella, 176, 206
Muerhy, Adolf, 8
Müller, Johannes, 47
Munich (Ger.), 116
Municipal Hospital (Phila.), 68
Muséum d'Histoire Naturelle, 14, 15

National Health Service (Great Britain),
    180–86, 199, 204, 211, 212, 217,
    223, 233–37
National Heart Association, 132
National Tuberculosis Association, 132
National Veneral Disease Control Act, 216
natural therapeutics, 91
Naturphilosophie, 47
Nazi regime, 96, 124–26, 198
Necker Hospital, 17
Neisser, Albert, 59, 108
nephrology, 193, 202
neurology, 75, 165, 193, 195, 202, 257
neurosurgery, 129, 132
New Jersey, 138
New York City, 69, 75, 88, 96, 99, 201,
    208, 257–58
New York Eye and Ear Infirmary, 67
New York Medical Practitioners, 100
New York State Medical Society, 77, 81
nose, 212
Noyes, Henry, 67

Oberlin, Serge, 159
Obstetrical Society of Philadelphia, 68
obstetrics, 203–9
    combined with gynecology, 193, 206,
        207
    in France, 5, 6–7, 8, 9, 204, 208–9
    in German-speaking world, 45, 46, 48,
        204, 207
    in Great Britain, 29, 40, 176–77, 204,
        206, 207
    specialists in U.S., France, and Ger-
        many, 257
    in U.S., 64, 65, 66, 130, 204, 205,
        207–8
ocular surgery, 4
oculists, 6, 8, 210, 211
Oken, Lorenz, 45
operateurs, 44–45
Ophthalmic Society of the United
    Kingdom, 37

ophthalmology, 210–12
    in Berlin, 55
    certification in, 136
    in France, 5, 7, 22, 211
    in German-speaking world, 53, 211
    in Great Britain, 30, 178, 211–12
    specialists in U.S., France, and Germany, 257
    in U.S., 67, 131, 132
    in Vienna, 48, 50, 53, 67, 211
    women practitioners, 195
ophthalmoscope, 211
Ordre des Médecins, 158, 159, 161, 209, 224, 228
orthopedics, 55, 123, 132, 137, 165–66, 176, 198, 199, 257
Osiander, F.B., 45
otolaryngology, 138, 170, 212, 257
otology, 55, 73, 212
otorhinolaryngology, 22, 213

Paris (France)
    as center of knowledge production, 13–14
    compared with Vienna, 50
    directories in, 87–88, 99, 100, 151
    early specialization in, xxi, 3–25
    hospitals in, 14, 16, 18, 23
    medical research community, xxii, 14
    obstetrics and gynecology in, 208
    population, 45
    specialists in, 257–58
    specialty chairs in, 147, 150, 204
    surgeons in, 197, 198
    venereology and dermatology in, 213–14
Paris Academy of Sciences, xx, 15
Paris College of Surgery, 4
Paris Faculty of Medicine, xxii, 14, 15, 20–23, 25, 46, 53, 54, 76, 147, 213, 224
patent medicines, 6
pathology, 123, 140, 192, 195, 258
pediatrics, 5–6, 193
    in France, 161
    in German-speaking world, 53, 106, 110–11, 116, 118, 119, 121, 202
    Infant Welfare Movement, 132
    and internal medicine, 53, 129
    specialists in U.S., France, and Germany, 257

specialty chairs in, 53, 116
    in U.S., 76, 129, 132
    women practitioners, 194, 195
Pennsylvania Almshouse Hospital, 68
Pennsylvania Hospital, 69
Pennsylvania Hospital for the Insane, 68
Pennsylvania Infirmary for Diseases of the Eye and Ear, 68
Pequignot, Henri, 162
pharmacology, 53
Philadelphia (Pa.), 68–70
Philadelphia Medical Register and Directory, The, 68
Philadelphia Polyclinic and College for Graduates of Medicine, 69–70
philanthropy xx, 29, 31, 68, 132, 211, 229
physical therapy, 140
physicians
    American Medical Association directory of, 93–94
    oversupply in France, 151
    overworked in Great Britain, 236
    in U.S., 74–75, 76, 253–54
    as users of directories, 96, 100
    women, 193–96, 233
    See also general practitioners; specialization
pictograms, 101, 212, 221
Pinel, Philippe, 18
Pipelet, François, 5
Polk and Company. See R.L. Polk and Company
polyclinics, 55, 62, 74
population, xxiv, 45
Pressman, Jack, 137
primary care, 201, 202, 203, 231, 233, 246, 247, 249–53
Prinzing, Friedrich, 119
professionalization theory, xiv
prostitution, 214
Prussia
    dentistry in, 220
    internists in, 200
    medical education in, 45
    ophthalmology in, 211
    pressure to create chairs of social medicine, 106
    regulation of specialists, 112, 113, 114

Prussia (*continued*)
　specialists in, 257–58
　surgeons and surgery in, 197, 198
　universities in, 51, 54
　venereology and dermatology in, 215
pseudo specialists, 108–9, 110, 133
psychiatry, 229
　in France, 10, 18
　in German-speaking world, 53,
　　55–56, 112, 193, 202
　and neurology, 193, 202
　specialists in U.S., France, and Ger-
　　many, 257
　in U.S., 67, 129, 132
　women doctors of, 195, 196
psychobiology, 137
public health, 132, 133, 134, 192, 196,
　258
public interest, 145, 146, 229
Puzos, N., 4

Quinke, Heinrich, 114
Quinze-Vingt asylum, 211

radiology
　in France, 149, 150
　in Germany, 122
　in Great Britain, 171, 177
　specialists in U.S., France, and Germany,
　　257
　in U.S., 129–30, 132, 141
Raige Delorme, M.J., 8, 19
Ramsey, Matthew, 4
Randolph, Jacob C., 65
Rayer, Pierre, 21, 34
RCP. *See* Royal College of Physicians
RCS. *See* Royal College of Surgeons
refraction, 67, 211
regulation, xxiii–xxix
　and American Medical Association,
　　139–45, 146
　of definitions of specialties, 91
　in France, 147–63, 238
　in Germany, 105–26, 153, 168, 169,
　　244
　in Great Britain, 164–87, 234–35
　in Prussia, 112, 113, 114
　in U.S., 127–46, 248
　See also certification

Reichs-Medizinal-Kalender (RMK)
　(Börner), 60, 95, 96, 97, 98–99,
　　101, 110, 207, 212, 214, 221
research. *See* medical research
*Revue des spécialités et innovations médi-
　cales et chirurgicales,* 7
rhinology, 212
rhinoscope, 212
Ricord, Philippe, 18, 20
R.L. Polk and Company, 94, 95, 96, 98
RMK. See Reichs-Medizinal-Kalender
Robin, Paul, 21
Robin, Pierre, 4
Rosen, George, xii–xiii, xix, xxv, 9, 11,
　50, 70, 89
Rosenwald, Lucien, 97
Rothstein, William, 145
Royal College of Medicine, 197
Royal College of Physicians (RCP), 29,
　30, 36, 41, 176, 236
Royal College of Surgeons (RCS), 29, 30,
　36, 41, 166, 171, 172, 176, 197,
　199, 222, 223
Royal Dental Hospital of London, 222
Royal Kalendar (Debrett), 92
Royal Society of London, xx, 28, 33
Royal Society of Medicine, 38, 41, 43,
　175, 207, 212

St. Anna Children's Hospital (Ger.), 48,
　49
St. Bartholomew's Hospital (Great
　Britain), 35
St. John's Hospital for Skin Diseases
　(Great Britain), 37–38
St. Joseph's Hospital (Phila.), 68
St. Louis Hospital (France), 16, 18
St. Mary's Hospital (Great Britain), 39,
　195
St. Mary's Hospital (Phila.), 68
St. Peter's Hospital for the Stone (Great
　Britain), 32
Salmon, Thomas, 137
Salpêtrière Hospital, 17, 18
Salvarsan, 213, 216
Saxony (Ger.), 113
Scheff, Julius, 220
Schellong, O., 118
Schleswig-Holstein (Ger.), 113

Schwalbe, Julius, 95, 101, 110
science, 73, 228
Seehofer reforms, 245
Ségalas, P.S., 9
segmentation, xiv
Semon, Felix, 212
sexually transmitted disease. *See* venereology and venereal disease
Simms, Marion, 66
skin diseases, 16, 17, 18, 23, 214
  See also dermatology
Skoda, Joseph, 49, 50
Smellie, William, 29
social medicine, 106
Société de Biologie, 21
Société de Stomatologie de Paris, 224
societies, xxv, 22, 38, 41, 57, 80, 81, 90
  See also specific societies
sociological models, xii
Solis-Cohen, Jacob, 70
Sorbonne (Paris), 14, 15
special branches, 72
specialization
  appearance of modern, 6–19
  categories of, 89–90, 98, 99
  certification, xxvi–xxvii, 105, 118,
    122, 123, 127, 134–39
  definitions of, 91, 98, 131, 152, 168,
    177–78
  in early nineteenth-century Paris, xxi,
    3–25
  in eighteenth century, 3–6
  emergence of, xviii–xxiii
  examinations for, 109, 110, 112, 114,
    127, 234
  fundamental justification for, 11, 12
  in German-speaking world, 44–63,
    105–26
  Gilibert on, 12
  in Great Britain, 26–43
  literature on, xii–xv
  of original branches of medicine,
    196–209
  "overdetermination" of, xii
  overview of, xviii–xxiii
  rapid expansion of, 87–92
  regulation and standardization of,
    xxiii–xxix, 91, 105–87
  Rosen on, 10, 89

social factors behind, xiii
sociological models of, xii
  under Nazis, 124–26
  in U.S., 63–83, 127–46
specialty chairs, 22–23, 53–57, 147, 150
specialty clinics, 51, 54, 55, 57
standardization, xxiii–xxix
*Standard Medical Directory of North
  America, The,* 94, 95, 101
Stevens, Rosemary, xiii–xiv, 82, 144, 145,
  184
stomatology, 153–54, 192, 218–25, 258
Storer, David Humphreys, 78
Storer, Horatio, 77, 80
Strauss, Paul, 24
Stuelp, Otto, 120
Stürtzbecher, Manfred, 53
surgery, xix, 196–99
  certification, 135
  elite status of, 193
  in France, 4, 5, 149, 156, 160, 197
  in German-speaking world, 45, 196,
    197, 198
  in Great Britain, 40, 182, 197, 198,
    199
  ocular, 4
  orthopedic, 123, 198
  specialists in U.S., France, and Ger-
    many, 257
  urological, 131
  in U.S., 64, 65, 66, 196, 197, 198
  in Vienna, 48
Sweden, 105, 153
Swieten, Gerhard van, 47
syphilis, 76, 106, 214, 215, 216
systemic humoralism, xviii–xix
system(s)
  definition of, xvii
  health-care, 228, 231, 248–55
  of professions, xvii, xviii
  of specialties, xvii, xviii, 229–30

technology, 231
teeth. *See* dentistry
Teicher, Wilfried, 56
teleological mechanism, 47
Tenon, Jacques, 16
Thomas, Hugh, 35
Thomson, St. Clair, 170

Tilley, Herbert, 171
Tocqueville, Alexis de, 64
Todd, Eli, 64
Todd Report, 234
training. *See* medical education
Trinity College Dublin, 40, 41
Trousseau, Armand, 20
true specialists, 108–9, 128, 143
tuberculosis, 258
Türck, Ludwig, 49
Türkheim, Ludwig Baron von, 34, 49
Turner, Steven, 51
Tweedy, John, 36

Union des Syndicats Médicaux, 150
United Kingdom. *See* Great Britain
United States
    certification in, xxvi–xxvii, 248, 251,
        255
    changing self-image of specialists, 132
    dentistry in, 219
    directories in, 93–95, 96, 97, 98, 101,
        104
    early history of specialties, 64–70
    enthusiasm for specialization in, xxiii
    general practitioners in, 74, 79, 81,
        132, 249, 250, 251
    health care in, 248–55
    internal medicine in, 199–201,
        202–3, 252–53
    medical education in, 69, 72, 75–76,
        250, 251, 254
    obstetrics and gynecology in, 64, 65,
        66, 130, 204, 205, 207–8
    philanthrophic activity in, xx
    regulation of specialists in, 127–46,
        248
    rise of specialties in, 63–83
    specialists compared with those in
        France and Germany, 257–58
    surgeons and surgery in, 64, 65, 66,
        196, 197, 198
    venereology and dermatology in, 75,
        215–16
    women doctors in, 194, 195, 196
unity of knowledge, 47
universities. *See* medical education;
    specific universities
University of Berlin, 54, 112
University of London, 39

University of Minnesota, 134
University of Pennsylvania, 69, 76, 134
urbanization, xiii
urological surgery, 131
urology, 257

Velpeau, Alfred, 211
venereology and venereal disease
    combined with dermatology, 193,
        213–18
    in France, 23, 24, 213–14
    in German-speaking world, 53, 116,
        214–15
    in Great Britain, 216–18
    Neisser on, 108
    rapid spread as specialty, 106
    specialists in U.S., France, and Germany,
        257
    in U.S., 215–16
    women practitioners, 195
Verein für Innere Medizin, 200
Versammlung der Deutschen Natur-
    forscher und Ärtze, 47, 52, 204,
    207, 214
Vienna (Austria)
    Allgemeine Krankenhaus, 16, 47, 48,
        49, 214
    compared with Paris, 50
    dentistry in, 219, 220
    early specialization in, xxi, xxii–xxiii,
        50–51
    hospitals in, 48
    medical education in, 46, 49, 55
    medical-scientific community, 47
    ophthalmology in, 48, 50, 53, 67, 211
    population, 45
    surgeons in, 48
Vienna Maternity House, 47
Vienna Society of Physicians, 49
Virchow, Rudolf, 51
von Stifft, Joseph Andreas, 49

Wakley, James, 35
Wakley, Thomas, 31–32, 33, 34, 93
Warner, John, 64, 72
Wassermann test, 213, 216
Watson-Williams, P., 170
Webster, Charles, 182, 185
Wenzel, Baron Michael de, 48
Wilbur, Ray Lyman, 141, 142, 146

Williams, David Innes, 41
Williams, J. Whitridge, 205, 207
Williams, Stephen W., 64
Wills Hospital (Phila.), 67, 68
Wilson, Adrian, 28
Wilson, Erasmus, 36
Wolff, Julius, 55
Woman's Hospital (N.Y.C.), 66

women, 193–96, 198, 233
writing, 72
Wunderlich, Carl, xxi, 9, 19, 48, 50
Württemberg (Ger.), 60

X-rays. *See* radiology

Yugoslavia, 153